Evidence-based Clinical Chinese Medicine

Volume 28
Endometriosis

Evidence-based Clinical Chinese Medicine

Print ISSN: 2529-7562
Online ISSN: 2529-7554

Series Co Editors-in-Chief

Charlie Changli Xue *(RMIT University, Australia)*
Chuanjian Lu *(Guangdong Provincial Hospital of Chinese Medicine, China)*

Published

Vol. 1 *Chronic Obstructive Pulmonary Disease*
by Charlie Changli Xue and Chuanjian Lu

Vol. 2 *Psoriasis Vulgaris*
Lead Authors: Claire Shuiqing Zhang and Jingjie Yu

Vol. 3 *Chronic Urticaria*
Lead Authors: Meaghan Coyle and Jingjie Yu

Vol. 4 *Adult Asthma*
Lead Authors: Johannah Shergis and Lei Wu

Vol. 5 *Allergic Rhinitis*
Lead Authors: Claire Shuiqing Zhang and Qiulan Luo

Vol. 6 *Herpes Zoster and Post-herpetic Neuralgia*
Lead Authors: Meaghan Coyle and Haiying Liang

Vol. 7 *Insomnia*
Lead Authors: Johannah Shergis and Xiaojia Ni

Vol. 8 *Alzheimer's Disease*
Lead Authors: Brian H May and Mei Feng

Vol. 9 *Vascular Dementia*
Lead Authors: Brian H May and Mei Feng

Vol. 10 *Diabetic Kidney Disease*
Lead Authors: Johannah Shergis and Lihong Yang

Vol. 11 *Acne Vulgaris*
Lead Authors: Meaghan Coyle and Haiying Liang

More information on this series can also be found at https://www.worldscientific.com/series/ebccm

(Continued at end of book)

Evidence-based Clinical Chinese Medicine

Co Editors-in-Chief

Charlie Changli Xue
RMIT University, Australia

Chuanjian Lu
Guangdong Provincial Hospital of Chinese Medicine, China

Volume 28

Endometriosis

Lead Authors

Meaghan Coyle
RMIT University, Australia

Yongxia Wang
Guangdong Provincial Hospital of Chinese Medicine, China

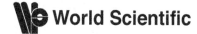

NEW JERSEY · LONDON · SINGAPORE · BEIJING · SHANGHAI · HONG KONG · TAIPEI · CHENNAI · TOKYO

Published by

World Scientific Publishing Co. Pte. Ltd.
5 Toh Tuck Link, Singapore 596224
USA office: 27 Warren Street, Suite 401-402, Hackensack, NJ 07601
UK office: 57 Shelton Street, Covent Garden, London WC2H 9HE

Library of Congress Cataloging-in-Publication Data
Names: Xue, Charlie Changli, author. | Lu, Chuan-jian, 1964–   author.
Title: Evidence-based clinical Chinese medicine / Charlie Changli Xue, Chuanjian Lu.
Description: New Jersey : World Scientific, 2016. | Includes bibliographical references and index.
Identifiers: LCCN 2015030389| ISBN 9789814723084 (v. 1 : hardcover : alk. paper) |
  ISBN 9789814723091 (v. 1 : paperback : alk. paper) |
  ISBN 9789814723121 (v. 2 : hardcover : alk. paper) |
  ISBN 9789814723138 (v. 2 : paperback : alk. paper) |
  ISBN 9789814759045 (v. 3 : hardcover : alk. paper) |
  ISBN 9789814759052 (v. 3 : paperback : alk. paper)
Subjects: | MESH: Medicine, Chinese Traditional--methods. | Clinical Medicine--methods. |
  Evidence-Based Medicine--methods. | Psoriasis. | Pulmonary Disease, Chronic Obstructive.
Classification: LCC RC81 | NLM WB 55.C4 | DDC 616--dc23
LC record available at http://lccn.loc.gov/2015030389

Volume 28: Endometriosis
ISBN 978-981-124-737-8 (hardcover)
ISBN 978-981-124-767-5 (paperback)
ISBN 978-981-124-738-5 (ebook for institutions)
ISBN 978-981-124-739-2 (ebook for individuals)

British Library Cataloguing-in-Publication Data
A catalogue record for this book is available from the British Library.

Copyright © 2022 by World Scientific Publishing Co. Pte. Ltd.

All rights reserved. This book, or parts thereof, may not be reproduced in any form or by any means, electronic or mechanical, including photocopying, recording or any information storage and retrieval system now known or to be invented, without written permission from the publisher.

For photocopying of material in this volume, please pay a copying fee through the Copyright Clearance Center, Inc., 222 Rosewood Drive, Danvers, MA 01923, USA. In this case permission to photocopy is not required from the publisher.

For any available supplementary material, please visit
https://www.worldscientific.com/worldscibooks/10.1142/12553#t=suppl

Printed in Singapore

Disclaimer

The information in this monograph is based on systematic analyses of the best available evidence for Chinese medicine interventions, both historical and contemporary. Every effort has been made to ensure accuracy and completeness of the data of this publication. This book is intended for clinicians, researchers, and educators. The practice of evidence-based medicine consists of consideration of the best available evidence, practitioners' clinical experience and judgement, and patients' preferences. However, it is important to note that not all interventions are acceptable in all countries, and some of the substances mentioned in this book may no longer be in use, may be toxic, or may be prohibited or restricted under the provisions of the Convention on International Trade in Endangered Species of Wild Fauna and Flora (CITES). Thus, practitioners, researchers, and educators are advised to comply with relevant regulations in their country and with the restrictions on the trade in species included in CITES appendices I, II, and III. This book is not intended as a guide for self-medication, so patients should seek professional advice from qualified Chinese medicine practitioners.

Foreword

Since the late 20th century, Chinese medicine, including acupuncture and herbal medicine, has been increasingly used throughout the world. The parallel development and spread of evidence-based medicine has provided challenges and opportunities for Chinese medicine.

The opportunities include evidence-based medicine's emphasis on the effective use of the best available clinical evidence alongside clinicians' clinical experience, subject to patients' preferences. Such a patient-focused approach reflects the historical nature of Chinese medicine practice. However, the challenges are also significant due to the fact that, despite the long-term development and very rich literature accumulated over 2,000 years, there is an overall lack of high-level clinical evidence for many of the interventions used in Chinese medicine.

To address this knowledge gap, we need to generate clinical evidence through high quality clinical studies and to evaluate this available evidence to enable their effective use in promoting evidence-based Chinese medicine practice.

Modern Chinese medicine is rooted in its classical literature and the legacies of ancient doctors, grounded in the practice of expert clinicians and increasingly informed by clinical and experimental research efforts. In recognition of the unique features of Chinese medicine, for each of the conditions in this series a 'whole-evidence' approach is used to provide a synthesis of different types and levels of evidence to enable practitioners to make clinical decisions informed by the current best evidence.

There are four main components of this 'whole-evidence' approach. Firstly, we present the current approaches to the diagnosis, differentiation, and treatment of each condition based on expert consensus in published textbooks and clinical guidelines. This provides an overview of how the condition is currently managed. The second section provides an analysis of the condition in historical context based on systematic searches of the *Zhong Hua Yi Dian* 中华医典, which includes the full texts of more than 1,000 classical medical books. These analyses provide objective views on how the condition has been treated over two millennia, reveal continuities and discontinuities between traditional and modern practice, and suggest avenues for future research.

The third component is the assessment of evidence derived from modern clinical studies of Chinese medicine interventions. The methods established by the Cochrane Collaboration are used as the basis for conducting systematic reviews and undertaking meta-analyses of outcome data for randomised controlled trials (RCTs). In addition, the clinical relevance of meta-analysis data is enhanced by examining the herbal formulae, individual herbs, and acupuncture treatments that were assessed in the RCTs, and the evidence base is broadened by the inclusion of data from controlled clinical trials and non-controlled studies. The fourth component is to determine how the herbal medicine interventions may achieve the effects indicated by the clinical trials. Thus, for each of the most frequently used herbs, we provide reviews of their effects in pre-clinical models and their likely mechanisms of action.

For each condition, this 'whole-evidence' approach links clinical expertise, historical precedents, and clinical and experimental research data to provide readers with assessments of the current state of the evidence of efficacy and safety for Chinese medicine interventions using herbal medicines, acupuncture, moxibustion, and other health care practices, such as *tai chi* 太极.

Since these books are available in Chinese and English, they can benefit patients, practitioners, and educators internationally and enable practitioners to make clinical decisions informed by the current best evidence.

Foreword

These publications represent a major milestone in Chinese medicine development and make a significant contribution to the global development of evidence-based Chinese medicine.

Co-editors-in-Chief
Distinguished Professor Charlie Changli Xue,
RMIT University, Australia

Professor Chuanjian Lu, Guangdong Provincial Hospital of Chinese Medicine, China

Purpose of the Monograph

This book is intended for clinicians, researchers, and educators. It can be used to inform tertiary education and clinical practice by providing systematic, multidimensional assessments of the best available evidence for the use of Chinese medicine to manage each common clinical condition.

How to Use This Monograph
Some Definitions
A glossary is included, containing terms and definitions that appear frequently in the book. It also describes the definitions of statistical tests, methodological terms, evaluation tools, and interventions. For example, in this book, integrative medicine refers to the combined use of a Chinese medicine treatment with conventional medical management, and combination therapies refer to two or more Chinese medicines from different therapy groups (Chinese herbal medicine, acupuncture, or other Chinese medicine therapies) administered together. Terminology used throughout the monograph is based on the World Health Organization's *Standard Terminologies on Traditional Medicine in the Western Pacific Region* (2007), where possible, or is from the cited reference.

Data Analysis and Interpretation of Results
In order to synthesise the clinical evidence, a range of statistical analysis approaches are used. In general, the effect size for dichotomous data is reported as a risk ratio (RR) with 95% confidence

intervals (CI), whereas continuous data are reported as mean difference (MD) scores with 95% CI. Statistically significant effects are indicated with an asterisk*. Readers should note that statistical significance does not necessarily correspond with a clinically important effect. Interpretation of results should take into consideration the clinical significance, quality of studies (expressed as high, low or unclear risk of bias in this book), and heterogeneity among studies. Tests for heterogeneity are conducted using the I^2 statistic. An I^2 score that is greater than 50% may indicate substantial heterogeneity.

Use of Evidence in Practice

The Grading of Recommendations Assessment, Development and Evaluation (GRADE) approach was used to summarise the quality and strength of the evidence ('certainty') for important comparisons and outcomes. Due to the diverse nature of Chinese medicine practice, treatment recommendations are not included in summary of findings tables. Therefore, readers will need to interpret the evidence with reference to the local practice environment.

Limitations

Readers should note some of the methodological limitations of the classical literature and clinical evidence.

- Terms used to search the *Zhong Hua Yi Dian* 中华医典 database may not include all terms that have been used for the condition, which may affect the findings.
- Chinese language has changed over time. Citations have been interpreted for analysis, and such interpretations may be subject to disagreement.
- Chinese medicine theory has evolved over time. As such, some concepts described in the classical Chinese medical literature may no longer be found in contemporary works.
- Symptoms described in classical literature citations may be common to many conditions, so a judgement is often required to

Purpose of the Monograph

determine the likelihood that the citation is related to the condition. This may have introduced some bias due to the subjective nature of the judgement.
- The vast majority of the clinical evidence for Chinese medicine treatments has come from China. The applicability of the findings to other populations and other countries requires further assessment.
- Many studies included participants with varying disease severity. Where possible, subgroup analyses were undertaken to examine the effects in different sub-populations. As this was not always possible, the findings may be limited to the population included, and not to sub-populations.
- The potential risk of bias found in many included studies suggests methodological limitations. The findings for GRADE assessments based on studies of very low- to moderate-certainty evidence should be interpreted accordingly.
- Nine major English and Chinese language databases were searched to identify clinical studies, in addition to clinical trial registers. Other studies may exist that were not identified through searches, which may alter the findings.
- The calculation of frequency of herbal formula use was based on formula names only. It is possible that studies evaluated herbal treatments with the same or similar herb ingredients, but which were given different formula names. Due to the complexity of herbal formulas, it was considered inappropriate to make judgements of the similarity of formulas for analysis. As such, the frequency of formulas reported in Chapter 5 may be underestimated.
- The most frequently utilised herbs that may have contributed to the treatment effect have been described in Chapter 5. These herbs may provide leads for further exploration. Calculation of the herbs with potential effects is based on frequency of formulas reported in the studies and does not account for the clinical implications and functions of every herb in a formula.

Authors and Contributors

CO-EDITORS-IN-CHIEF
Distinguished Prof. Charlie Changli Xue *(RMIT University, Australia)*
Prof. Chuanjian Lu *(Guangdong Provincial Hospital of Chinese Medicine, China)*

CO-DEPUTY EDITORS-IN-CHIEF
Assoc. Prof. Anthony Lin Zhang *(RMIT University, Australia)*
Dr. Brian H. May *(RMIT University, Australia)*
Prof. Xinfeng Guo *(Guangdong Provincial Hospital of Chinese Medicine, China)*
Prof. Zehuai Wen *(Guangdong Provincial Hospital of Chinese Medicine, China)*

LEAD AUTHORS
Dr. Meaghan Coyle *(RMIT University, Australia)*
Dr. Yongxia Wang *(Guangdong Provincial Hospital of Chinese Medicine, China)*

CO-AUTHORS:
RMIT University (Australia):
Dr. Mary Xinmei Zhang
Assoc. Prof. Anthony Lin Zhang
Distinguished Prof. Charlie Changli Xue
Guangdong Provincial Hospital of Chinese Medicine (China):
Prof. Xuefang Liang
Prof. Dongfang Xiang
Prof. Xinfeng Guo
Prof. Chuanjian Lu

Members of Advisory Committee and Panel

CO-CHAIRS OF PROJECT PLANNING COMMITTEE
Prof. Peter J. Coloe *(RMIT University, Australia)*
Prof. Yubo Lyu *(Guangdong Provincial Hospital of Chinese Medicine, China)*
Prof. Dacan Chen *(Guangdong Provincial Hospital of Chinese Medicine, China)*

CENTRE ADVISORY COMMITTEE (ALPHABETICAL ORDER)
Prof. Keji Chen *(The Chinese Academy of Sciences, China)*
Prof. Aiping Lu *(Hong Kong Baptist University, China)*
Prof. Caroline Smith *(Western Sydney University, Australia)*
Prof. David F. Story *(RMIT University, Australia)*

METHODOLOGY EXPERT ADVISORY PANEL (ALPHABETICAL ORDER)
Prof. Zhaoxiang Bian *(Hong Kong Baptist University, China)*
The Late Prof. George Lewith *(University of Southampton, United Kingdom)*
Prof. Lixing Lao *(The University of Hong Kong, China)*
Prof. Jianping Liu *(Beijing University of Chinese Medicine, China)*
Prof. Frank Thien *(Monash University, Australia)*
Prof. Jialiang Wang *(Sichuan University, China)*

CONTENT EXPERT ADVISORY PANEL (ALPHABETICAL ORDER)
Dr Mike Armour (*Western Sydney University, Australia*)
Prof. Neil Johnson (*University of Adelaide, Australia*)
Prof. Ruihua Zhao (*China Academy of Chinese Medical Sciences, China*)
Prof. Ruining Liang (*Affiliated Hospital of Jiangxi University of Traditional Chinese Medicine, China*)

Distinguished Professor Charlie Changli Xue, PhD

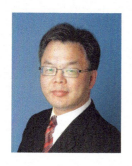

Distinguished Professor Charlie Changli Xue holds a Bachelor of Medicine (majoring in Chinese Medicine) from Guangzhou University of Chinese Medicine, China (1987), and a PhD from RMIT University, Australia (2000). He has been an academic, researcher, regulator, and practitioner for over three decades. Distinguished Professor Xue has made significant contributions to evidence-based educational development, clinical research, regulatory framework and policy development, and provision of high-quality clinical care to the community. Distinguished Professor Xue is recognised internationally as an expert in evidence-based traditional medicine and integrative healthcare.

Distinguished Professor Xue was appointed by the Australian Health Workforce Ministerial Council in 2011 as the Inaugural National Chair of the Chinese Medicine Board of Australia, and he was reappointed in 2014 and 2017 for second and third terms. Since 2007, he has been a Member of the World Health Organization's (WHO) Expert Advisory Panel for Traditional and Complementary Medicine, Geneva. Distinguished Professor Xue is also an Honorary Senior Principal Research Fellow at the Guangdong Provincial Academy of Chinese Medical Sciences, China.

At RMIT, Distinguished Professor Xue is an Associate Deputy Vice-Chancellor (International). He is also the Director of WHO's Collaborating Centre for Traditional Medicine.

Between 1995 and 2010, Distinguished Professor Xue was Discipline Head of Chinese Medicine at RMIT University. He leads the development of five successful undergraduate and postgraduate degree programs in Chinese Medicine at RMIT University, which is now a global leader in Chinese medicine education and research.

Distinguished Professor Xue's research has been supported by over AU$15 million in research grants, including six project grants from the Australian Government's National Health and Medical Research Council (NHMRC) and two Australian Research Council (ARC) grants. He has contributed over 200 publications and has been frequently invited as keynote speaker for numerous national and international conferences. Distinguished Professor Xue has contributed to over 300 media interviews on issues related to complementary medicine education, research, regulation, and practice.

Professor Chuanjian Lu, MD

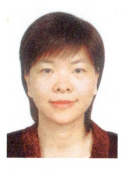

Professor Chuanjian Lu, Doctor of Medicine, is the Vice President of Guangdong Provincial Hospital of Chinese Medicine (Guangdong Provincial Academy of Chinese Medical Sciences, Second Clinical Medical College of Guangzhou University of Chinese Medicine). She is also the Chair of the Guangdong Traditional Chinese Medicine (TCM) Standardization Technical Committee and the Vice-Chair of the Immunity Specialty Committee of the World Federation of Chinese Medicine Societies.

Professor Lu has engaged in scientific research in TCM, clinical practice, and teaching for some 25 years. Her research has been devoted to integrated traditional and conventional medicine, and she has edited and published 12 monographs and 120 academic research articles as first author and corresponding author, with over 30 articles being included in SCI journals.

Professor Lu has received widespread recognition for her achievements with awards for Excellent Teacher of South China, National Outstanding Women TCM Doctor, and National Outstanding Young Doctor of TCM. She also received The Science and Technology Star of the Association of Chinese Medicine, the National Excellent Science and Technology Workers of China Award, and the Five-Continent Women's Scientific Awards of China Medical Women's Association.

Professor Lu has won the Award of Science and Technology Progress more than 10 times from the Guangdong Provincial Government, China Association of Chinese Medicine, and Chinese Hospital Association.

Acknowledgements

The authors and contributors would like to acknowledge the valuable contributions of the following people who assisted with database searches, data extraction, data screening, data assessment, translation of documents, editing, and/or administrative tasks: Dr Kevin Kaiyi Wang, Mr Edward Caruso, Prof. Yi Situ, Prof. Lixing Cao, and Yiyuan Chen.

5. Clinical Evidence for Chinese Herbal Medicine	**89**
Introduction	89
Chapter Structure	89
Previous Systematic Reviews	90
Systematic Reviews of Chinese Herbal Medicine for Endometriosis	90
Systematic Reviews of Chinese Herbal Medicine Formulas for Endometriosis	92
Systematic Reviews of Chinese Herbal Medicine for Adenomyosis	95
Identification of Clinical Studies	95
Part 1. Endometriosis	95
Oral Chinese Herbal Medicine for Endometriosis	97
Randomised Controlled Trials of Oral Chinese Herbal Medicine for Endometriosis	97
Risk of bias assessment	101
Outcomes	102
Dysmenorrhoea	104
Oral Chinese herbal medicine versus no treatment	104
Oral Chinese herbal medicine versus placebo	105
Oral Chinese herbal medicine versus pharmacotherapy	105
Oral Chinese herbal medicine plus pharmacotherapy versus pharmacotherapy	108
Oral Chinese herbal medicine plus hormone therapy versus placebo plus hormone therapy	111
Pelvic pain	111
Oral Chinese herbal medicine versus no treatment	111
Oral Chinese herbal medicine versus pharmacotherapy	112
Oral Chinese herbal medicine plus hormone therapy versus hormone therapy	112
Dyspareunia	113
Oral Chinese herbal medicine versus no treatment	113

Contents

Treatment with Oral Chinese Herbal Medicine	53
Most frequent oral use formulas in possible endometriosis citations	54
Most frequent oral use herbs in possible endometriosis citations	58
Most frequent oral use formulas in most likely endometriosis citations	60
Most frequent oral use herbs in most likely endometriosis citations	61
Treatment with Topical Chinese Herbal Medicine	62
Discussion of Chinese Herbal Medicine for Endometriosis	63
Acupuncture and Other Chinese Medicine Therapies	65
Classical Literature in Perspective	66
References	69

4. Methods for Evaluating Clinical Evidence — 71

Introduction	71
Search Strategy	72
Inclusion Criteria	73
Exclusion Criteria	76
Outcomes	76
Pain	77
Recurrence	78
Uterine and Cyst Volume	78
Menstrual Volume	79
Pregnancy Outcomes	79
Health-related Quality of Life	79
Other Outcomes	81
Risk of Bias Assessment	82
Statistical Analyses	83
Assessment Using Grading of Recommendations Assessment, Development and Evaluation	84
References	86

2. Endometriosis in Chinese Medicine — 23

Introduction — 23
Aetiology and Pathogenesis — 24
Syndrome Differentiation and Treatments — 24
Oral Chinese Herbal Medicine Treatment
   Based on Syndrome Differentiation — 26
   Qi Stagnation and Blood Stasis 气滞血瘀 — 27
   Kidney Deficiency and Blood Stasis 肾虚血瘀 — 28
   Cold Congealing and Blood Stasis 寒凝血瘀 — 29
   Qi Deficiency and Blood Stasis 气虚血瘀 — 30
   Phlegm and Stasis Binding 痰瘀互结 — 31
   Dampness-heat and Stasis Obstructing the Uterus 湿热瘀阻 — 32
External Chinese Herbal Medicine Treatment — 33
   Topical Chinese Herbal Medicine — 33
   Chinese Herbal Medicine Enema — 34
Acupuncture Therapies — 34
   Acupuncture — 35
   Ear Acupuncture — 36
   Abdominal Acupuncture — 37
   Moxibustion — 37
Other Management Strategies — 37
References — 38

3. Classical Chinese Medicine Literature — 41

Introduction — 41
Search Terms — 42
Procedures for Search, Data Coding, and Data Analysis — 44
Search Results — 47
Citations Related to Endometriosis — 48
Definitions of Endometriosis — 49
Descriptions of the Aetiology of Endometriosis — 50
Chinese Herbal Medicine — 52
   Frequency of Treatment Citations by Dynasty — 52

Contents

Disclaimer	v
Foreword	vii
Purpose of the Monograph	xi
Authors and Contributors	xv
Members of Advisory Committee and Panel	xvii
Distinguished Professor Charlie Changli Xue	xix
Professor Chuanjian Lu	xxi
Acknowledgements	xxiii
List of Figures	xlv
List of Tables	xlvii

1. Introduction to Endometriosis   **1**

Definition of Endometriosis	1
Clinical Presentation	2
Epidemiology	3
Burden	4
Risk Factors	5
Pathological Processes	6
Diagnosis	9
Management	11
Surgical Management	12
Medical Management	12
Management of Endometriosis-related Infertility	13
Complementary and Alternative Medicine	14
Prognosis	14
References	14

Contents

Oral Chinese herbal medicine versus pharmacotherapy	114
Oral Chinese herbal medicine plus hormone therapy versus hormone therapy	114
Oral Chinese herbal medicine plus hormone therapy versus placebo plus hormone therapy	115
Recurrence	116
Oral Chinese herbal medicine versus no treatment	116
Oral Chinese herbal medicine versus hormone therapy	117
Oral Chinese herbal medicine plus hormone therapy versus hormone therapy	120
Ovarian cyst size	121
Oral Chinese herbal medicine versus no treatment	121
Oral Chinese herbal medicine versus placebo	121
Oral Chinese herbal medicine versus hormone therapy	121
Oral Chinese herbal medicine plus hormone therapy versus hormone therapy	122
Uterine volume	123
Menstrual volume	123
Oral Chinese herbal medicine versus hormone therapy	123
Oral Chinese herbal medicine plus hormone therapy versus placebo plus hormone therapy	123
Pregnancy outcomes	123
Oral Chinese herbal medicine versus no treatment	124
Oral Chinese herbal medicine versus pharmacotherapy	125
Oral Chinese herbal medicine plus pharmacotherapy versus pharmacotherapy	126
Fatigue	128
Health-related quality of life	128
Oral Chinese herbal medicine versus no treatment	128

Oral Chinese herbal medicine versus hormone therapy … 130
Kupperman Index … 133
Bone density … 133
Assessment using Grading of Recommendations Assessment, Development and Evaluation … 133
Oral Chinese herbal medicine versus placebo … 135
Oral Chinese herbal medicine versus hormone therapy … 136
Oral Chinese herbal medicine plus hormone therapy versus hormone therapy … 139
Shao fu zhu yu tang 少腹逐瘀汤 plus hormone therapy versus hormone therapy … 142
Xue fu zhu yu tang 血府逐瘀汤 versus hormone therapy … 142
Xue fu zhu yu tang 血府逐瘀汤 plus hormone therapy versus hormone therapy … 143
Gui zhi fu ling jiao nang 桂枝茯苓胶囊 versus hormone therapy … 146
Gui zhi fu ling jiao nang 桂枝茯苓胶囊 plus hormone therapy versus hormone therapy … 147
Randomised controlled trial evidence for individual oral formulas … 147
Frequently reported orally used herbs in meta-analyses showing favourable effect … 149
Safety of oral Chinese herbal medicine in randomised controlled trials … 153
Controlled Clinical Trials of Oral Chinese Herbal Medicine for Endometriosis … 154
Outcomes … 157
Dysmenorrhoea … 157
Oral Chinese herbal medicine versus no treatment … 157
Oral Chinese herbal medicine versus pharmacotherapy … 158
Oral Chinese herbal medicine plus pharmacotherapy versus pharmacotherapy … 158

Pelvic pain	158
Dyspareunia	159
Recurrence	159
Oral Chinese herbal medicine versus no treatment	159
Oral Chinese herbal medicine versus hormone therapy	160
Oral Chinese herbal medicine plus hormone therapy versus hormone therapy	161
Pregnancy outcomes	161
Oral Chinese herbal medicine versus no treatment	162
Oral Chinese herbal medicine plus hormone therapy versus hormone therapy	162
Ovarian cyst size	162
Oral Chinese herbal medicine versus hormone therapy	162
Oral Chinese herbal medicine plus hormone therapy versus hormone therapy	163
Uterine volume	163
Safety of oral Chinese herbal medicine in controlled clinical trials	163
Non-controlled Studies of Oral Chinese Herbal Medicine for Endometriosis	164
Safety of oral Chinese herbal medicine in non-controlled studies	167
Topical Chinese Herbal Medicine for Endometriosis	168
Randomised Controlled Trials of Topical Chinese Herbal Medicine for Endometriosis	168
Risk of bias assessment	169
Outcomes	170
Dysmenorrhoea	170
Topical Chinese herbal medicine versus pharmacotherapy	171
Topical Chinese herbal medicine plus hormone therapy versus hormone therapy	171
Pelvic pain	171
Dyspareunia	172

Recurrence	172
Topical Chinese herbal medicine versus no treatment	172
Topical Chinese herbal medicine versus hormone therapy	172
Topical Chinese herbal medicine plus hormone therapy versus hormone therapy	173
Ovarian cyst size	173
Topical Chinese herbal medicine versus hormone therapy	173
Topical Chinese herbal medicine plus hormone therapy versus hormone therapy	173
Safety of topical Chinese herbal medicine in randomised controlled trials	174
Controlled Clinical Trials of Topical Chinese Herbal Medicine for Endometriosis	174
Outcomes	175
Pregnancy outcomes	175
Safety of topical Chinese herbal medicine in controlled clinical trials	175
Non-controlled Studies of Topical Chinese Herbal Medicine for Endometriosis	176
Oral plus Topical CHM for Endometriosis	176
Randomised Controlled Trials of Oral plus Topical Chinese Herbal Medicine for Endometriosis	176
Risk of bias assessment	177
Outcomes	179
Dysmenorrhoea	179
Dyspareunia	180
Recurrence	180
Oral plus topical Chinese herbal medicine versus hormone therapy	180
Oral plus topical Chinese herbal medicine plus hormone therapy versus hormone therapy	181
Ovarian cyst volume	181

Pregnancy outcomes	181
Health-related quality of life	181
Safety of oral plus topical Chinese herbal medicine in randomised controlled trials	182
Controlled Clinical Trials of Oral plus Topical Chinese Herbal Medicine for Endometriosis	182
Outcomes	183
Dysmenorrhoea	183
Recurrence	183
Pregnancy outcomes	184
Safety of oral plus topical Chinese herbal medicine in controlled clinical trials	184
Non-controlled Studies of Oral plus Topical Chinese Herbal Medicine for Endometriosis	184
Part 2. Adenomyosis	185
Oral Chinese Herbal Medicine for Adenomyosis	186
Randomised Controlled Trials of Oral Chinese Herbal Medicine for Adenomyosis	186
Risk of bias assessment	187
Outcomes	190
Dysmenorrhoea	190
Oral Chinese herbal medicine versus no treatment	190
Oral Chinese herbal medicine versus placebo	191
Oral CHM versus pharmacotherapy	191
Oral Chinese herbal medicine plus hormone therapy versus hormone therapy	193
Dyspareunia	195
Oral Chinese herbal medicine versus hormone therapy	195
Oral Chinese herbal medicine plus hormone therapy versus hormone therapy	195
Uterine volume	195
Oral Chinese herbal medicine versus no treatment	195
Oral Chinese herbal medicine versus hormone therapy	196

Oral Chinese herbal medicine plus hormone therapy versus hormone therapy	196
Menstrual volume	197
Oral Chinese herbal medicine versus no treatment	198
Oral Chinese herbal medicine versus hormone therapy	198
Oral Chinese herbal medicine plus hormone therapy versus hormone therapy	198
Pregnancy outcomes	200
Fatigue	200
Health-related quality of life	200
Randomised controlled trial evidence for individual oral formulas	201
Frequently reported herbs in meta-analyses showing favourable effect	204
Safety of oral Chinese herbal medicine for adenomyosis in randomised controlled trials	206
Controlled Clinical Trials of Oral Chinese Herbal Medicine for Adenomyosis	207
Dysmenorrhoea	208
Oral Chinese herbal medicine versus hormone therapy	208
Oral Chinese herbal medicine plus hormone therapy versus hormone therapy	208
Uterine volume	209
Oral Chinese herbal medicine versus pharmacotherapy	209
Oral Chinese herbal medicine plus hormone therapy versus hormone therapy	209
Menstrual volume	209
Safety of oral Chinese herbal medicine in controlled clinical trials for women with adenomyosis	210
Non-controlled Studies of Oral Chinese Herbal Medicine for Adenomyosis	210
Topical Chinese Herbal Medicine for Adenomyosis	212

Contents

Randomised Controlled Trials of Topical Chinese Herbal Medicine for Adenomyosis	212
Risk of bias assessment	212
Dysmenorrhoea	213
Topical Chinese herbal medicine versus hormone therapy	213
Topical Chinese herbal medicine plus ultrasound therapy versus ultrasound therapy	213
Uterine volume	214
Ovarian cyst volume	214
Menstrual volume	214
Safety of topical Chinese herbal medicine in randomised controlled trials for women with adenomyosis	214
Non-controlled Studies of Topical Chinese Herbal Medicine for Adenomyosis	214
Oral plus Topical Chinese Herbal Medicine for Adenomyosis	215
Randomised Controlled Trials of Oral plus Topical Chinese Herbal Medicine for Adenomyosis	215
Non-controlled Studies of Oral plus Topical Chinese Herbal Medicine for Adenomyosis	216
Part 3. Endometriosis and Adenomyosis	217
Oral Chinese Herbal Medicine for Endometriosis and Adenomyosis	217
Randomised Controlled Trials of Oral Chinese Herbal Medicine for Endometriosis and Adenomyosis	217
Risk of bias assessment	218
Dysmenorrhoea	219
Oral Chinese herbal medicine versus pharmacotherapy	219
Oral Chinese herbal medicine plus hormone therapy versus hormone therapy	219
Safety of oral Chinese herbal medicine in randomised controlled trials for endometriosis and adenomyosis	220

Controlled Clinical Trials of Oral Chinese Herbal
   Medicine for Endometriosis and Adenomyosis   220
   Outcomes   222
   Dysmenorrhoea   222
      Oral Chinese herbal medicine versus hormone
         therapy   222
      Oral Chinese herbal medicine plus hormone
         therapy versus hormone therapy   222
   Recurrence   223
   Safety of oral Chinese herbal medicine in controlled
      clinical trials for endometriosis and adenomyosis   223
Non-controlled Studies of Oral Chinese Herbal
   Medicine for Endometriosis and Adenomyosis   223
Oral plus Topical Chinese Herbal Medicine for
   Endometriosis and Adenomyosis   225
Randomised Controlled Trials of Oral plus Topical
   Chinese Herbal Medicine for Endometriosis and
   Adenomyosis   225
Non-controlled Studies of Oral plus Topical Chinese
   Herbal Medicine for Endometriosis and Adenomyosis   226
Part 4. Side Effects of Gonadotropin-releasing Hormone
   Agonists   226
Randomised Controlled Trials of Oral Chinese Herbal
   Medicine for Side Effects of Gonadotropin-releasing
   Hormone Agonists   226
Risk of Bias Assessment   228
Outcomes   229
Dysmenorrhoea   230
Recurrence   230
Endometriosis Health Profile-5   230
Menopausal Symptoms   231
   Oral Chinese herbal medicine versus no treatment   231
   Oral Chinese herbal medicine versus
      pharmacotherapy   233
   Oral Chinese herbal medicine plus pharmacotherapy
      versus pharmacotherapy   233

Bone Density	235
Safety of Oral Chinese Herbal Medicine for Side Effects of Gonadotropin-releasing Hormone Agonists in Randomised Controlled Trials	235
Controlled Clinical Trials of Oral Chinese Herbal Medicine for Side Effects of Gonadotropin-releasing Hormone Agonists	236
Outcomes	237
Dysmenorrhoea	237
Recurrence	237
Menopausal Symptoms	237
Oral Chinese herbal medicine versus placebo	238
Oral Chinese herbal medicine versus hormone therapy	238
Oral Chinese herbal medicine plus hormone therapy versus hormone therapy	238
Bone Density	238
Safety of Oral Chinese Herbal Medicine for Side Effects of Gonadotropin-releasing Hormone Agonists	239
Part 5. Endometriosis Outside the Pelvic Cavity	239
Clinical Evidence for Commonly Used Chinese Herbal Medicine Treatments	240
Ge xia zhu yu tang 膈下逐瘀汤	241
Xue fu zhu yu tang 血府逐瘀汤	242
Shao fu zhu yu tang 少腹逐瘀汤	243
Li chong tang 理冲汤	244
Qing re tiao xue tang 清热调血汤	244
San jie zhen tong jiao nang 散结镇痛胶囊	245
Endometriosis	245
Adenomyosis	247
Endometriosis and Adenomyosis	248
Gui zhi fu ling jiao nang 桂枝茯苓胶囊	249
Endometriosis	249
Adenomyosis	250
Summary of Chinese Herbal Medicine Clinical Evidence	251

Key Findings for Endometriosis	254
Key Findings for Adenomyosis	256
Key Findings for Endometriosis and Adenomyosis	257
Key Findings for Side Effects of Gonadotropin-releasing Hormone Agonists	258
Limitations of the Evidence	258
Safety of Chinese Herbal Medicine	259
References	260
References for Included Chinese Herbal Medicine Clinical Studies	263

6. Pharmacological Actions of Frequently Used Herbs — 291

Introduction	291
Methods	292
Experimental Studies on *Chi Shao* 赤芍	293
Anti-endometriosis Actions	293
Analgesic Actions	294
Hormone Regulation	295
Immunomodulatory Actions	295
Experimental Studies on *Chuan Xiong* 川芎	295
Anti-endometriosis Actions	295
Analgesic Actions	296
Hormone Regulation	297
Immunomodulatory Actions	298
Experimental Studies on *Dan Shen* 丹参	298
Anti-endometriosis Actions	298
Analgesic Actions	299
Hormone Regulation	300
Immunomodulatory Actions	300
Experimental Studies on *Dang Gui* 当归	300
Anti-endometriosis Actions	300
Analgesic Actions	301
Hormone Regulation	301
Immunomodulatory Actions	302
Experimental Studies on *E Zhu* 莪术	302
Anti-endometriosis Actions	302

Analgesic Actions	303
Hormone Regulation	304
Immunomodulatory Actions	304
Experimental Studies on *Gan Cao* 甘草	304
Anti-endometriosis Actions	305
Analgesic Actions	306
Hormone Regulation	306
Immunomodulatory Actions	306
Experimental Studies on *San Leng* 三棱	307
Anti-endometriosis Actions	307
Analgesic Actions	308
Hormone Regulation	308
Experimental Studies on *Tao Ren* 桃仁	308
Anti-endometriosis Actions	308
Analgesic Action	310
Hormone Regulation	310
Immunomodulatory Actions	310
Experimental Studies on *Xiang Fu* 香附	310
Anti-endometriosis Actions	311
Analgesic Actions	311
Hormone Regulation	312
Experimental Studies on *Yan Hu Suo* 延胡索	312
Anti-endometriosis Actions	312
Analgesic Actions	313
Hormone Regulation	314
Experimental Studies on Herbal Formulas	314
Shao Fu Zhu Yu Tang 少腹逐瘀汤	314
Gui Zhi Fu Ling Wan 桂枝茯苓丸	315
Summary of the Pharmacological Actions of the Common Herbs	316
References	317

7. Clinical Evidence for Acupuncture and Related Therapies   329

Introduction	329
Previous Systematic Reviews	330
Identification of Clinical Studies	331

Endometriosis	331
Acupuncture	331
Randomised Controlled Trials of Acupuncture for Endometriosis	333
Risk of bias assessments	335
Outcomes	336
Dysmenorrhoea	337
Acupuncture versus sham acupuncture	337
Acupuncture versus hormone therapy	337
Warm needle acupuncture versus hormone therapy	337
Pelvic pain	338
Acupuncture versus sham acupuncture	338
Acupuncture plus moxibustion and electroacupuncture versus placebo acupuncture	338
Dyspareunia	339
Acupuncture versus sham acupuncture	339
Acupuncture versus hormone therapy	339
Recurrence	339
Ovarian cyst size	339
Quality of life	340
Acupuncture versus sham acupuncture	340
Acupuncture plus moxibustion versus gestrinone	341
Acupuncture plus moxibustion and electroacupuncture versus placebo acupuncture	341
Warm needle acupuncture versus hormone therapy	343
Assessment using Grading of Recommendations Assessment, Development and Evaluation	343
Acupuncture versus sham acupuncture	344
Acupuncture versus hormone therapy	344
Controlled Clinical Trials of Acupuncture for Endometriosis	345
Non-controlled Studies of Acupuncture for Endometriosis	346
Safety of Acupuncture for Endometriosis	347
Moxibustion	348
Risk of Bias Assessment	348

Contents

Outcomes	349
Assessment Using Grading of Recommendations Assessment, Development and Evaluation	350
Moxibustion versus hormone therapy	350
Moxibustion plus hormone therapy versus hormone therapy	351
Safety of Moxibustion for Endometriosis	352
Adenomyosis	352
Moxibustion	352
Randomised Controlled Trials of Moxibustion for Adenomyosis	352
Controlled Clinical Trials of Moxibustion for Adenomyosis	353
Safety of Moxibustion for Adenomyosis	353
Clinical Evidence for Commonly Used Acupuncture and Related Therapies	354
Summary of Acupuncture and Related Therapies Clinical Evidence	354
References	356
References for Included Acupuncture Therapies Clinical Studies	357

8. Clinical Evidence for Combination Therapies — 359

Introduction	359
Identification of Clinical Studies	359
Endometriosis	360
Randomised Controlled Trials of Combination Therapies for Endometriosis	360
Risk of Bias Assessment	364
Outcomes	364
Clinical Evidence for Combination Chinese Medicine Therapies	365
Chinese herbal medicine plus moxibustion	365
Chinese herbal medicine plus electroacupuncture	365
Chinese herbal medicine plus acupuncture point stimulator	366

xli

Chinese herbal medicine plus acupuncture and moxibustion	366
Chinese herbal medicine plus acupuncture, tuina 推拿 and hormone therapy	366
Chinese herbal medicine plus acupuncture, moxibustion, and plum-blossom needle therapy	367
Controlled Clinical Trials of Combination Therapies for Endometriosis	367
Non-controlled Studies of Combination Therapies for Endometriosis	368
Safety of Combination Therapies for Endometriosis	369
Adenomyosis	369
Randomised Controlled Trials of Combination Therapies for Adenomyosis	370
Risk of Bias Assessment	371
Clinical Evidence for Combination Chinese Medicine Therapies	371
Chinese herbal medicine plus acupuncture and hormone therapy	371
Chinese herbal medicine plus moxibustion	372
Non-controlled Studies of Combination Therapies for Adenomyosis	372
Safety of Combination Therapies for Adenomyosis	373
Endometriosis and Adenomyosis	373
Summary of Combination Therapies Evidence	374
References	375
References for Included Combination Therapies Clinical Studies	375

9. Summary and Conclusions   377

Introduction	377
Chinese Medicine Syndrome Differentiation	378
Chinese Herbal Medicine	379
Chinese Herbal Medicine Formulas in Key Clinical Guidelines and Textbooks, Classical Literature and Clinical Studies	384

Contents

Acupuncture and Related Therapies	387
Acupuncture Therapies in Key Clinical Guidelines and Textbooks, Classical Literature and Clinical Studies	388
Limitations of Evidence	392
Classical Literature	392
Clinical Studies	394
Experimental Studies	396
Implications for Practice	396
Implications for Research	398
References	401
Glossary	405
Index	415

List of Figures

Figure 3.1.	Classical literature citations.	45
Figure 5.1.	Flowchart of study selection process: Chinese herbal medicine.	96
Figure 7.1.	Flowchart of study selection process: Acupuncture and related therapies.	332
Figure 8.1.	Flowchart of study selection process: Combination therapies.	361

List of Tables

Table 2.1.	Summary of Chinese Herbal Medicines for Endometriosis	26
Table 2.2.	Summary of Acupuncture Therapies for Endometriosis	36
Table 3.1.	Search Terms	43
Table 3.2.	Criteria for Rating Citations	45
Table 3.3.	Hit Frequency by Search Term Group	47
Table 3.4.	Dynastic Distribution of Chinese Herbal Medicine Treatment Citations	53
Table 3.5.	Most Frequent Oral Use Formulas in Possible Endometriosis Citations	54
Table 3.6.	Most Frequent Oral Use Herbs in Possible Endometriosis Citations	58
Table 3.7.	Most Frequent Formulas in Most Likely Endometriosis Citations	60
Table 3.8.	Most Frequent Herbs in Most Likely Endometriosis Citations	61
Table 3.9.	Most Frequent Topical Use Herbs in Possible Endometriosis Citations	63
Table 4.1.	Chinese Medicine Interventions Included in Clinical Evidence Evaluation	74
Table 4.2.	Pre-specified Outcomes	75
Table 5.1.	Frequently Reported Oral Formulas in Randomised Controlled Trials	99
Table 5.2.	Frequently Reported Orally Used Herbs in Randomised Controlled Trials	101
Table 5.3.	Risk of Bias Assessment of Randomised Controlled Trials: Oral CHM	102

Table 5.4.	Oral Chinese Herbal Medicine versus Pharmacotherapy for Endometriosis: Dysmenorrhoea Visual Analogue Scale	106
Table 5.5.	Oral Chinese Herbal Medicine versus Pharmacotherapy for Endometriosis: 1993 Guideline at End of Treatment	107
Table 5.6.	Oral Chinese Herbal Medicine versus Pharmacotherapy for Endometriosis: 1993 Guideline at Follow-up Assessment	107
Table 5.7.	Oral Chinese Herbal Medicine plus Pharmacotherapy versus Pharmacotherapy for Endometriosis: Dysmenorrhoea Visual Analogue Scale	109
Table 5.8.	Oral Chinese Herbal Medicine versus No Treatment for Endometriosis: Recurrence	116
Table 5.9.	Oral Chinese Herbal Medicine versus Hormone Therapy for Endometriosis: Recurrence	118
Table 5.10.	Oral Chinese Herbal Medicine versus Hormone Therapy for Endometriosis: Recurrence	120
Table 5.11.	Oral Chinese Herbal Medicine versus Hormone Therapy for Endometriosis: Ovarian Cyst Size	122
Table 5.12.	Oral Chinese Herbal Medicine versus No Treatment for Endometriosis: Pregnancy Outcomes	124
Table 5.13.	Oral Chinese Herbal Medicine versus Pharmacotherapy for Endometriosis: Pregnancy Outcomes	125
Table 5.14.	Oral Chinese Herbal Medicine plus Pharmacotherapy versus Pharmacotherapy for Endometriosis: Pregnancy Rate	127
Table 5.15.	Oral Chinese Herbal Medicine plus Pharmacotherapy versus Pharmacotherapy for Endometriosis: Miscarriage Rate	128
Table 5.16.	Oral Chinese Herbal Medicine versus No Treatment for Endometriosis: SF-36	129

List of Tables

Table 5.17.	Oral Chinese Herbal Medicine versus Hormone Therapy for Endometriosis: WHOQOL-BREF	131
Table 5.18.	GRADE: Oral Chinese Herbal Medicine versus Placebo	135
Table 5.19.	GRADE: Oral Chinese Herbal Medicine versus Hormone Therapy	137
Table 5.20.	GRADE: Oral Chinese Herbal Medicine plus Hormone Therapy versus Hormone Therapy	140
Table 5.21.	GRADE: *Xue fu zhu yu tang* 血府逐瘀汤 versus Hormone Therapy	143
Table 5.22.	GRADE: *Xue fu zhu yu tang* 血府逐瘀汤 plus Hormone Therapy versus Hormone Therapy	144
Table 5.23.	GRADE: *Gui zhi fu ling jiao nang* 桂枝茯苓胶囊 versus Hormone Therapy	146
Table 5.24.	GRADE: *Gui zhi fu ling jiao nang* 桂枝茯苓胶囊 plus Hormone Therapy versus Hormone Therapy	148
Table 5.25.	Oral CHM Formulas plus Pharmacotherapy versus Pharmacotherapy for Endometriosis: Dysmenorrhoea Visual Analogue Scale	148
Table 5.26.	Frequently Reported Orally Used Herbs in Meta-Analyses Showing Favourable Effect for Dysmenorrhoea	150
Table 5.27.	Frequently Reported Orally Used Herbs in Meta-Analyses Showing Favourable Effect for Recurrence	151
Table 5.28.	Frequently Reported Orally Used Herbs in Meta-Analyses Showing Favourable Effect for Pregnancy Outcomes	152
Table 5.29.	Frequently Reported Orally Used Herbs in Meta-Analyses Showing Favourable Effect for Sonographic Measures	152
Table 5.30.	Frequently Reported Orally Used Herbs in Meta-Analyses Showing Favourable Effect for Health-related Quality of Life	153

Table 5.31.	Frequently Reported Oral Formulas in Controlled Clinical Trials	156
Table 5.32.	Frequently Reported Orally Used Herbs in Controlled Clinical Trials	156
Table 5.33.	Frequently Reported Oral Formulas in Non-controlled Studies	165
Table 5.34.	Frequently Reported Orally Used Herbs in Non-controlled Studies	167
Table 5.35.	Frequently Reported Topically Used Herbs in Randomised Controlled Trials	169
Table 5.36.	Risk of Bias Assessment of Randomised Controlled Trials: Topical CHM	170
Table 5.37.	Frequently Reported Oral plus Topical Herbs in Randomised Controlled Trials	178
Table 5.38.	Risk of Bias Assessment of Randomised Controlled Trials: Oral plus Topical CHM	178
Table 5.39.	Frequently Reported Orally plus Topically Used Herbs in Non-controlled Studies	185
Table 5.40.	Frequently Reported Oral Formulas in Randomised Controlled Trials for Adenomyosis	188
Table 5.41.	Frequently Reported Herbs in Randomised Controlled Trials for Adenomyosis	189
Table 5.42.	Risk of Bias Assessment of Randomised Controlled Trials for Adenomyosis: Oral CHM	189
Table 5.43.	Oral Chinese Herbal Medicine versus Pharmacotherapy for Adenomyosis: Dysmenorrhoea	192
Table 5.44.	Oral Chinese Herbal Medicine plus Pharmacotherapy versus Pharmacotherapy for Adenomyosis: Dysmenorrhoea	194
Table 5.45.	Oral Chinese Herbal Medicine plus Hormone Therapy versus Hormone Therapy for Adenomyosis: Uterine Volume at the End of Treatment	197

List of Tables

Table 5.46.	Oral Chinese Herbal Medicine plus Hormone Therapy versus Hormone Therapy for Adenomyosis: Uterine Volume at Follow-up	197
Table 5.47.	Oral Chinese Herbal Medicine plus Hormone Therapy versus Hormone Therapy for Adenomyosis: Pictorial Blood Loss Assessment Chart	199
Table 5.48.	Oral Chinese Herbal Medicine plus Pharmacotherapy versus Pharmacotherapy for Adenomyosis: Dysmenorrhoea	202
Table 5.49.	Oral Chinese Herbal Medicine plus Hormone Therapy versus Hormone Therapy for Adenomyosis: Pictorial Blood Loss Assessment Chart	203
Table 5.50.	Oral Chinese Herbal Medicine plus Hormone Therapy versus Hormone Therapy for Adenomyosis: Uterine Volume at End of Treatment	203
Table 5.51.	Oral Chinese Herbal Medicine plus Hormone Therapy versus Hormone Therapy for Adenomyosis: Uterine Volume at Follow-up	204
Table 5.52.	Frequently Reported Orally Used Herbs in Meta-Analyses Showing Favourable Effect for Dysmenorrhoea	205
Table 5.53.	Frequently Reported Orally Used Herbs in Meta-Analyses Showing Favourable Effect for Sonographic Measures	205
Table 5.54.	Frequently Reported Orally Used Herbs in Non-controlled Studies for Adenomyosis	211
Table 5.55.	Frequently Reported Herbs in Controlled Clinical Trials for Endometriosis and Adenomyosis	221
Table 5.56.	Frequently Reported Orally Used Herbs in Randomised Controlled Trials for Endometriosis and Adenomyosis	224

Table 5.57.	Frequently Reported Herbs in Randomised Controlled Trials for Side Effects of Gonadotropin-releasing Hormone Agonists	228
Table 5.58.	Risk of Bias Assessment of Randomised Controlled Trials for Side Effects of Gonadotropin-releasing Hormone Agonists	229
Table 5.59.	Oral Chinese Herbal Medicine versus Gonadotropin-releasing Hormone Agonists: Endometriosis Health Profile-5	232
Table 5.60.	Oral Chinese Herbal Medicine plus Pharmacotherapy versus Pharmacotherapy Alone: Kupperman Index	234
Table 7.1.	Frequently Used Points in Acupuncture Randomised Controlled Trials	334
Table 7.2.	Risk of Bias of Randomised Controlled Trials: Acupuncture	336
Table 7.3.	GRADE: Acupuncture versus Sham Acupuncture	345
Table 7.4.	GRADE: Moxibustion versus Hormone Therapy	350
Table 7.5.	GRADE: Moxibustion plus Hormone Therapy versus Hormone Therapy	351
Table 8.1.	Summary of Interventions in Combination Therapies Studies	360
Table 8.2.	Frequently Reported Orally Used Herbs in Randomised Controlled Trials of Combination Therapies for Endometriosis	363
Table 8.3.	Risk of Bias of Randomised Controlled Trials: Combination Therapies for Endometriosis	364
Table 9.1.	Summary of Oral Chinese Herbal Medicine Traditional Formulas	385
Table 9.2.	Summary of Oral Chinese Herbal Medicine Manufactured Products	386
Table 9.3.	Summary of Acupuncture and Related Therapies	389
Table 9.4.	Summary of Acupuncture Points	390

1

Introduction to Endometriosis

OVERVIEW

Endometriosis is a common gynaecological condition affecting women of reproductive age. The key symptoms are pain that can coincide with menstrual cycles, abnormal menstruation, and infertility. This chapter reviews the definition, prevalence, diagnosis, burden, and risk factors for endometriosis and describes conventional medical management of symptoms.

Definition of Endometriosis

Endometriosis is a chronic medical condition usually found in women of reproductive age.[1,2] Lesions consisting of endometrial-like tissue grows outside the uterus and induces an inflammatory response.[3,4] Endometrial-like tissue is usually found in the pelvic cavity, but can also be found in the thorax and, to a lesser extent, the skin and brain.[5,6] The eutopic endometrium (endometrium in the uterus) contains both endometrial glands and stroma. The ectopic endometrium (endometrial tissue outside of the uterus) displays the same characteristics, but also contains blood, fibrous tissue, and cysts.[7]

Three main phenotypes exist: superficial endometriosis, ovarian endometrioma, and deep infiltrating endometriosis.[8] Superficial endometriosis, including implanted lesions and adhesions, vary in size and appearance.[7] Ovarian endometriomas, a type of cyst, develop when endometrial tissue inside the ovary bleeds, creating a haematoma. The old blood from repeated haemorrhages turns a chocolate colour[8,9]; ovarian endometriomas are often referred to as 'chocolate cysts'. Deep infiltrating endometriosis has been described as endometriosis that infiltrates the peritoneum by five millimetres or more[10], although Koninckx et al. (2012)[11] later acknowledged the difficulties in accurate assessment of lesion depth and suggested that deep endometriosis should involve a pathological diagnosis of adenomyosis externa. The World Endometriosis Society (WES) suggests the following definition: 'deep endometriosis should be defined as lesions extending deeper than 5 mm under the peritoneal surface or those involving or distorting bowel, bladder, ureter, or vagina'.[4, p.318]

Adenomyosis (growth of endometrial tissue in the uterine myometrium), peritoneal endometrioma, deep infiltrating endometrioma, ovarian endometrioma, and adenomyosis (growth of endometrial tissue in the uterine myometrium) were considered types of 'adenomyoma' until the 1920s, when adenomyosis and endometriosis were considered two different but related conditions.[12] Adenomyosis presents with similar symptoms endometriosis, including dysmenorrhoea, dyspareunia, chronic pelvic pain, abnormal uterine bleeding, and subfertility.[13]

Clinical Presentation

Pelvic pain and/or infertility are the key symptoms of endometriosis.[2,4] The OXYGENE study, which included 1,000 women with endometriosis, showed that 78.7% of women experienced menstrual pain (dysmenorrhoea) and 26.2% experienced infertility.[14] Pain can include dysmenorrhoea, cyclical or non-cyclical pelvic pain; pain during sexual intercourse (dyspareunia), defaecation (dyschezia), or urination (dysuria); lower abdominal pain; low back pain; and loin pain.[2]

As endometriosis is an oestrogen-dependent condition,[7] symptoms are often cyclical. Other symptoms include nausea, vomiting, abdominal bloating, changes in bowel movements,[2] and fatigue.[7] Nodules or masses on physical examination, tenderness on vaginal examination, and immobility of the uterus or cervix may suggest endometriosis.[15] Some women do not experience symptoms; the number of asymptomatic women has been estimated at 2%.[14]

Some symptoms, or clusters of symptoms, can suggest the type of endometriosis. For example, dyspareunia is often suggestive of deep infiltrating endometriosis,[7] while urinary symptoms can suggest bladder endometriosis,[16] bowel symptoms suggest bowel endometriosis,[17] and cyclical chest pain, haemoptysis, or pneumothorax may suggest thoracic endometriosis.[18]

Epidemiology

While pelvic endometriosis has been reported to affect 6–10% of women,[19] estimates of prevalence vary according to the population under study and the way in which endometriosis is diagnosed.[20] Findings from the Global Burden of Disease Study 2013 suggest that the prevalence of endometriosis was 4.8% between 2006 and 2013.[21] Actual prevalence may be higher, particularly when considering that delays between the onset of symptoms and diagnosis may be up to 11 years.[22] Incidence of endometriosis is higher in women aged 25 to 35 years and lowest in women over 44 years.[23]

Estimates of prevalence vary globally. A cross-sectional survey of 59,411 women in the United States (US) found that the prevalence of diagnosed endometriosis was 6.1%.[24] Prevalence in Germany was higher than the US (8.1%),[25] while prevalence in other European countries was lower: 2% in Italy[26] and 2.1% in the United Kingdom (UK).[27] Australian estimates of the prevalence of endometriosis appear to be lower than global estimates. In a cross-sectional survey, Reid et al.[28] found that 3.4% of 2,025 Australian women reported endometriosis, while findings from the Australian Longitudinal Study on Women's Health, involving 7,427 women, estimated prevalence at 3.7%.[29] More recent data from a population-based cohort study found the prevalence to be higher: cumulative prevalence of confirmed endometriosis was 6.0%, and was as high as 11.4% when suspected endometriosis cases were added.[30]

Prevalence of endometriosis is considerably higher in women with subfertility or infertility, with several studies suggesting prevalence as high as 47%.[31,32] Not all women with endometriosis will have symptoms, however. A small study of 86 asymptomatic women undergoing laparoscopy, who did not report typical symptoms, found that 45.3% had visualised pelvic endometriosis.[33]

Burden

Endometriosis carries significant burden in terms of cost and impact on health-related quality of life (HRQoL).[3] The cost of laparoscopic diagnosis in the UK exceeded £46 million in 2003[34]; costs would be higher if treatment were provided at the time of surgery. Direct annual costs of treatment per person, including cost of inpatient and outpatient admissions, medications, and use of healthcare services, range from $1,109 in Canada to $12,118 in the US.[35] Much of the direct costs relate to surgical procedures.

Indirect costs, including absenteeism, lost productivity due to missed work, and loss of leisure time, have been more challenging to estimate.[35] Indirect costs appear to be greater than direct costs of care (indirect costs: €6298.3 per person; direct costs: €3281.0).[36] Research from the UK Endometriosis All Party Parliamentary Group found that women missed 5.3 days of work per month on average due to endometriosis, at a potential population cost of €30 billion.[37] Women with endometriosis incur direct and indirect costs that are at least three times greater than women without endometriosis.[38]

Annual costs vary according to the method of calculation, population size, and social and financial contexts.[35] Simoens et al. (2012)[36] estimated that the total annual cost per person was €9579. Total costs for Australian women appear to be higher than for women in the US, UK, and Europe ($20,898 International dollars).[39] Annual costs were comparable to other chronic diseases, such as diabetes, rheumatoid arthritis, and Crohn's disease.[36,40] Total costs have been found to increase as HRQoL decreases[36] and as a pain severity worsens.[39]

In addition to the financial costs of diagnosis and treatment, the emotional burden from side effects of treatment, frustration from recurrence, uncertainty about the future, and impaired fertility can be considerable.[2] Women also report that endometriosis negatively affects their social, academic, and romantic relationships.[41] A cross-sectional study of 1,269 women with endometriosis found moderate impairment in HRQoL measured with the Endometriosis Health Profile 30-item questionnaire; HRQoL further deteriorated as the number of symptoms and symptom severity increased.[42] An earlier study by Nnoaham et al. (2011)[43] showed a similar finding: women with endometriosis had poorer HRQoL on the bodily pain, physical function, role function due to physical problems, and role function due to emotional problems domains of the 36-item Short Form Health Survey (second version) than symptomatic women without endometriosis. Endometriosis had the third highest number of disability-adjusted life years of all gynaecological diseases in China in 2016, with 23.3 healthy years lost to disability per 100,000 women.[44]

Endometriosis can affect activities of daily living. Simoens et al. (2012)[36] found that more than half of the 909 survey respondents (56%) reported pain or discomfort at the beginning of the study, and over one-third of women (36%) experienced anxiety or depression. Twenty-nine per cent of women reported difficulty with daily activities, 16% reported mobility problems, and three per cent reported problems with self-care. Endometriosis has also been found to reduce sleep quality and heighten perceived stress.[45]

Risk Factors

Endometriosis tends to develop after menarche and is less common after menopause.[46] Several risk factors have been identified that relate to the menstrual cycle, including menstrual flow obstruction,[3] short menstrual cycles, and heavy menstruation.[46] Women with low birth weight are more likely to develop endometriosis,[47] and having a mother or sister with endometriosis also appears to increase the risk of developing the disease.[46] Nulliparous women have a higher risk of developing endometriosis; conversely, multiple pregnancies and extended lactation appear to have a protective effect against endometriosis.[46]

Education level has been found to be positively associated with endometriosis.[48] Higher social class has also been associated with greater prevalence of endometriosis, although this may be attributed to 'diagnostic bias'.[46] The chance of developing endometriosis is nine-fold higher in Asian women than in European-American women.[49] Environmental factors that induce oxidative stress, alter the immune response, and change hormonal balance also increase the risk, including endocrine disrupting hormones (EDCs) such as phthalate esters, perfluorochemicals,[49] and exposure to cigarette smoke[49] or diethylstilbesterol[47] in utero. Lower genital tract infections may also increase the risk of developing endometriosis.[50]

Dietary and lifestyle risk factors include greater consumption of trans-unsaturated fats and red meat/animal fat.[51] Evidence is mixed for the potential risk from cigarette smoking, use of oral contraceptive pills, and caffeine and alcohol consumption.[46] A diet rich in fruits, green vegetables, and long-chain fatty acids may reduce the risk of developing endometriosis.[52]

Pathological Processes

The pathogenesis of endometriosis has not been clearly elucidated.[53] The eutopic endometrium in women with endometriosis is different to that of women without the disease, suggesting that functional traits may contribute to the development of endometriosis.[54] Other factors suggested to contribute to the development of endometriosis include changes in hormone and immune function, genetic predisposition, and environmental factors.[54] Several mechanisms have been proposed; none, however, fully explain the development of endometriosis.

The most robust and generally accepted theory is the retrograde menstruation phenomenon.[8] Retrograde menstruation refers to reflux of endometrial fragments through the fallopian tubes to the pelvic cavity.[8] This may arise due to lack of coordination of uterine contractions to effectively expel sloughed endometrial cells or tissue.[55] This phenomenon alone does not fully explain the development of endometriosis — many women will have retrograde menstruation but not all will develop endometriosis.[56]

In the retrograde menstruation phenomenon, endometrial fragments adhere to the peritoneal surfaces and/or the ovary, begin cell proliferation, invade surrounding tissue, and begin secreting oestradiol (E_2) and prostaglandin E_2 (PGE_2).[3] This stimulates an inflammatory response involving monocyte chemotactic protein 1 (MCP-1) macrophages, matrix metalloproteinases (MMPs, enzymes for tissue remodelling), tissue inhibitors of MMPs (TIMPs), nerve growth factor, and substances that promote the development of new blood vessels (angiogenesis) such as vascular endothelial growth factor and interleukin (IL)-8.[3] Other proinflammatory cytokines secreted by lesions, such as IL-1β, IL-6, and tumour necrosis factor (TNF)-α, are abundant in the peritoneal fluid of women with endometriosis.[3] Oestradiol stimulates production of PGE_2, which in turn stimulates activation of pain fibres and promotes growth of nociceptors, leading to chronic pain.[3]

The retrograde menstruation theory is extended in the endometrial stem cell implantation theory.[8] In addition to movement of endometrial cells and tissue, this theory proposes the spread of endometrial progenitor cells and mesenchymal stem-cell-like cells, thought to be present in the basalis layer of the endometrium,[57] into the pelvic cavity.[55] Further, it has been suggested that endometrial progenitor cells may translocate to the peritoneal cavity during uterine bleeding in neonatal girls (Huber [1976], cited in Brosens et al.[58]) to be reactivated in the presence of ovarian hormones prior to menarche.[58] Research is ongoing to determine whether stem or progenitor cells from bone marrow may also differentiate into endometrial tissue.[59]

The coelomic metaplasia theory suggests that cells outside the uterus, typically in the peritoneal or visceral mesothelium, differentiate abnormally or develop into endometrial cells.[55] This theory seems most relevant for ovarian endometriosis, where coelomic epithelium can transform into endometrium.[8] The reasons for abnormal differentiation are not well-defined, but may involve 'an endogenous inductive stimulus',[53; p. 512] such as factors released from the degenerating endometrium,[60] EDCs, or immunological factors.[53] It is thought that this inductive process leads to metaplasia of ovarian serosal epithelium.[61] A similar theory is that of embryonic Müllerian rests, where embryonic cells from Müllerian ducts are stimulated by oestrogen and develop into endometriotic lesions.[53]

Endometrial tissue in the peritoneal cavity is usually removed by the immune system, leading to suggestions that immune dysfunction may be involved in implantation and growth of endometrial cells and tissue outside the uterus.[53] Further, it has been suggested that the immune system function of clearing endometrial tissue, which is seen in non-human primates, may have been lost in women during evolution.[62] Other factors that contribute to the survival of endometrial cells in the peritoneal cavity include suppression of apoptosis of endometrial cells and upregulation of antiapoptotic genes,[55] as well as greater expression of antiapoptotic factors by the endometrium in women with endometriosis.[63]

Endometrial tissue growth outside the uterus is thought to be regulated by steroid hormones, particularly as endometrial tissue expresses oestrogen receptors.[64] In the eutopic endometrium, progesterone regulates oestrogen-induced proliferation.[55] Progesterone resistance has also been suggested as a factor in the development of endometriosis due to decreased progesterone receptors, particularly progesterone receptor B, and lower levels of the enzyme 12beta-hydroxysteroid dehydrogenase type 2 (12beta-HSD-2), which metabolises E_2 to estrone (E_1).[65] A stromal cell defect in endometriotic tissue prevents progesterone from inducing expression of 12beta-HSD-2; this 'resistance' to progesterone results in increased levels of un-metabolised E_2 and decreased apoptosis.[65]

Oxidative stress during menstruation may cause genetic or epigenetic changes.[66] The genetic/epigenetic theory described by Koninckx et al.[67] suggests that the combination of 1) endometrial, stem, or bone marrow cells with inherited genetic/epigenetic defects and 2) an abnormal environment with inflammation, oxidative stress, and immunological cytokines interact to create the right environment for endometrial tissue to grow outside the uterus.

In addition to contributing to endometrial tissue growth, several of these factors affect fertility. Increased number of macrophages and proinflammatory cytokines in the peritoneal fluid, impaired apoptosis, and oxidative stress can affect fusion of oocytes and sperm.[68] Products of inflammation have deleterious effects on gametes and embryos, and progesterone resistance can impair embryo implantation.[3] Increased pelvic pain, particularly dyspareunia, can prevent regular sexual intercourse, thereby affecting fertility.[68]

Diagnosis

Women often experience delay in diagnosis of endometriosis,[22] although research from Australia suggests that the time to diagnosis has decreased since clinical guidelines were introduced in 2005.[41] Definitive diagnosis is made through visualisation and histological confirmation of endometriosis using laparoscopic surgery.[8,37] Not all women will undergo laparoscopic surgery, however, and delays exist in the time from onset of symptoms and surgical diagnosis.[22] In the absence of laparoscopic or histological confirmation, symptoms such as chronic pelvic pain, cyclical pain including dysmenorrhoea, dyspareunia, dyschezia, and dysuria, and subfertility in adolescent girls and women, are suggestive of endometriosis.[69,70]

Evaluation includes an assessment of medical history, family history, and surgical history; pelvic examination is indicated for women with chronic pelvic pain.[3] Tenderness on pelvic examination has been found to be associated with endometriosis in 66% of women.[71] Rectovaginal nodules, pelvic mass and immobile pelvic organs,[3] and bluish lesions visible during vaginal examination[70] also suggest endometriosis, but should not be considered as a reliable diagnostic tool.

The specificity of imaging, including ultrasound and magnetic imaging resonance, in detecting peritoneal and ovarian lesions is low.[72] Nevertheless, transvaginal ultrasound may be useful to detect ovarian endometriomas of two centimetres or greater in diameter[72] and deep nodular disease.[40] Biological markers, such as the cancer antigen 125 (CA-125), may be elevated in women with endometriosis but are not specific to the disease; most clinical practice guidelines recommend against the use of these indicators for diagnosis.[69,73,74]

The most well-known and established staging system for describing surgical findings for endometriosis is the revised American Society for Reproductive Medicine (rASRM, also referred to as the revised American Fertility Society [rAFS]),[4,75] which was developed to predict recurrence of endometriosis after surgery.[76] The system considers the appearance of the lesion, type of lesion, lesion location, depth of implantation, and extent of disease and adhesions visualised during laparoscopy. Points are allocated according to lesion size and adhesions and are summed to provide a total score that indicates the extent of endometriosis[77]:

- Stage I: minimal disease (score 1–5);
- Stage II: mild disease (score 6–15);
- Stage III: moderate disease (score 16–40);
- Stage IV: severe disease (score > 40).[75]

Criticisms of the rASRM staging system are that it does not include assessment of subjective pain, nor does it provide information about morphology of endometriosis lesions,[77] predict treatment response,[75] or adequately describe deep infiltrating endometriosis.[4] Further, disease stage does not correlate with pain severity or impact on quality of life.[75]

Another way of classifying endometriosis, which can be used for both superficial and deep endometriosis and which supplements the rASRM, is the revised Enzian system.[78] This system grades severity according to the depth of endometrial tissue invasion for each of three compartments: compartment a (vagina and rectovaginal septum), compartment b (sacro-uterine ligament to pelvic wall), and compartment c (rectum and sigmoid colon).[77] Additional assessments can be made for adenomyosis as well as the involvement of the bladder, ureter, bowel, or other locations.[77] Grade 0 is used when no endometrial lesions are found in the compartment, grade 1 is used for invasion less than one centimetre, grade 2 is used for invasion between one and three centimetres, and grade 3 is used for invasion greater than three centimetres.[77] The grading is reported as the letter and number (e.g., A0 B2 C1).

A further classification system, the Endometriosis Fertility Index (EFI),[79] is used to predict the chance of pregnancy for women with surgically confirmed endometriosis who wish to conceive without undergoing *in vitro* fertilisation. The index considers the function of the fallopian tube, fimbria, and ovary after surgery (scored from zero for absent or non-functional to four for normal function), age, number of infertile years, previous pregnancy, rASRM endometriosis score,

Introduction to Endometriosis

and rASRM total score to calculate a total EFI score in the range of zero to 10 (higher score means greater chance of conception).

Until better classification systems are available, the WES recommends the rASRM classification for use in all cases, the Enzian system for women with deep endometriosis, and the EFI for women who may wish to conceive in the future.[4]

Management

The American Society for Reproductive Medicine states that 'endometriosis should be viewed as a chronic disease that requires a lifelong management plan with the goal of maximising the use of medical treatment and avoiding repeated surgical procedures'.[80, p. 932] The selection of medical or surgical management of suspected or confirmed endometriosis should consider women's expectations of treatment, desire to conceive, the severity of endometriosis and endometriosis-related pain, potential side effects of treatment,[70] cost, and availability.[73] Generally, asymptomatic endometriosis in women who do not wish to conceive do not require medical or surgical management.[74,81]

Nine clinical practice guidelines (CPGs) were reviewed to summarise the management of endometriosis with conventional medicine. These included guidelines of the WES,[1] American College of Obstetricians and Gynecologists (ACOG),[82] French National Authority for Health (HAS)/College of Gynaecologists and Obstetricians (CNGOF),[70] European Society of Human Reproduction and Embryology (ESHRE),[73] Korean Society of Endometriosis,[74] National Institute for Health and Care Excellence (NICE),[69,83] Society of Obstetricians and Gynaecologists of Canada (SOGC),[84] the National German Guideline (S2k),[81] and the Australasian Certificate of Reproductive Endocrinology and Infertility Consensus Expert Panel on Trial evidence (ACCEPT).[85] As has been described elsewhere,[86,87] variation exists among clinical guidelines in recommendations for diagnosis and treatment. The information presented hereafter provides a brief overview of conventional medical management; readers are encouraged to consult individual guidelines for further information.

Surgical Management

Peritoneal endometriosis should be treated when found on laparoscopy.[73] Laparoscopy is preferred to laparotomy due to reduced recovery time, shorter hospital stay, and less pain associated with the procedure.[73] Guidelines recommend excision over ablation for removal of endometrial lesions, despite lack of evidence of superiority.[1] Women, particularly young women who are yet to complete a family, should be advised of the potential for loss of ovarian function with cystectomy of ovarian endometriomas greater than three centimetres in diameter.[1,74,84]

Guidelines vary in their recommendations for deep infiltrating endometriosis. Complete resection of deep infiltrating endometriosis is recommended in the S2k guideline,[81] while the ESHRE CPG suggests surgical removal of deep infiltrating endometriosis to be considered in light of the high rate of complications.[73] Cystectomy is recommended for endometriosis infiltrating the bladder,[70] laparotomy or laparoscopy for colorectal endometriosis,[70] and surgical treatment for women experiencing symptoms from parietal, thoracic, or diaphragmatic endometriosis.[70]

The use of hormone therapy prior to surgery does not reduce the risk of recurrence or prevent surgical complications and is not recommended.[70,74] Hormone therapy after surgery may be considered to prevent recurrence and improve quality of life for women who do not wish to become pregnant.[70,73,74,81,84] Hysterectomy may be appropriate for women with adenomyosis who have completed their family.[81] Where possible, second-line surgical treatment should be avoided when endometriosis has recurred after the initial surgery.[74]

Medical Management

Patient preferences, potential side effects, contraindications, and previous treatments should be considered when selecting hormonal treatments for endometriosis-related pain.[70] The CPGs are generally consistent in recommending the use of combined oral contraceptives (containing both oestrogen and progesterone), progestins (synthetic progestogens), and gonadotropin-releasing hormone (GnRHa) agonists (e.g., goserelin, leuprorelin) for endometriosis-related pain.[1,70,73,74,81,84] Commonly used progestins include medroxyprogesterone acetate, dienogest, cyproterone, norethisterone acetate, and danazol.

Analgesics, including paracetamol and non-steroidal anti-inflammatory drugs (NSAIDs), are recommended in the WES,[1] ESHRE,[73] and NICE[69] guidelines. Both the combined oral contraceptive pill and NSAIDs are effective, have few side effects, and are low risk.[88] Analgesics, progestins, and combined oral contraceptives are generally recommended as first-line treatments (where indicated in CPGs). Stronger analgesics, such as opioids, may be used as second-line treatment.[1,84]

Gonadotropin-releasing hormone agonists may be considered for women who do not receive adequate relief from first-line treatments,[1,70,81,84] and should be combined with add-back therapy (use of oestrogen and progestin to reduce hypoestrogenic symptoms).[1,74,81,82,84] Levonorgestrel-releasing intrauterine systems (LNG-IUS) may also be considered for women refractory to analgesics and/or combined oral contraceptives.[1,70,73,74,84] Other hormonal treatments that can be considered for women with endometriosis include anti-progestogens (gestrinone),[73] and aromatase inhibitors in combination with other hormonal treatments when usual therapy does not relieve symptoms.[74]

Management of Endometriosis-related Infertility

All CPGs made recommendations about the management of endometriosis-related infertility. Evidence shows that laparoscopic removal of endometriosis lesions in stages I and II improves fertility,[1,73,81,82,84,85] while hormonal suppression of ovarian function does not increase the chance of spontaneous pregnancy.[1,69,70,73,81,85] Treatment with GnRHa for three to six months before *in vitro* fertilisation or intracytoplasmic sperm injection is effective at improving pregnancy outcomes.[1,70,84] Several guidelines provided detailed recommendations about the management of assisted conception that can provide additional information for interested readers.[1,73,81,84,85]

Complementary and Alternative Medicine

Women may look to complementary and alternative medicines (CAMs) when the response to conventional medical treatments and/or surgery is inadequate. Indeed, women with endometriosis were found to be more likely to have visited a massage therapist or acupuncturist and to have used vitamin supplements, yoga, meditation, or Chinese medicines than women without endometriosis.[29]

In advocating for a multidisciplinary team to meet expectations for women with endometriosis, D'Hooghe and Hummelshoj (2006)[2] suggest that such a team may include traditional Chinese medicine practitioners, acupuncturists, and homeopaths. Several CPGs state that there is limited evidence for CAMs, including Chinese medicine, and therefore do not recommend their use.[1,69,73,81] The ESHRE clinical practice guidelines acknowledge that some women may obtain benefit from CAMs, despite the lack of robust evidence.[73]

Prognosis

Endometriosis is a chronic condition. Endometriosis lesions may resolve spontaneously, remain stable, or progress.[89] As it is common to experience recurrence of pain within 12 months of surgery,[90] women should be supported with information on how to live with endometriosis and manage pain.[2] Providing realistic information about treatment success can greatly assist the management of patient expectations.[2]

References

1. Johnson NP, Hummelshoj L. (2013) Consensus on current management of endometriosis. *Hum Reprod* **28**(6): 1552–1568.
2. D'Hooghe T, Hummelshoj L. (2006) Multi-disciplinary centres/networks of excellence for endometriosis management and research: A proposal. *Hum Reprod* **21**(11): 2743–2748.
3. Giudice LC. (2010) Clinical practice. Endometriosis. *N Engl J Med* **362**(25): 2389–2398.

4. Johnson NP, Hummelshoj L, Adamson GD, et al. (2017) World Endometriosis Society consensus on the classification of endometriosis. *Hum Reprod* **32**(2): 315–324.
5. Bagan P, Berna P, Assouad J, et al. (2008) Value of cancer antigen 125 for diagnosis of pleural endometriosis in females with recurrent pneumothorax. *Eur Respir J* **31**(1): 140–142.
6. Jubanyik KJ, Comite F. (1997) Extrapelvic endometriosis. *Obstet Gynecol Clin North Am* **24**(2): 411–440.
7. Schenken R. (2019) Endometriosis: Pathogenesis, clinical features, and diagnosis 2019 [cited 2019 28th July]. Available from: https://www.uptodate.com/contents/endometriosis-pathogenesis-clinical-features-and-diagnosis.
8. Vercellini P, Vigano P, Somigliana E, et al. (2014) Endometriosis: pathogenesis and treatment. *Nat Rev Endocrinol* **10**(5): 261–275.
9. Andres MP, Borrelli GM, Abrao MS. (2018) Endometriosis classification according to pain symptoms: Can the ASRM classification be improved? *Best Pract Res Clin Obstet Gynaecol* **51**: 111–118.
10. Koninckx PR, Martin DC. (1992) Deep endometriosis: A consequence of infiltration or retraction or possibly adenomyosis externa? *Fertil Steril* **58**(5): 924–928.
11. Koninckx PR, Ussia A, Adamyan L, et al. (2012) Deep endometriosis: Definition, diagnosis, and treatment. *Fertil Steril* **98**(3): 564–571.
12. Benagiano G, Brosens I, Lippi D. (2014) The history of endometriosis. *Gynecol Obstet Invest* **78**(1): 1–9.
13. Gordts S, Grimbizis G, Campo R. (2018) Symptoms and classification of uterine adenomyosis, including the place of hysteroscopy in diagnosis. *Fertil Steril* **109**(3): 380–388.e1.
14. Sinaii N, Plumb K, Cotton L, et al. (2008) Differences in characteristics among 1,000 women with endometriosis based on extent of disease. *Fertil Steril* **89**(3): 538–545.
15. Hickey M, Ballard K, Farquhar C. (2014) Endometriosis. *BMJ* **348**: g1752.
16. Berlanda N, Vercellini P, Carmignani L, et al. (2009) Ureteral and vesical endometriosis. Two different clinical entities sharing the same pathogenesis. *Obstet Gynecol Surv* **64**(12): 830–842.
17. Ballard K, Lane H, Hudelist G, et al. (2010) Can specific pain symptoms help in the diagnosis of endometriosis? A cohort study of women with chronic pelvic pain. *Fertil Steril* **94**(1): 20–27.

18. Hwang SM, Lee CW, Lee BS, et al. (2015) Clinical features of thoracic endometriosis: A single center analysis. *Obstet Gynecol Sci* **58**(3): 223–231.
19. Giudice LC, Kao LC. (2004) Endometriosis. *The Lancet* **364**(9447): 1789–1799.
20. Laufer M. Endometriosis in adolescents: Diagnosis and treatment 2019 [cited 2019 28th July]. Available from: https://www.uptodate.com/contents/endometriosis-in-adolescents-diagnosis-and-treatment.
21. Vos T, Barber R, Bell B, et al. (2015) Global, regional, and national incidence, prevalence, and years lived with disability for 301 acute and chronic diseases and injuries in 188 countries, 1990–2013: A systematic analysis for the Global Burden of Disease Study 2013. *Lancet* **386**(9995): 743–800.
22. Hudelist G, Fritzer N, Thomas A, et al. (2012) Diagnostic delay for endometriosis in Austria and Germany: Causes and possible consequences. *Hum Reprod* **27**(12): 3412–3416.
23. Missmer SA, Hankinson SE, Spiegelman D, et al. (2004) Incidence of laparoscopically confirmed endometriosis by demographic, anthropometric, and lifestyle factors. *Am J Epidemiol* **160**(8): 784–796.
24. Fuldeore MJ, Soliman AM. (2017) Prevalence and symptomatic burden of diagnosed endometriosis in the United States: National estimates from a cross-sectional survey of 59,411 women. *Gynecol Obstet Invest* **82**(5): 453–461.
25. Abbas S, Ihle P, Koster I, et al. (2012) Prevalence and incidence of diagnosed endometriosis and risk of endometriosis in patients with endometriosis-related symptoms: Findings from a statutory health insurance-based cohort in Germany. *Eur J Obstet Gynecol Reprod Biol* **160**(1): 79–83.
26. Morassutto C, Monasta L, Ricci G, et al. (2016) Incidence and estimated prevalence of endometriosis and adenomyosis in northeast Italy: A data linkage study. *PLoS One* **11**(4): e0154227.
27. Cea Soriano L, Lopez-Garcia E, Schulze-Rath R, et al. (2017) Incidence, treatment and recurrence of endometriosis in a UK-based population analysis using data from The Health Improvement Network and the Hospital Episode Statistics database. *Eur J Contracept Reprod Health Care* **22**(5): 334–343.
28. Reid R, Steel A, Wardle J, et al. (2019) The prevalence of self-reported diagnosed endometriosis in the Australian population: Results from a nationally-representative survey. *BMC Res Notes* **12**(1): 88.

29. Fisher C, Adams J, Hickman L, et al. (2016) The use of complementary and alternative medicine by 7427 Australian women with cyclic perimenstrual pain and discomfort: A cross-sectional study. *BMC Complement Altern Med* **16**: 129.
30. Rowlands IJ, Abbott JA, Montgomery GW, et al. (2020) Prevalence and incidence of endometriosis in Australian women: A data linkage cohort study. *BJOG*: 1–9.
31. Balasch J, Creus M, Fabregues F, et al. (1996) Visible and non-visible endometriosis at laparoscopy in fertile and infertile women and in patients with chronic pelvic pain: A prospective study. *Hum Reprod* **11**(2): 387–391.
32. Meuleman C, Vandenabeele B, Fieuws S, et al. (2009) High prevalence of endometriosis in infertile women with normal ovulation and normospermic partners. *Fertil Steril* **92**(1): 68–74.
33. Rawson JM. (1991) Prevalence of endometriosis in asymptomatic women. *J Reprod Med* **36**(7): 513–515.
34. Pearson S, Pickersgill A. (2004) The cost of endometriosis. *Gynaecology Forum* **9**(4): 23–27.
35. Soliman AM, Yang H, Du EX, et al. (2016) The direct and indirect costs associated with endometriosis: A systematic literature review. *Hum Reprod* **31**(4): 712–722.
36. Simoens S, Dunselman G, Dirksen C, et al. (2012) The burden of endometriosis: Costs and quality of life of women with endometriosis and treated in referral centres. *Hum Reprod* **27**(5): 1292–1299.
37. Hummelshoj L, Prentice A, Groothuis P. (2006) Update on endometriosis. *Womens Health (Lond)* **2**(1): 53–56.
38. Soliman AM, Surrey E, Bonafede M, et al. (2018) Real-world evaluation of direct and indirect economic burden among endometriosis patients in the United States. *Adv Ther* **35**(3): 408–423.
39. Armour M, Lawson K, Wood A, et al. (2019) The cost of illness and economic burden of endometriosis and chronic pelvic pain in Australia: A national online survey. *PLoS One* **14**(10): e0223316.
40. Zondervan KT, Becker CM, Koga K, et al. (2018) Endometriosis. *Nat Rev Dis Primers* **4**(1): 9.
41. Armour M, Sinclair J, Ng CM, et al. (2020) Endometriosis and chronic pelvic pain have similar impact on women, but time to diagnosis is decreasing: An Australian survey. *medRxiv*: 2020.06.16.20133231.
42. Soliman AM, Coyne KS, Zaiser E, et al. (2017) The burden of endometriosis symptoms on health-related quality of life in women in the

United States: A cross-sectional study. *J Psychosom Obstet Gynaecol* **38**(4): 238–248.
43. Nnoaham KE, Hummelshoj L, Webster P, *et al.* (2011) Impact of endometriosis on quality of life and work productivity: A multicenter study across ten countries. *Fertil Steril* **96**(2): 366–373.e8.
44. 吉宁, 刘世炜, 曾新颖, *et al.* (2016) 2016年中国妇科疾病的疾病负担研究. 中华妇产科杂志 **53**(5): 313–318.
45. Marinho MCP, Magalhaes TF, Fernandes LFC, *et al.* (2018) Quality of life in women with endometriosis: An integrative review. *J Womens Health (Larchmt)* **27**(3): 399–408.
46. Vigano P, Parazzini F, Somigliana E, *et al.* (2004) Endometriosis: Epidemiology and aetiological factors. *Best Pract Res Clin Obstet Gynaecol* **18**(2): 177–200.
47. Missmer SA, Hankinson SE, Spiegelman D, *et al.* (2004) In utero exposures and the incidence of endometriosis. *Fertil Steril* **82**(6): 1501–1508.
48. Hemmings R, Rivard M, Olive DL, *et al.* (2004) Evaluation of risk factors associated with endometriosis. *Fertil Steril* **81**(6): 1513–1521.
49. Dai Y, Li X, Shi J, *et al.* (2018) A review of the risk factors, genetics and treatment of endometriosis in Chinese women: A comparative update. *Reprod Health* **15**(1): 82.
50. Lin WC, Chang CY, Hsu YA, *et al.* (2016) Increased risk of endometriosis in patients with lower genital tract infection: A nationwide cohort study. *Medicine (Baltimore)* **95**(10): e2773.
51. Missmer SA, Chavarro JE, Malspeis S, *et al.* (2010) A prospective study of dietary fat consumption and endometriosis risk. *Hum Reprod* **25**(6): 1528–1535.
52. Parazzini F, Esposito G, Tozzi L, *et al.* (2017) Epidemiology of endometriosis and its comorbidities. *Eur J Obstet Gynecol Reprod Biol* **209**: 3–7.
53. Burney RO, Giudice LC. (2012) Pathogenesis and pathophysiology of endometriosis. *Fertil Steril* **98**(3): 511–519.
54. Brosens I, Brosens JJ, Benagiano G. (2012) The eutopic endometrium in endometriosis: are the changes of clinical significance? *Reprod Biomed Online* **24**(5): 496–502.
55. Sourial S, Tempest N, Hapangama DK. (2014) Theories on the pathogenesis of endometriosis. *Int J Reprod Med* **2014**: 179515.
56. Halme J, Hammond MG, Hulka JF, *et al.* (1984) Retrograde menstruation in healthy women and in patients with endometriosis. *Obstet Gynecol* **64**(2): 151–154.

57. Padykula HA. (1991) Regeneration in the primate uterus: the role of stem cells. *Ann N Y Acad Sci* **622**: 47–56.
58. Brosens I, Gordts S, Benagiano G. (2013) Endometriosis in adolescents is a hidden, progressive and severe disease that deserves attention, not just compassion. *Hum Reprod* **28**(8): 2026–2031.
59. Sasson IE, Taylor HS. (2008) Stem cells and the pathogenesis of endometriosis. *Ann N Y Acad Sci* **1127**: 106–115.
60. Nap AW, Groothuis PG, Demir AY, *et al.* (2004) Pathogenesis of endometriosis. *Best Pract Res Clin Obstet Gynaecol* **18**(2): 233–244.
61. Ohtake H, Katabuchi H, Matsuura K, *et al.* (1999) A novel in vitro experimental model for ovarian endometriosis: The three-dimensional culture of human ovarian surface epithelial cells in collagen gels. *Fertil Steril* **71**(1): 50–55.
62. Donnez O, Van Langendonckt A, Defrere S, *et al.* (2013) Induction of endometriotic nodules in an experimental baboon model mimicking human deep nodular lesions. *Fertil Steril* **99**(3): 783–789.e3.
63. Taniguchi F, Kaponis A, Izawa M, *et al.* (2011) Apoptosis and endometriosis. *Front Biosci (Elite Ed)* **3**: 648–662.
64. Fujimoto J, Hirose R, Sakaguchi H, *et al.* (1999) Expression of oestrogen receptor-alpha and -beta in ovarian endometriomata. *Mol Hum Reprod* **5**(8): 742–747.
65. Bulun SE, Cheng YH, Yin P, *et al.* (2006) Progesterone resistance in endometriosis: Link to failure to metabolize estradiol. *Mol Cell Endocrinol* **248**(1–2): 94–103.
66. Donnez J, Binda MM, Donnez O, *et al.* (2016) Oxidative stress in the pelvic cavity and its role in the pathogenesis of endometriosis. *Fertil Steril* **106**(5): 1011–1017.
67. Koninckx PR, Ussia A, Adamyan L, *et al.* (2019) Pathogenesis of endometriosis: The genetic/epigenetic theory. *Fertil Steril* **111**(2): 327–340.
68. de Ziegler D, Borghese B, Chapron C. (2010) Endometriosis and infertility: Pathophysiology and management. *Lancet* **376**(9742): 730–738.
69. Kuznetsov L, Dworzynski K, Davies M, *et al.* (2017) Diagnosis and management of endometriosis: Summary of NICE guidance. *BMJ* **358**: j3935.
70. Collinet P, Fritel X, Revel-Delhom C, *et al.* (2018) Management of endometriosis: CNGOF/HAS clinical practice guidelines — Short version. *J Gynecol Obstet Hum Reprod* **47**(7): 265–274.
71. Ripps BA, Martin DC. (1991) Focal pelvic tenderness, pelvic pain and dysmenorrhea in endometriosis. *J Reprod Med* **36**(7): 470–472.

72. Brosens I, Puttemans P, Campo R, et al. (2004) Diagnosis of endometriosis: Pelvic endoscopy and imaging techniques. *Best Pract Res Clin Obstet Gynaecol* **18**(2): 285–303.
73. Dunselman GA, Vermeulen N, Becker C, et al. (2014) ESHRE guideline: Management of women with endometriosis. *Hum Reprod* **29**(3): 400–412.
74. Hwang H, Chung YJ, Lee SR, et al. (2018) Clinical evaluation and management of endometriosis: Guideline for Korean patients from Korean Society of Endometriosis. *Obstet Gynecol Sci* **61**(5): 553–564.
75. American Society for Reproductive Medicine. (1997) Revised American Society for Reproductive Medicine classification of endometriosis: 1996. *Fertil Steril* **67**(5): 817–821.
76. Wang W, Li R, Fang T, et al. (2013) Endometriosis fertility index score maybe more accurate for predicting the outcomes of in vitro fertilisation than r-AFS classification in women with endometriosis. *Reprod Biol Endocrinol* **11**: 112.
77. Haas D, Shebl O, Shamiyeh A, et al. (2013) The rASRM score and the Enzian classification for endometriosis: Their strengths and weaknesses. *Acta Obstet Gynecol Scand* **92**(1): 3–7.
78. Tuttlies F, Keckstein J, Ulrich U, et al. (2005) [ENZIAN-score, a classification of deep infiltrating endometriosis]. *Zentralbl Gynakol* **127**(5): 275–281.
79. Adamson GD, Pasta DJ. (2010) Endometriosis Fertility Index: The new, validated endometriosis staging system. *Fertil Steril* **94**(5): 1609–1615.
80. Practice Committee of the American Society for Reproductive Medicine. (2014) Treatment of pelvic pain associated with endometriosis: A committee opinion. *Fertil Steril* **101**(4): 927–935.
81. Ulrich U, Buchweitz O, Greb R, et al. (2014) National German Guideline (S2k): Guideline for the diagnosis and treatment of endometriosis: Long version — AWMF Registry No. 015-045. *Geburtshilfe Frauenheilkd* **74**(12): 1104–1118.
82. The American College of Obstetricians and Gynecologists (2010) Practice bulletin no. 114: Management of endometriosis. *Obstet Gynecol* **116**(1): 223–236.
83. NICE. (2017) Endometriosis: Diagnosis and management 2017 [cited 2018 2nd October]. Available from: nice.org.uk/guidance/ng73.
84. Leyland N, Casper R, Laberge P, et al. (2010) Endometriosis: Diagnosis and management. *J Obstet Gynaecol Can* **32**(7 Suppl 2): S1–32.

85. Koch J, Rowan K, Rombauts L, et al. (2012) Endometriosis and infertility — a consensus statement from ACCEPT (Australasian CREI Consensus Expert Panel on Trial evidence). *Aust N Z J Obstet Gynaecol* **52**(6): 513–522.
86. Hirsch M, Begum MR, Paniz E, et al. (2018) Diagnosis and management of endometriosis: A systematic review of international and national guidelines. *BJOG* **125**(5): 556–564.
87. Kho RM, Andres MP, Borrelli GM, et al. (2018) Surgical treatment of different types of endometriosis: Comparison of major society guidelines and preferred clinical algorithms. *Best Pract Res Clin Obstet Gynaecol* **51**: 102–110.
88. Schenken R. (2019) Endometriosis: Treatment of pelvic pain 2019 [cited 2019 28th July]. Available from: https://www.uptodate.com/contents/endometriosis-treatment-of-pelvic-pain.
89. Sutton CJG, Pooley AS, Ewen SP, et al. (1997) Follow-up report on a randomized controlled trial of laser laparoscopy in the treatment of pelvic pain associated with minimal to moderate endometriosis. *Fertil Steril* **68**(6): 1070–1074.
90. Practice Committee of the American Society for Reproductive Medicine. (2008) Treatment of pelvic pain associated with endometriosis. *Fertil Steril* **90**(5): S260–S269.

2

Endometriosis in Chinese Medicine

OVERVIEW

This chapter introduces the aetiology and pathogenesis, syndrome differentiation, and management of endometriosis in contemporary Chinese medicine. The main treatments for endometriosis recommended by Chinese medicine guidelines and textbooks are summarised in this chapter; these include oral and topical Chinese herbal medicine, acupuncture and related therapies, and dietary therapy.

Introduction

The Chinese conventional medical term for endometriosis is *zi gong nei mo yi wei zheng* 子宫内膜异位症. Diseases related to endometriosis, such as adenomyosis, are called *zi gong nei mo yi wei xing ji bing* 子宫内膜异位性疾病. Endometriosis and adenomyosis are different but related uterine diseases. They are considered to have different aetiology and pathogenesis, but manifest with similar symptoms such as dysmenorrhoea, chronic pelvic pain, pain during intercourse (dyspareunia), and infertility.

As endometriosis is a recently defined disease, there is no specific term for endometriosis in Chinese medicine (CM). Instead, endometriosis is usually described according to signs and symptoms. For example, *tong jing* 痛经 refers to dysmenorrhoea, *zheng jia* 癥瘕 refers to abdominal mass, *bu yun zheng* 不孕症 refers to infertility, and *yue jing bu tiao* 月经不调 refers to irregular menstruation.

Aetiology and Pathogenesis

The aetiology of endometriosis is complex. Causes of endometriosis include external contraction of any of the six pathogenic factors (cold, wind, damp, heat, fire, and dryness), internal damage due to any of the seven emotions (joy, anger, worry, fear, sadness, shock, and anxiety), and other causes that are neither external nor internal, such as overexertion, fatigue, weak constitution, previous history of miscarriage, and surgery. These causes can impair the circulation of *qi* and Blood, damage the *Chong* 冲 and *Ren* 任 meridians, and lead to the escape of menses from the vessels and retention of Blood in the lower abdomen, in turn further obstructing the circulation of *qi* and Blood in the *Chong* 冲 and *Ren* 任 meridians, uterus meridian (*Bao mai* 胞脉), and collaterals.[1]

As a result, Blood stasis is considered the main syndrome, and the most commonly seen endometriosis symptoms are all related to Blood stasis. Blood stasis obstructs the uterus meridian and induces dysmenorrhoea. Blood stasis also obstructs the *Chong* 冲 and *Ren* 任 meridians, causing Blood to 'leak' from the meridian and resulting in menstrual problems such as menorrhagia, prolonged menstruation, and abnormal uterine bleeding. The location of endometriosis is commonly around the *Chong* 冲 and *Ren* 任 meridians, uterus meridian, and collaterals. Blockage of the uterus meridian and collaterals prevents female and male essence (*jing* 精) from interacting, leading to infertility. Long-term Blood stasis may lead to abdominal mass.[1]

Syndrome Differentiation and Treatments

The first national standard of diagnosis, syndrome differentiation, and assessment of treatment efficacy of endometriosis was established in *The Clinical Guideline of Chinese Herbal Medicine and New Medication* 中药新药临床指导原则, published by the Ministry of Health of the People's Republic of China in 1993.[2] Four syndromes were listed for endometriosis: *qi* stagnation and Blood stasis 气滞血瘀, cold congealing and Blood stasis 寒凝血瘀, Kidney deficiency and Blood stasis 肾虚血瘀, and dampness-heat and stasis obstructing the uterus 湿热瘀阻. In the 2012 *Guidelines for Diagnosis and Treatment of Common Diseases of Gynaecology in Traditional Chinese Medicine* 中医妇科常见病诊疗指南 by the China Association of Chinese Medicine,[3] two additional syndromes were added for endometriosis: *qi* deficiency and Blood stasis 气虚血瘀 and phlegm and stasis binding 痰瘀互结.

The prevalence of these six syndromes was examined in a recent Chinese cross-sectional study of 450 women with endometriosis. The most frequent syndrome was *qi* stagnation and Blood stasis (36.2%) followed by Kidney deficiency and Blood stasis (17.8%), cold congealing and Blood stasis (16.9%), *qi* deficiency and Blood stasis (12.2%), dampness-heat and stasis obstructing the uterus (8.7%), and phlegm and stasis binding (8.2%).[4] These six syndromes have been widely adopted in contemporary CM guidelines, textbooks, and monographs.

In this chapter, the treatment principle, Chinese herbal medicine (CHM) formulas and herbs, and manufactured medicines are summarised from the following CM textbooks, guidelines, and monographs:

- *Chinese Medicine of Gynaecology* 中医妇科学;[1,5,6]
- *Integrated Medicine of Gynaecology and Obstetrics* 中西医结合妇产科学;[7-9]
- *Chinese Medicine Management for Twenty-two Specialties and Ninety-five Diseases (Dysmenorrhoea)* 22 个专业 95 个病种中医诊疗方案 (痛经);[10]
- *Chinese Medicine Management for Twenty-four Specialties and One Hundred and Five Diseases (Endometrioma)* 24 个专业 105 个病种中医诊疗方案 (巧囊);[11]
- *Guidelines for Diagnosis and Treatment of Common Diseases of Gynaecology in Traditional Chinese Medicine* 中医妇科常见病诊疗指南;[3]
- *The Research Progress of Gynaecology in Integrated Medicine* 中西医结合妇科学研究新进展;[12]
- *The Chinese Medicine Diagnosis and Management of Gynaecology 3rd Edition* 中医临床诊治-妇科专病 (第三版);[13]

- The Integrated Medicine of Diagnosis and Management for Common Diseases 常见病中西医结合诊疗常规.[14]

The use of some herbs may be restricted in some countries. In addition, some herbs are restricted under the provisions of the Convention on International Trade in Endangered Species of Wild Fauna and Flora (CITES). Readers are advised to comply with relevant regulations.

Oral Chinese Herbal Medicine Treatment Based on Syndrome Differentiation

The following syndromes describe symptoms that occur in women with endometriosis that are both related and unrelated to the menstrual cycle. As Blood stasis is considered the key mechanism in endometriosis, the treatment principle for many of the syndromes is to activate Blood and dispel stasis. Chinese herbal medicine formulas are selected according to syndrome differentiation and are summarised in Table 2.1.

Table 2.1. Summary of Chinese Herbal Medicines for Endometriosis

Syndrome	Treatment Principle	Oral Chinese Herbal Medicine	
		Traditional Formula	Manufactured Medicine
Qi stagnation and Blood stasis	Regulate qi, activate Blood, resolve stasis, and relieve pain.	Ge xia zhu yu tang 膈下逐瘀汤 or Xue fu zhu yu tang 血府逐瘀汤.	San jie zhen tong jiao nang 散结镇痛胶囊, Dan e kang fu jian gao 丹莪妇康煎膏.
Kidney deficiency and Blood stasis	Tonify Kidney, regulate menstruation, activate Blood, and resolve stasis.	Gui shen wan 归肾丸 plus Tao hong si wu tang 桃红四物汤.	None

(Continued)

Table 2.1 (Continued)

Syndrome	Treatment Principle	Oral Chinese Herbal Medicine	
		Traditional Formula	Manufactured Medicine
Cold congealing and Blood stasis	Warm the meridian to dissipate cold, resolve stasis, and relieve pain.	Shao fu zhu yu tang 少腹逐瘀汤.	Gui zhi fu ling jiao nan g桂枝茯苓胶囊, Ai fu nuan gong wan 艾附暖宫丸.
Qi deficiency and Blood stasis	Tonify qi, activate Blood, resolve stasis, and relieve pain.	Li chong tang 理冲汤, Ju yuan jian 举元煎 plus Tao hong si wu tang 桃红四物汤, Ju yuan jian 举元煎 plus Shi xiao san 失笑散, and san qi 三七.	None
Phlegm and stasis binding	Resolve phlegm, dissipate binds, activate Blood, and resolve stasis.	Cang fu dao tan wan 苍附导痰丸 plus Tao hong si wu tang 桃红四物汤.	San jie zhen tong jiao nang 散结镇痛胶囊.
Dampness-heat and stasis obstructing the uterus	Clear heat, harmonise the ying 营, activate Blood, and resolve stasis.	Qing re tiao xue tang 清热调血汤.	None

Qi Stagnation and Blood Stasis 气滞血瘀

Clinical manifestations: Distending pain in the lower abdomen during menstruation with difficulty expelling the blood, accompanied by dark, clotty menses. Pain may be alleviated after expelling the blood clot. Other symptoms include menorrhagia, abdominal mass, sensation of heaviness and distension in the anus and/or urethra, distending breast pain before the menstrual period, and infertility. The patient may report depression or irritability. The tongue will be dark with spots and the pulse will be thin, string-like, or rough.

Treatment principle: Regulate *qi*, activate Blood, resolve stasis, and relieve pain.

Formula: *Ge xia zhu yu tang* 膈下逐瘀汤[1,3,5,8–10,13,14] or *Xue fu zhu yu tang* 血府逐瘀汤.[1,3]

Herbs: *Zhi qiao* 枳壳, *wu yao* 乌药, *xiang fu* 香附, *dang gui* 当归, *chuan xiong* 川芎, *chi shao* 赤芍, *tao ren* 桃仁, *hong hua* 红花, *mu dan pi* 牡丹皮, *yan hu suo* 延胡索, *wu ling zhi* 五灵脂, *gan cao* 甘草, *sheng di* 生地, *niu xi* 牛膝, *jie geng* 桔梗, and *chai hu* 柴胡.

Main actions of herbs: *Tao ren* 桃仁, *hong hua* 红花, *dang gui* 当归, *chuan xiong* 川芎, and *chi shao* 赤芍 activate Blood and resolve stasis. *Dang gui* 当归 and *sheng di* 生地 nourish Blood and remove stasis; *chai hu* 柴胡 and *zhi ke* 枳壳 soothe the Liver and regulate *qi*. *Niu xi* 牛膝 resolves stasis, unblocks the meridians, and guides Blood stasis downwards; *jie geng* 桔梗 diffuses the Lung and guides the herbs upwards. *Gan cao* 甘草 relaxes tension and harmonises all herbs. All herbs are used to activate Blood and regulate *qi*.

Manufactured medicines: *San jie zhen tong jiao nang* 散结镇痛胶囊,[10,11] *Dan e kang fu jian gao* 丹莪妇康煎膏.[8,10,11]

Kidney Deficiency and Blood Stasis 肾虚血瘀

Clinical manifestations: Sensation of cold and pain, stabbing pain, or heaviness in the lower abdomen. The pain radiates to the lumbosacral area and the location is fixed. There may be menstrual period disorders, such as lighter menstrual flow and light-coloured menses with clots. Other symptoms include abdominal mass, sensation of heaviness and distension in the anus, infertility and miscarriage, lower back and knee pain, dizziness and tinnitus, dark colour around the eye, frequent enuresis, and sexual hypoactivity. The tongue will be dark with spots and a white thin coat, while the pulse will be thin, sunken, and rough.

Treatment principle: Tonify the Kidneys, regulate menstruation, activate Blood, and resolve stasis.

Formula: *Gui shen wan* 归肾丸 plus *Tao hong si wu tang* 桃红四物汤.[1,3,8,9]

Herbs: *Shu di huang* 熟地黄, *shan yao* 山药, *gou qi zi* 枸杞子, *shan zhu yu* 山茱萸, *fu ling* 茯苓, *dang gui* 当归, *du zhong* 杜仲, *tu si zi* 菟丝子, *tao ren* 桃仁, *hong hua* 红花, *chuan xiong* 川芎, *chi shao* 赤芍, *yan hu suo* 延胡索, *san qi* 三七, etc.

Main actions of herbs: *Shan zhu yu* 山茱萸, *tu si zi* 菟丝子, and *shan yao* 山药 warm and nourish Kidney essence; *tao ren* 桃仁, *hong hua* 红花, *dang gui* 当归, *chi shao* 赤芍, and *san qi* 三七 activate Blood and resolve stasis. *Gou qi zi* 枸杞子 and *shu di huang* 熟地黄 nourish *yin* and Blood, *chuan xiong* 川芎 regulates *qi* to remove Blood stasis, and *fu ling* 茯苓 drains dampness and expels pathogens via urination.

Cold Congealing and Blood Stasis 寒凝血瘀

Clinical manifestations: Lower abdominal mass, sensation of cold, pain before or during the menstrual period, and refusal to be touched. The pain may be relieved by warmth. Menstrual flow may be lighter with dark-coloured menstrual blood and metrorrhagia. Other signs and symptoms include a pale face, aversion to cold, and sensation of cold all over the body. The tongue will be dark with a thin white coat and the pulse will be sunken and tight.

Treatment principle: Warm the meridian to dissipate cold, resolve stasis, and relieve pain.

Formula: *Shao fu zhu yu tang* 少腹逐瘀汤.[1,3,5,8–11,13,14]

Herbs: *Xiao hui xiang* 小茴香, *gan jiang* 干姜, *rou gui* 肉桂, *dang gui* 当归, *chuan xiong* 川芎, *chi shao* 赤芍, *mo yao* 没药, *pu huang* 蒲黄, *wu ling zhi* 五灵脂, *yan hu suo* 延胡索, *san leng* 三棱, *e zhu* 莪术, *wu yao* 乌药, and *ba ji tian* 巴戟天.

Main actions of herbs: *Dang gui* 当归, *chuan xiong* 川芎, and *chi shao* 赤芍 activate Blood and dispel stasis, nourish Blood, and regulate menstruation. *Xiao hui xiang* 小茴, *gan jiang* 干姜, and *rou gui* 肉桂 expel cold, unblock *yang,* and warm the *Chong* and *Ren* meridians. *Pu huang* 蒲黄, *wu ling zhi* 五灵脂, *yan hu suo* 延胡索, and *mo yao* 没药 activate Blood and dispel stasis, dissipate binds, and alleviate pain.

Manufactured medicines: *Gui zhi fu ling jiao nang* 桂枝茯苓胶囊,[10,11] *Ai fu nuan gong wan* 艾附暖宫丸.[10,11]

Qi Deficiency and Blood Stasis 气虚血瘀

Clinical manifestations: Intolerable pain with a sensation of heaviness and distension in the lower abdomen; some patients will have lower abdominal mass. Menstrual changes can include heavy menstrual flow or prolonged menstruation and light-coloured, thin menses. Other symptoms include a pale and dull face, fatigue, lack of desire to speak, poor appetite, and diarrhoea. The tongue will be enlarged and pale with spots on the tip and margins of the tongue, and the coat will be white and thin. The pulse will be sunken and tight.

Treatment principle: Tonify *qi*, activate Blood, resolve stasis, and relieve pain.

Formula: *Li chong tang* 理冲汤,[8,9] *Ju yuan jian* 举元煎 plus *Tao hong si wu tang* 桃红四物汤,[1,5] *Ju yuan jian* 举元煎 plus *Shi xiao san* 失笑散, and *san qi* 三七.[7,13]

Herbs: *Sheng huang qi* 生黄芪, *ren shen* 人参, *bai zhu* 白术, *shan yao* 山药, *tian hua fen* 天花粉, *zhi mu* 知母, *san leng* 三棱, *e zhu* 莪术, *sheng ji nei jin* 生鸡内金, *sheng ma* 升麻, *gan cao* 甘草, *pu huang* 蒲黄, *wu ling zhi* 五灵脂, *san qi* 三七, *tao ren* 桃仁, *hong hua* 红花, *shu di huang* 熟地黄, *dang gui* 当归, *bai shao* 白芍, and *chuan xiong* 川芎.

Main actions of herbs: *Tao ren* 桃仁, *hong hua* 红花, *pu huang* 蒲黄, *wu ling zhi* 五灵脂, *san leng* 三棱, and *e zhu* 莪术 remove Blood stasis; *ren shen* 人参, *huang qi* 黄芪, *bai zhu* 白术, and *shan yao* 山药 nourish *qi*. *Shu di huang* 熟地黄, *dang gui* 当归, and *bai shao* 白芍 nourish *yin* and Blood. *Tian hua fen* 天花粉 and *zhi mu* 知母 nourish *yin* and clear heat; *sheng ji nei jin* 生鸡内金 nourishes the Spleen to promote digestion; *sheng ma* 升麻 and *chuan xiong* 川芎 regulate *qi* and resolve Blood stasis in the meridians.

Phlegm and Stasis Binding 痰瘀互结

Clinical manifestations: Lower abdominal pain before or during the menstrual period, lower abdominal mass with sensation of distention, and aversion to being touched. Other symptoms include infertility, obesity, dizziness, chest tightness, poor appetite, heavy and sticky vaginal discharge, and diarrhoea. The tongue will be dark with a thick and slimy coat, and the pulse will be fine and slippery.

Treatment principle: Resolve phlegm, dissipate binds, activate Blood, and resolve stasis.

Formula: *Cang fu dao tan wan* 苍附导痰丸 plus *Tao hong si wu tang* 桃红四物汤.[3,8]

Herbs: *Cang zhu* 苍术, *xiang fu* 香附, *chen pi* 陈皮, *nan xing* 南星, *zhi qiao* 枳壳, *ban xia* 半夏, *chuan xiong* 川芎, *hua shi* 滑石, *fu ling* 茯苓, *shen qu* 神曲, *dang gui* 当归, *tao ren* 桃仁, *hong hua* 红花, *shu di* 熟地, *bai shao* 白芍, etc.

Main actions of herbs: *Xiang fu* 香附 regulates *qi*, resolves stagnation, and harmonises Blood; *cang zhu* 苍术 drains dampness and nourishes the Spleen. *Chen pi* 陈皮, *ban xia* 半夏, *fu ling* 茯苓, *gan cao* 甘草, *hua shi* 滑石, *shen qu* 神曲, and *tian nan xing* 天南星 dry dampness to expel phlegm, regulate *qi*, and harmonise the Middle Energiser; *zhi ke* 枳壳 and *chuan xiong* 川芎 guide the *qi* downwards to dissipate binds. *Tao ren* 桃仁 and *hong hua* 红花 activate Blood to remove stasis; *shu di* 熟地, *bai shao* 白芍, and *dang gui* 当归 nourish Blood.

Manufactured medicines: *San jie zhen tong jiao nang* 散结镇痛胶囊.[11,13]

Dampness-heat and Stasis Obstructing the Uterus 湿热瘀阻

Clinical manifestations: Distending or burning lower abdominal pain before or during the period, heavy and sticky red or dark red menses, and lower abdominal mass. Patients may also report a large amount of yellow, sticky vaginal discharge. Other symptoms may include a sticky or slimy sensation in the mouth, poor appetite, diarrhoea, and yellow or dark urine. The tongue will be dark with a slimy yellow coat and the pulse will be rapid and slippery or soggy.

Treatment principle: Clear heat, harmonise the *ying* 营, activate Blood, resolve stasis.

Formula: *Qing re tiao xue tang* 清热调血汤.[3]

Herbs: *Dan pi* 丹皮, *huang lian* 黄连, *dang gui* 当归, *chuan xiong* 川芎, *sheng di* 生地, *chi shao* 赤芍, *hong hua* 红花, *tao ren* 桃仁, *e zhu* 莪术, *xiang fu* 香附, *yan hu suo* 延胡索, *huang bai* 黄柏, *hong teng* 红藤, *yi yi ren* 薏苡仁, *san leng* 三棱, etc.

Main actions of herbs: *Huang lian* 黄连 and *yi yi ren* 薏苡仁 clear heat and dampness; *hong teng* 红藤 and *bai jiang cao* 败酱草 clear heat and detoxify. *Dang gui* 当归, *chuan xiong* 川芎, *tao ren* 桃仁,

hong hua 红花, and *mu dan pi* 牡丹皮 activate Blood, remove stasis, and unblock the meridians. *E zhu* 莪术, *xiang fu* 香附, and *yang hu suo* 延胡索 regulate *qi*, activate Blood, and alleviate pain; *sheng di* 生地 and *bai shao* 白芍 cool Blood, clear heat, and relax tension to alleviate pain.

External Chinese Herbal Medicine Treatment

External CHM can provide symptomatic relief and can be used to treat endometriosis. The most common forms of external CHM are topical application and CHM enema.

Topical Chinese Herbal Medicine

Topical CHM can be used for all syndrome types; herbs can be added or removed according to the syndrome. The herb(s) can be made into a powder, mixed with boiling water and honey, and applied to the abdomen, painful areas, or acupuncture points. Topical treatments are contraindicated for patients with skin conditions and those allergic to herbs or surgical tape. Two commonly used topical prescriptions include:

1) *Hong hua* 红花, *ru xiang* 乳香, *mo yao* 没药, *ze lan* 泽兰, *chi shao* 赤芍, *dan shen* 丹参, *dang gui* 当归, *san leng* 三棱, and *e zhu* 莪术: After grinding herbs into a powder, make a paste with boiling water and honey and apply to the abdomen. This treatment is suitable for all patients.[9]
2) *Da huang* 大黄, *ce bo ye* 侧柏叶, *bo he* 薄荷, *huang bai* 黄柏 and *ze lan* 泽兰: grind 1 kg of *da huang* 大黄 and *ce bo ye* 侧柏叶 and 500 g of *bo he* 薄荷, *huang bai* 黄柏 and *ze lan* 泽兰 and mix with boiling water and honey to make a paste. This treatment is suitable for patients with damp-heat and phlegm.[13]

She xiang dysmenorrhoea cream 麝香痛经膏 (a commercially manufactured product) can be applied to the acupuncture point SP6

Sanyinjiao 三阴交 for three days before the menstrual period or during dysmenorrhoea.[6] Chinese medicine clinicians may consider applying a mixture of zhong ru shi 钟乳石, ru xiang 乳香, and mo yao 没药 to the posterior vaginal fornix if nodules are detected during pelvic examination.[5]

Chinese Herbal Medicine Enema

Chinese herbal medicine enemas can be used for each syndrome described in clinical guidelines and textbooks.[1,5,6,8–11,13,14] The decoction or manufactured CHM is mixed with warm water to make 100 mL; the temperature of the liquid should be between 39 and 41°C. Lubricate the anal canal with paraffin oil, drain the liquid, insert the tube 10–15 cm and slowly inject the herbal solution. The rate of injection can be slower for older women or those with specific medical conditions. The patient should try to retain the enema for two hours before voiding.

Chinese herbal medicine enema is contraindicated during menstruation and when there is a high risk of rectal perforation. Commonly used herbs include dan shen 丹参, chi shao 赤芍, dan pi 丹皮, san leng 三棱, e zhu 莪术, xi cao gen 紫草根, feng fang 蜂房, yan hu suo 延胡索, zao jiao ci 皂角刺, chuan lian zi 川楝子, hong teng 红藤, bai jiang cao 败酱草, bai zhi 白芷, and huang bai 黄柏; herbs can be modified according to the CM syndrome.

Acupuncture Therapies

Several acupuncture therapies have been recommended in clinical guidelines and clinical textbooks, including acupuncture, ear acupuncture, abdominal acupuncture (a microsystem of acupuncture), and moxibustion (Table 2.2). Acupuncture points can be selected according to syndrome differentiation. Acupuncture points that can be used with any of these interventions include CV3 Zhongji 中极,

CV4 *Guanyuan* 关元, and SP6 *Sanyinjiao* 三阴交. Their actions are described below[15]:

- CV3 *Zhongji* 中极: regulates *qi* and menstruation, drains dampness, benefits the uterus and Lower Energiser, and tonifies the Kidneys.
- CV4 *Guanyuan* 关元: tonifies *yuan qi* 元氣 and *jing* 精, tonifies the Kidneys, strengthens the Spleen, benefits the uterus, and regulates the Lower Energiser.
- SP6 *Sanyinjiao* 三阴交: resolves dampness, tonifies the Stomach, Spleen, and Kidneys, harmonises the Lower Energiser, regulates menstruation, and invigorates Blood.

Acupuncture

Treatment with acupuncture involves a core set of acupuncture points supplemented with additional points selected according to CM syndrome differentiation. The main points for manual acupuncture include CV4 *Guanyuan* 关元, CV3 *Zhongji* 中极, SP6 *Sanyinjiao* 三阴交, SP10 *Xuehai* 血海, EX-CA1 *Zigong* 子宫, and ST36 *Zusanli* 足三里.[11] Supplementary points according to syndromes include:

- LR3 *Taichong* 太冲 and BL32 *Ciliao* 次髎 for *qi* stagnation and Blood stasis;
- SP8 *Diji* 地机, LR2 *Xingjian* 行间, and ST29 *Guilai* 归来 for cold congealing and Blood stasis (use both acupuncture and moxibustion);
- SP9 *Yinlingquan* 阴陵泉, BL34 *Xialiao* 下髎, LR3 *Taichong* 太冲, and LI11 *Quchi* 曲池 for damp-heat and phlegm;
- ST40 *Fenglong* 丰隆 and SP9 *Yinlingquan* 阴陵泉 for phlegm and stasis binding;
- BL23 *Shenshu* 肾俞, KI3 *Taixi* 太溪, and BL18 *Ganshu* 肝俞 for Kidney deficiency and Blood stasis.

Table 2.2. Summary of Acupuncture Therapies for Endometriosis

Intervention	Acupuncture Points/Body Area	Treatment Frequency
Acupuncture	Main points: CV4 *Guanyuan* 关元, CV3 *Zhongji* 中极, SP6 *Sanyinjiao* 三阴交, SP10 *Xuehai* 血海, EX-CA1 *Zigong* 子宫, and ST36 *Zusanli* 足三里.	Start 3–5 days before onset of dysmenorrhoea and treat on alternate days during menstruation. Treat twice daily for severe pain.
Ear acupuncture	TF2 *Zigong* 子宫 (Uterus), TF2 *Luanchao* 卵巢 (Ovary), CO18 *Neifenmi* 内分泌 (Endocrine), TF4 *Shenmen* 神门, AT4 *Pizhixia* 皮质下 (Subcortex), CO12 *Gan* 肝 (Liver), and CO10 *Shen* 肾 (Kidney).	Retain press needles for up to three days.
Abdominal acupuncture	CV3 *Zhongji* 中极, ST26 *Wailing* 外陵, *Xiafengshidian* 下风湿点.	Not specified.
Moxibustion	Ginger moxibustion: CV8 *Shenque* 神阙, CV4 *Guanyuan* 关元, and SP6 *Sanyinjiao* 三阴交.	5–7 moxa cones on alternate days.

Acupuncture should be applied using neutral supplementation and draining needle techniques 采取平补平泻法. Start treatment 3–5 days before the onset of menstrual pain and treat once or twice daily when the pain is severe. During menstruation, treatment can be provided on alternate days. Warm needle (moxibustion on the needle handle) can be used for cold coagulation.

Ear Acupuncture

Common acupuncture points include TF2 *Zigong* 子宫 (Uterus), TF2 *Luanchao* 卵巢 (Ovary), CO18 *Neifenmi* 内分泌 (Endocrine), TF4 *Shenmen* 神门, AT4 *Pizhixia* 皮质下 (Subcortex), CO12 *Gan* 肝 (Liver), and CO10 *Shen* 肾 (Kidney).[3] After locating acupuncture points on the ear, disinfect the area and use either acupuncture needles or short press needles that remain *in situ* for up to three days to stimulate the acupuncture points.[3]

Abdominal Acupuncture

Abdominal acupuncture is a microsystem that uses meridian and non-meridian points on the abdomen to treat disease. In this system, Dr Cheng describes three levels in each acupuncture point: 'sky' (upper level), 'human' (middle level), and 'earth' (lower level). Treatment aims to direct *qi* back to the centre (abdomen), and acupuncture points include CV3 *Zhongji* 中极, ST26 *Wailing* 外陵, and *Xiafengshidian* 下风湿点 ('lower rheumatic point'; a point in the abdominal acupuncture microsystem located 2.5 cun lateral to CV6 *Qihai* 气海). Insert the needle into the 'human' level of ST26 *Wailing* 外陵 and into the 'earth' level of the other points and retain for 30 minutes.[13]

Moxibustion

Different types of moxibustion can be selected according to the condition and syndrome type, including moxibustion, warm box moxibustion, 'thunder fire' moxibustion, and other methods.[11] 'Thunder fire' moxibustion is a strong, concentrated treatment method using a cigar-shaped roll made from medicinal herbs such as *chen xiang* 沉香, *mu xiang* 木香, *ru xiang* 乳香, and others.[16] Ginger moxibustion, the application of moxa cones on a slice of ginger over an acupuncture point, can be used for the syndrome cold congealing with Blood stasis. Use between five and seven moxa cones on CV8 *Shenque* 神阙, CV4 *Guanyuan* 关元, and SP6 *Sanyinjiao* 三阴交, with treatment administered on alternate days.[14]

Other Management Strategies

Women can be advised about CM strategies that may alleviate symptoms or prevent recurrence. Patient education can include advice about appropriate self-care during menstruation and the puerperium, avoiding strenuous exercise during menstruation, and avoiding sexual intercourse from three days prior to three days after the menstrual period.[5] Women can be supported with appropriate family planning advice and advice about contraceptive methods to avoid surgical termination of pregnancy.⁷ If hysteroscopy or surgery is required, these can be scheduled between three and seven days after the end of menstruation.⁶

Clinicians can provide dietary advice according to CM principles, including avoiding spicy or fried foods and foods considered 'cold', 'dry', or 'hot' in CM.[13] For women with *qi* stagnation and Blood stasis 气滞血瘀 dysmenorrhoea, *Xiong gui shao tang cha* 芎归芍糖茶 (herbal tea) and *Ji dan xiong jiu yin* 鸡蛋芎酒饮 (herbal drink) are suggested; for body deficient 体虚 patients, *Dang gui yang rou tang* 当归羊肉汤 (herbal soup) is recommended; for cold congealing and Blood stasis 寒凝血瘀 patients, *Da mi gui xin zhou* 大米桂心粥 (a rice porridge made with *gui xin* 桂心 [cinnamon bark]) could be used.[13]

Patients can be counselled to keep a healthy state of mind with stable emotions and to avoid excessive feelings of sorrow and anger, especially for women with endometriosis as the main complaint. Patients can be advised to maintain work–life balance to strengthen the body's constitution with regular exercise and to seek psychological therapy, if required.[13,14]

References

1. 罗颂平, 刘雁峰主编. (2016) 中医妇科学 (第三版). 北京: 人民卫生出版社, pp. 270–276.
2. 郑筱萸. (1993) 中药新药临床研究指导原则 (第一辑). 中国医药科技出版社; 北京.
3. 中华中医药学会. (2012) 中医妇科常见病诊疗指南. 北京: 中国中医药出版社, pp. 120–126.
4. 余燚薇, 赵瑞华, 张润顺, *et al.* (2017) 子宫内膜异位症中医证候要素分布特点多元分析. 环球中医药 **10**(11): 1242–1247.
5. 张玉珍. (2002) (新世纪) 中医妇科学. 北京: 中国中医药出版社, pp. 130–136.
6. 欧阳惠卿. (2002) 中医妇科学. 北京: 人民卫生出版社, pp. 101–103.
7. 司徒仪主编. (2008) 中西医结合妇产科学 (第二版). 北京: 科学出版社, pp. 271–279.
8. 欧阳惠卿. (2012) 中西医结合妇产科学 (新世纪第二版). 北京: 中国中医药出版社, pp. 169–179.

9. 王小云, 黄建玲主编. (2018) 中西医结合妇产科学 (第三版). 北京: 科学出版社, pp. 326–334.
10. 国家中医药管理局医政司. (2010) *22个专业95个病种中医诊疗方案-痛经 (子宫内膜异位症, 子宫腺肌病) 诊疗方案*. 国家中医药管理局医政司; 北京.
11. 国家中医药管理局医政司. (2011) *24个专业105个病种中医诊疗方案-癥瘕病（卵巢巧克力样囊肿）中医诊疗方案*. 国家中医药管理局医政司; 北京.
12. 王小云主编. (2017) 中西医结合妇科学研究新进展. 北京: 人民卫生出版社, pp. 29–52.
13. 王小云, 黄建玲主编. (2013) 中医临床诊治-妇科专病 (第三版). 北京: 人民卫生出版社, pp. 361–388.
14. 罗云坚, 张英哲. (2003) 常见病中西医结合诊疗常规. 广州: 广东科技出版社, pp. 432–439.
15. Deadman P, Al-Khafaji M, Baker K. (2000) *A manual of acupuncture*. Journal of Chinese Medicine Publications, East Sussex, England.
16. World Health Organization. (2007) *WHO International Standard Terminologies of Traditional Medicine in the Western Pacific Region*. World Health Organization, Geneva, Switzerland.

3

Classical Chinese Medicine Literature

OVERVIEW

Treatments for endometriosis-like symptoms have been described in classical Chinese medicine texts. This chapter presents the findings of an analysis of endometriosis-like symptoms found through a search of the *Zhong Hua Yi Dian*, one of the largest digitalised collections of Chinese medical texts. Terms related to dysmenorrhoea, menstruation, mass, and infertility were used. In total, 707 citations that met the inclusion criteria were analysed. Chinese herbal medicine was the most common treatment for endometriosis-like symptoms in past eras. The symptoms, aetiology, and treatments are discussed.

Introduction

Chinese medicine (CM) has a long history. Some of the earliest written records that describe concepts such as *yin* and *yang* can be dated back to the Spring and Autumn (770–476 BCE) and Warring states (474–221 BCE) periods. Passages from these records also describe therapeutic methods such as herbal decoctions, acupuncture, and mugwort (*ai* 艾) used for moxibustion.[1]

As endometriosis is a relatively modern disease, there is no equivalent term to describe the various symptoms experienced by women in past eras. Symptoms such as dysmenorrhoea and abdominal mass may have related to a range of gynaecological conditions. Thus, a systematic search using specific criteria was required to understand how symptoms typical of endometriosis were viewed and treated in past eras. We conducted electronic searches of *Zhong Hua*

Yi Dian (ZHYD) 中华医典, 'Encyclopedia of Traditional Chinese Medicine', a CD of more than 1,100 medical books.[2] This collection is the largest currently available and is considered to be representative of other large collections of classical and pre-modern CM literature.[3,4]

Search Terms

The modern medical term for endometriosis in Chinese is *zi gong nei mo yi wei zheng* 子宫内膜异位症, while *zi gong nei mo yi wei xing ji bing* 子宫内膜异位性疾病 is used for diseases related to endometriosis, such as adenomyosis. Considering that endometriosis and adenomyosis were separated as distinct entities in the 1920s (Cullen 1920, cited in Benagiano, Brosens and Lippi, 2014),[5] it is highly unlikely that either of these terms would be found in the classical CM literature. Further, as the 'gold standard' for diagnosis of endometriosis is laparoscopic confirmation, such cases could not be found in the classical CM literature.

Instead, the most appropriate approach to identify citations that describe conditions similar to endometriosis is to search for the symptoms associated with the condition. While pelvic pain during menstruation is a characteristic symptom of endometriosis, many women experience a variety of symptoms, such as abdominal mass and infertility, and some experience no symptoms at all. Further, several of the typical symptoms, such as abdominal mass or infertility, are not gender or disease specific. This presented a challenge when selecting search terms to identify symptoms associated with endometriosis in women from past eras.

A variety of sources was consulted to identify terms used for endometriosis symptoms in the classical CM literature. These included textbooks on CM, integrated CM, and conventional medicine; gynaecology;[6-17] a CM dictionary;[18] the World Health Organization's *International Standard Terminologies on Traditional Medicine in the Western Pacific Region*;[19] a specialist monograph on dysmenorrhoea;[20] and the contemporary literature.[21] Terms described in these sources were collated and pilot searches were conducted in

Classical Chinese Medicine Literature

the ZHYD. Terms such as *yue jing bu tiao* 月经不调 (irregular menstruation), *yue jing guo duo* 月经过多 (hypermenorrhoea), and *jing qi yan chang* 经期延长 (menostaxis) produced few relevant results and were not used in the final search. Similarly, terms related to male infertility were excluded.

The terms used in the final search are listed in Table 3.1. Terms for dysmenorrhoea (group 1) and menstruation (group 4) would naturally be limited to this symptom in women. With the exception of *chang qin* 肠覃, which is specific to women, terms for 'mass' (group 2) may be used to describe symptoms in men or women. These terms were searched in combination with terms for women (*fu ren* 妇人, *nv zhi* 女子, and *nv ren* 女人) to increase specificity. In these searches, the Boolean operator 'and' was used to allow detection of passages

Table 3.1. Search Terms

Symptom Group	Terms
1. Dysmenorrhoea	*Tong jing* 痛经, *jing xing fu tong* 经行腹痛, *jing qi fu tong* 经期腹痛, *yue shui lai fu tong* 月水来腹痛, *jing qian fu tong* 经前腹痛, *jing hou fu tong* 经后腹痛, *yue jing lai fu tong* 月经来腹痛, *yue jie lai fu tong* 月节来腹痛, *jing xing qi fu tong* 经行脐腹痛, *jing lai xie qi tong* 经来胁气痛
2. Mass (combined with woman *fu ren* 妇人, girl *nv zhi* 女子, and female *nv ren* 女人)	*Zheng jia* 癥瘕, *zheng jia* 症瘕, *zheng jia* 徵瘕, *zheng ji* 癥积, *jia ju* 瘕聚, *shi zheng* 石癥, *xue jia* 血瘕, *zheng pi* 癥痞, *ba jia* 八瘕, *qi zheng* 七癥, *zheng ju* 癥聚, *jia pi* 瘕癖, *rou zheng* 肉癥, *chang qin* 肠覃
3. Infertility	*Bu yun* 不孕, *wu zi* 无子, *quan bu chan* 全不产, *duan xu* 断续, *jue chan* 绝产, *bu shou yun* 不受孕, *jue yi* 绝子, *jue si* 绝嗣, *jue yun* 绝孕, *qiu si* 求嗣, *zhong zi* 种子, *si yu* 嗣育
4. Menstruation (combined with abdominal pain *fu tong* 腹痛)	*Yue shi* 月事, *yue jie* 月节, *yue shui* 月水, *xing jing* 行经, *yue jing* 月经, *yue xin* 月信
5. Abdominal pain in women	*Fu ren fu tong* 妇人腹痛, *fu ren fu zhong zhu teng tong* 妇人腹中诸疼痛, *fu ren fu zhong tong* 妇人腹中痛, *sha xue xin tong* 杀血心痛

of text that contained terms for mass and woman in close proximity (but not necessarily together).

The same approach was used for menstruation (group 4) and abdominal pain (fu tong 腹痛). This identified citations that contained both terms but which did not appear together. Terms in groups 1, 3, and 5 were searched as a single phrase, and results of searches were for exact matches.

Procedures for Search, Data Coding, and Data Analysis

Search of the ZHYD utilised both the heading and text search fields. Search terms were entered into the fields and the results were downloaded into spreadsheets for further review of eligibility. A 'citation' was defined as a distinct passage of text referring to one or more of the search terms. Codes were allocated for types of citations, books, and dynasties in which they were written to facilitate data analysis, following the procedures described in May et al. (2013).[3] Books written after 1949 (the beginning of the People's Republic of China) were excluded. The process for identifying, classifying, and analysing information from classical literature books is illustrated in Figure 3.1.

The number of hits for each term was recorded and the results were added together to provide the total number of hits. Citations found by multiple search terms were considered duplicates. The terms that identified the citation were noted and the duplicate citation was removed from the data set. Irrelevant citations were excluded if they did not relate to key symptoms of endometriosis or were CM dictionary citations. Many citations were pharmacopoeia-style herb or acupuncture point entries. For example, one citation described endometriosis symptoms as an indication for the use of a particular herb or acupuncture point, with no additional information about endometriosis. Such citations were excluded from further analysis.

The remaining citations were assessed against eligibility criteria to identify those that were possibly or most likely related to endometriosis. Criteria were developed in consultation with expert CM

Classical Chinese Medicine Literature

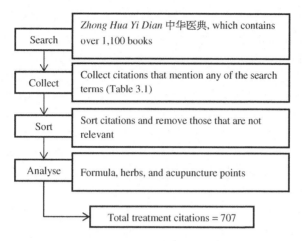

Figure 3.1. Classical literature citations.

Table 3.2. Criteria for Rating Citations

Likelihood of Relating to Endometriosis	Group Criteria
Most likely to be endometriosis	Group A + (B1 + B2; +/– any term from B3)
	Group A + (B1 + B2 + B3 + B4)
	Group S
Possibly related to endometriosis	Group A alone
	Group A + (B1 or B2 or B3 or B4)
	Group A + (B2 + B3)
	Group A + (B2 + B3 + B4)
	Group A + (B3 + B4)

Group A: dysmenorrhoea; Group B1: mass; Group B2: infertility; Group B3: menstrual changes; Group B4: abdominal mass in women; Group S: special types of endometriosis such as haematuria (*xue niao* 血尿), haematochezia (*bian xue* 便血), or haemoptysis (*ka xue* 咯血).

gynaecologists familiar with the classical literature. The criteria used to judge whether citations were possible or most likely endometriosis are described in Table 3.2. Citations that described dysmenorrhoea alone (any term from Group 1 in Table 3.1, or the combination of abdominal pain and menstruation) or with at least one symptom of mass (Group B1), infertility (Group B2), menstrual changes (Group

B3), or abdominal pain in women (Group B4) was considered to possibly relate to endometriosis. Citations that described dysmenorrhoea, mass, and infertility (with or without descriptions of menstrual changes or abdominal pain) were considered the best examples of endometriosis and were judged most likely to be endometriosis.

Endometriosis can also develop outside the pelvic cavity and present with different symptoms. Blood in the urine (haematuria, *xue niao* 血尿), passing of blood per rectum (haematochezia, *bian xue* 便血), or coughing up blood (haemoptysis, *ka xue* 咯血) that is related to the menstrual cycle can suggest endometriosis in the bladder, bowel, or lungs, respectively (Group S in Table 3.2), although cyclical chest pain or cyclical pneumothorax are more common presentations in thoracic endometriosis. Citations that described these symptoms in relation to the menstrual cycle were considered to be most likely cases of special types of endometriosis. Finally, citations that described the gradual onset of dysmenorrhoea after menarche were also considered typical of endometriosis and were judged as most likely to be endometriosis.

Citations that described a specific cause for dysmenorrhoea, such as induced by eating cold food, and those that reported dysmenorrhoea at menarche were considered not likely to be endometriosis and were excluded. Similarly, citations that did not describe the primary symptom of endometriosis, dysmenorrhoea, were also considered unlikely to relate to endometriosis and were excluded.

Some citations described the name of a Chinese herbal medicine (CHM) formula but not the herb ingredients. The book sections and books where such citations were found were searched to identify other instances of the formula. If found, herb ingredients were used for analysis. If herb ingredients could not be found, the data were marked as 'missing'. Descriptive statistics were used to analyse the number of books, publication years, and types of treatments. Data are presented for the most frequently found CHM formulas, herbs, and acupuncture points for citations judged as 'possible' and 'most likely' cases of endometriosis.

Search Results

In total, 30,201 hits were identified by the terms and combinations of terms (Table 3.3). The combination of terms for mass and women identified more than 15,000 hits; 2,789 (9.2%) of the hits for mass and women were found by the combination of zheng jia 癥瘕 and

Table 3.3. Hit Frequency by Search Term Group

Search Term Group	Terms	Hit Frequency (n, %)
Dysmenorrhoea	Tong jing 痛经, jing xing fu tong 经行腹痛, jing qi fu tong 经期腹痛, yue shui lai fu tong 月水来腹痛, jing qian fu tong 经前腹痛, jing hou fu tong 经后腹痛, yue jing lai fu tong 月经来腹痛, yue jie lai fu tong 月节来腹痛, jing xing qi fu tong 经行脐腹痛, jing lai xie qi tong 经来胁气痛	388 (1.3)
Mass (combined with fu ren 妇人, nv zhi 女,子 and nv ren 女人)	Zheng jia 癥瘕, zheng jia 症瘕, zheng jia 徵瘕, zheng ji 癥积, jia ju 瘕聚, shi zheng 石癥, xue jia 血瘕, zheng pi 癥痞, ba jia 八瘕, qi zheng 七癥, zheng ju 癥聚, jia pi 瘕癖, rou zheng 肉癥, chang qin 肠覃	15,676 (51.9)
Infertility	Bu yun 不孕, wu zi 无子, quan bu chan 全不产, duan xu 断续, jue chan 绝产, bu shou yun 不受孕, jue yi 绝子, jue si 绝嗣, jue yun 绝孕, qiu si 求嗣, zhong zi 种子, si yu 嗣育	5,874 (19.4)
Menstruation (combined with fu tong 腹痛)	Yue shi 月事, yue jie 月节, yue shui 月水, xing jing 行经, yue jing 月经, yue xin 月信	8,165 (27.0)
Abdominal pain in women	Fu ren fu tong 妇人腹痛, fu ren fu zhong zhu teng tong 妇人腹中诸疼痛, fu ren fu zhong tong 妇人腹中痛, sha xue xin tong 杀血心痛	98 (0.3)
Total		30,201

fu ren 妇人. The largest number of hits for any single term or combination of terms was found with the terms *yue shui* 月水 (menstruation) and *fu tong* 腹痛 (abdominal pain; 3,195 hits, 10.6%). Other combinations that identified more than 1,000 hits included the following: *zheng jia* 癥瘕 and *fu ren* 妇人 (2,789 hits, 9.2%); *xue jia* 血瘕 and *fu ren* 妇人 (2,550 hits, 8.4%); *yue jing* 月经 and *fu tong* 腹痛 (2,235 hits, 7.4%); *zheng jia* 症瘕 and *fu ren* 妇人 (1,996 hits, 6.6%); *xing jing* 行经 and *fu tong* 腹痛 (1,517 hits, 5.0%); and *jia ju* 瘕聚 and *fu ren* 妇人 (1,028 hits, 3.4%). Terms for abdominal pain in women produced comparatively fewer hits (98 hits, 0.3%).

Over 40% of the hits were duplicate citations (12,844 hits, 42.5%). After these were removed, the number of citations that remained were reviewed against the eligibility criteria. Some of the best examples that described endometriosis-like symptoms and aetiology were selected for discussion, and citations that described treatment were analysed.

Citations Related to Endometriosis

After exclusion of duplicates, irrelevant citations, and those with insufficient information to make a judgment, 306 citations were considered 'possibly' related to endometriosis. Among these, 27 citations met the inclusion criteria and were judged as 'most likely' to refer to endometriosis. All but seven citations described treatment. These seven citations described symptoms similar to endometriosis, or the aetiology and pathogenesis of endometriosis without describing symptoms, and were judged as possible cases of endometriosis. These citations provide insight into how endometriosis was conceptualised in past eras.

One hundred and twenty-four of the 306 citations (40.5%) described multiple treatments, and each treatment described was separated as a separate citation to allow analysis of CHM, acupuncture, and other CM therapies. This process resulted in 700 treatment citations considered to possibly relate to endometriosis. Thus, the final data set included 707 citations, of which 685 described orally administered CHM formulas or single herbs, six described topical use of CHM, seven described acupuncture therapies, two described other CM therapies (massage), and seven did not describe any treatment for symptoms. All 44 treatment citations that were judged most likely to be endometriosis described treatment with oral CHM.

Among the included 707 citations, more than half were found by terms relating to menstruation and *fu tong* 腹痛 (abdominal pain; 416 citations, 58.8%), and almost one-third (229 citations, 32.4%) were found by terms for mass and women. Menstrual pain and abdominal mass are two of the key symptoms of endometriosis. Other terms that identify a smaller number of included citations were those for infertility (38 citations, 5.4%) and dysmenorrhoea (16 citations, 2.3%). Terms for abdominal pain in women produced the smallest number of citations possibly related to endometriosis (two citations, 0.3%).

Definitions of Endometriosis

In past eras, books included descriptions of the characteristic symptoms of endometriosis, such as pelvic pain, dysmenorrhoea and abdominal mass, and possible sequelae, such as impaired fertility. Symptoms that were less common and more specific, including vomiting or coughing up blood during menstruation, appear to be indicative of the less common thoracic endometriosis.

In the book *Qi Shi Yi An* 齐氏医案 (c. 1806), Qi Binghui noted that he often saw women who suffered from *nijing* 逆经, which can be translated as 'reverse menstruation'. Symptoms of *nijing* 逆经 were explained as the Blood travelling upwards, causing vomiting of blood or nasal bleeding. Such symptoms were caused by women not taking care of themselves during menstruation, which allowed external pathogens to invade the uterus. (慧常见妇女因月信来日不善调养,其六淫外邪乘隙而入血室,经期一至,血不下行,上逆吐衄,名曰逆经。)

Another passage from the same book described the 'strange condition' of a woman who presented with premenstrual abdominal pain that radiated to her perineum. During menstruation, the woman bled from the anus rather than the vagina; this occurred every menstrual cycle. (曾治一妇,患奇证,每当经期,腹中痛连少腹,引入阴中,其经血不行于前阴,反从后阴而行,三日则腹痛诸证自己。次月当期,亦复如是.) Dr Qi diagnosed cold stagnation in the three lower *yin* meridians (Spleen, Liver, and Kidney); this blocked the flow of menstrual blood to the vagina and resulted in blood flowing to the large intestine. (其证总为三阴寒结,阻截前阴,经血不能归于冲任,而直趋大肠.)

Some of the more typical symptoms were described in case reports. For example, in the recent text *Liu Xuan Si Jia Yi An* 柳选四家医案 (c. 1900), Liu Baoyi recorded the case of a woman with dysmenorrhoea for several years who was unable to conceive. Her symptoms included pain starting three days before menstruation and abdominal mass similar to food stagnation. She also had poor appetite, a thin body, and a tired appearance. (痛经数年,不得孕育,经来三日前必腹痛,腹中有块凝滞,状似癥瘕伏梁之类,纳减运迟,形瘦神羸,调经诸法,医者岂曰无之.) Other case reports described women with irregular menstruation (经血循环失其常度, *Wang Jiu Feng Yi An* 王九峰医案 (一), c. 1889), and irritability and a cold abdomen (自述嗔怒病加 …下焦时冷, *Ye Shi Yi An Cun Zhen* 叶氏医案存真, c. 1832).

Descriptions of the Aetiology of Endometriosis

The aetiology of endometriosis was predominantly viewed as a disease of external origin in past eras. Women were seen as vulnerable to external pathogens invading the uterus when they did not practise proper care during menstruation. A citation from the Ming dynasty book *Wan Bing Hui Chun* 万病回春 (c. 1587) stated that external fire was the main external pathogen contributing to *ni jing* 逆经; abnormal movement of Blood was the result of fire drawing the Blood upward, resulting in bleeding from the mouth and nose. Menstruation can be regulated by nourishing and replenishing (tonifying) *yin*, eliminating fire, and regulating *qi* and the meridians. Chinese herbs include *dang gui* 当归, *chuan xiong* 川芎, *bai shao* 白芍, *sheng di huang* 生地黄, *huang qin* 黄芩, *shan zhi* 山栀, *mu dan pi* 牡丹皮,

Classical Chinese Medicine Literature

e jiao 阿胶, *xi jiao* 犀角, *fu ling* 茯苓, *mai dong* 麦冬, and *chen pi* 陈皮. (六淫中,火被认为是逆经的重要原因.《万病回春》中指出: 错经妄行于口鼻者,是火载血上,气之乱也,治当滋阴降火,顺气调经,经自准也. 用当归,川芎,白芍,生地黄,黄芩,山栀,牡丹皮,阿胶(炒),犀角,白茯苓,(去皮),麦门冬,(去心),陈皮,锉一剂,水煎服.)

Inappropriate timing of sexual intercourse was also considered a cause of dysmenorrhoea. As described in *Jia Yong Liang Fang* 家用良方 (c. 1859), women who did not have dysmenorrhoea before marriage but developed it after marriage did so because of sexual intercourse immediately prior to menstruation or when menstruation was not completely finished. Such activity damaged the *Chong* 冲 and *Ren* 任 Vessels, leading to *ni jing* 逆经, dysmenorrhoea, and infertility. (月经前后性生活可能是导致子宫内膜异位症的原因. 例如,家用良方中提到凡闺女行经无疼,嫁后经痛,此乃不和禁忌,或经水将来,或经行未尽,遂而交媾,震动血海,损及冲任,致成逆经疼痛,难以受孕,非投以培养通络不可.)

Other doctors considered internal causes of endometriosis-like symptoms. Liver *qi* uprising was considered the cause of vomiting blood during menstruation by Chen Shiduo. In the book *Bian Zheng Qi Wen* 辨证奇闻 (c. 1687), Chen described the case of a woman who reported sudden abdominal pain and vomiting blood. Chen explained that rather than being caused by internal fire, as was thought by others at the time, these symptoms resulted from disturbance of the free flow of *qi* that led to Liver *qi* uprising. Chen also considered that Kidney and Liver fire caused vomiting of blood. The treatment principle was to tonify the Kidney and regulate *qi* movement using formulas such as *Shun jing tang* 顺经汤. (肝气上逆也是经行吐血的重要原因. 陈世铎在《辨证奇闻》中指出: 经前一二日,忽腹痛吐血,人谓火盛极,谁知肝逆血不下行而上吐乎. 肝气最急,顺则安,逆则动. 血随气而俱行,气安则安,气动则动. 但经逆在肾不在肝,何随血妄行,竟从口出? 不知少阴火,急如奔马,得肝中龙雷合冲,其势更捷,反经为血又至便,正不必肝不藏血始吐也. 然各经吐血乃内伤,逆经乃火气内溢,激之使出. 症不同,逆则一. 似宜治逆以平肝,不必益精以补肾. 然逆经而吐血虽不损血,反复倾倒,必伤肾气血,又上泄过多,肾水亦亏,须于补肾中行顺气. 用顺经汤.)

Chen Shiduo elaborated on his ideas in another passage in *Bian Zheng Qi Wen* 辨证奇闻, where he suggested that people may not realise that blood in the stool is actually menstrual blood. Chen considered bleeding from the anus during menstruation to be a sign of disharmony of the Heart and Kidney. When the uterus, Heart, and Kidney are not in harmony, the uterus [menstrual] blood will be out of control and may go into the stool. Treatment should not only focus on stopping bleeding, but it should also include tonifying the *qi* of the Heart and Kidney. The CHM formula *Gui jing liang an tang* 归经两安汤 can be used. (陈世铎还提出,心肾不交是大便出血的原因.《辨证奇闻》云: 经前大便出血,人谓血崩,谁知经入大肠乎. 大肠与经路别,何能入？不知胞胎之系,上通心,下通肾,心肾不交,胞胎之血两无可归,心肾气不照摄,听其自走大便. 若单止便血,则愈止愈多,反击动三焦气,拂乱不止. 盖原因心肾不交,今不补心肾,使心肾气按,胞胎气不散,血自不乱行. 用 归经两安汤.)

Chinese Herbal Medicine

Chinese herbal medicine was the main treatment method described in classical CM books for endometriosis-like symptoms. Six citations described topical application of CHM, while 685 described CHM for oral use. The 691 CHM citations came from 134 books, with 20 books providing 10 or more citations. The book that provided the greatest number of citations was *Sheng Ji Zong Lu* 圣济总录 (c. 1117), with 51 citations. Other books that provided large numbers of citations included the formulary *Pu Ji Fang* 普济方 (c. 1406; 46 citations), the gynaecology book *Jin Gui Qi Yao — Fu Ke* 金匮启钥-妇科 (c. 1804; 30 citations), and *Nv Ke Zheng Zhi Zhun Sheng* 女科证治准绳 (c. 1607; 30 citations).

Frequency of Treatment Citations by Dynasty

The vast majority of citations came from the Ming and Qing dynasties (569 citations, 82.3%; Table 3.4). The earliest citations came from two Tang and Five dynasty books that are dated as 682 CE: *Hua Tuo Shen Fang* 华佗神方 and *Qian Jin Yi Fang* 千金翼方. Both citations

Classical Chinese Medicine Literature

Table 3.4. Dynastic Distribution of Chinese Herbal Medicine Treatment Citations

Dynasty	No. of Treatment Citations
Before Tang Dynasty (before 618)	0
Tang and Five Dynasties (618–960)	5
Song and Jin Dynasties (961–1271)	100
Yuan Dynasty (1272–1368)	2
Ming Dynasty (1369–1644)	257
Qing Dynasty (1645–1911)	312
Min Guo/Republic of China (1912–1949)	13
Total	**689***

*The publication year for one book that provided two citations was not able to be determined.

described dysmenorrhoea alone or with menstrual changes and were judged as possible cases of endometriosis. The most recent citations were also found in two books published in 1949: *Fu Ke Wen Da* 妇科问答 and *Zhang Shi Fu Ke* 张氏妇科. Citations from these recent books described dysmenorrhoea and were also considered possible cases of endometriosis.

Treatment with Oral Chinese Herbal Medicine

Oral CHM was used for endometriosis-like symptoms in 685 citations; a subset of 44 citations described oral CHM for symptoms considered most likely to refer to endometriosis. Chinese herbal medicine formulas and herb ingredients were analysed for all citations and for the subset judged most likely to be endometriosis. Oral CHM formulas were described in their traditional, unmodified form or were modified by adding or removing herb ingredients according to the patient's clinical presentation. Modified and unmodified formulas were grouped for frequency analyses.

Review of oral CHM formulas found several instances of formulas with either 1) the same or similar herb ingredients but with a different formula name or 2) formulas with the same name with very different clinical actions based on herb ingredients. For each instance, a consensus was reached as to whether formulas should be grouped or kept separate for analysis.

Most frequent oral use formulas in possible endometriosis citations

In total, 195 named formulas and 130 unnamed formulas were included in the 685 oral CHM treatment citations. Analysis of named formulas showed that *Si wu tang* 四物汤 was the most frequently described oral CHM used for endometriosis-like symptoms (Table 3.5).

Table 3.5. Most Frequent Oral Use Formulas in Possible Endometriosis Citations

Formula Name	Herb Ingredients	No. of Citations
Si wu tang/Si wu tang jia jian 四物汤/四物汤加减	Dang gui 当归, bai shao 白芍, chuan xiong 川芎, sheng di huang 生地黄 (*Fu Ren Da Quan Liang Fang* 妇人大全良方 c. 1237).	88
Ba zhen tang/Ba zhen tang jia jian/ Ba wu tang 2/Ba zhen san/Ba zhen san jia jian 八珍汤/八珍汤加减/八物汤2/八珍散/八珍散加减	Dang gui 当归, shu di huang 熟地黄, chuan xiong 川芎, bai shao 白芍, ren shen 人参, fu ling 茯苓, bai zhu 白术, zhi gan cao 炙甘草 (*Yi Xue Zheng Zhuan* 医学正传 c. 1515).	19
Jue jin jian/Jue jin jian jia jian 决津煎/决津煎加减	Dang gui 当归, ze xie 泽泻, niu xi 牛膝, rou gui 肉桂, shu di huang 熟地黄, wu yao 乌药 (*Fu Ren Gui* 妇人规 c. 1624).	16
Tao ren gui zhi tang/ Gui zhi tao ren tang 1 桃仁桂枝汤/桂枝桃仁汤1	Gui zhi 桂枝, bai shao 白芍, sheng di huang 生地黄, tao ren 桃仁, gan cao 甘草, sheng jiang 生姜 (*Jiao Zhu Fu Ren Liang Fang* 校注妇人良方 c. 1558).	15
Dang gui tang/san/ wan 当归汤/散/丸	Dang gui 当归, hu po 琥珀, an lu zi 菴蔄子, yi mu cao 益母草, wu zhu yu 吴茱萸, rou gui 肉桂, chuan jiao 川椒, niu xi 牛膝, shui zhi 水蛭, chuan xiong 川芎, yan hu suo 延胡索, mo yao 没药 (*Tai Ping Sheng Hui Fang* 太平圣惠方 c. 992 CE).	13

Table 3.5. (Continued)

Formula Name	Herb Ingredients	No. of Citations
Hu po san/Tong jing hu po san/Yan shi hu po san 琥珀散/痛经琥珀散/严氏琥珀散	Liu ji nu 刘寄奴, mu dan pi 牡丹皮, shu di huang 熟地黄, yan hu suo 延胡索, wu yao 乌药, chi shao 赤芍, e zhu 莪术, san leng 三棱, dang gui 当归, rou gui 肉桂, hei dou 黑豆, sheng jiang 生姜, cu 醋 (Yu Ji Wei Yi 玉机微义 c. 1396).	13
Wen jing tang 1/ Da wen jing tang/ Wen jing tang jia jian 温经汤1/大温经汤/温经汤加减	Variant 1: Ren shen 人参, tu chao bai zhu 土炒白术, dang gui 当归, bai shao 白芍, chuan xiong 川芎, shu di huang 熟地黄, sha ren 砂仁, xiao hui xiang 小茴香, fu ling 茯苓, gan cao 甘草, xiang fu 香附, chen pi 陈皮, chen xiang 沉香, wu zhu yu 吴茱萸, yan hu suo 延胡索, lu rong 鹿茸. Variant 2: E jiao 阿胶, bai shao 白芍, chuan xiong 川芎, dang gui 当归, ren shen 人参, rou gui 肉桂, mu dan pi 牡丹皮, wu zhu yu 吴茱萸, gan cao 甘草, ban xia 半夏, mai men dong 麦门冬, sheng jiang 生姜 (both variants from Yi Xue Ru Men 医学入门 c. 1575).	12
Tiao jing yin/Tiao jing yin jia jian 调经饮/调经饮加减	Dang gui 当归, niu xi 牛膝, zhi xiang fu 制香附, yan hu suo 延胡索, shan zha 山楂, fu ling 茯苓, chen pi 陈皮, jiu 酒 (Fu Ren Gui 妇人规 c. 1624).	12
Ba wu tang 八物汤 1	Shu di huang 熟地黄, dang gui 当归, bai shao 白芍, chuan xiong 川芎, yan hu suo 延胡索, ku lian zi 苦楝子, bin lang 槟榔, mu xiang 木香 (Su Wen Bing Ji Qi Yi Bao Ming Ji 素问病机气宜保命集 c. 1186).	11
Fu long gan san 伏龙肝散	Fu long gan 伏龙肝, yu yu liang 禹余粮, chi shao 赤芍, sheng di huang 生地黄, di yu 地榆, bai mao gen 白茅根, long gu 龙骨, dang gui 当归, zhi gan cao 炙甘草, xue jie 血竭 (Sheng Ji Zong Lu 圣济总录 c. 1117).	10

Note: The use of some herbs may be restricted in some countries. Readers are advised to comply with relevant regulations.

The four ingredients of *Si wu tang* 四物汤 are *dang gui* 当归, *shu di huang* 熟地黄, *bai shao* 白芍, and *chuan xiong* 川芎; the key action of this formula is to nourish and invigorate Blood.[22] Eleven of the 88 citations described the use of these four ingredients. Seventy-seven citations included modifications, and many renamed the formulas according to the addition of a particular herb or herbs. For example, some citations that described the addition of important herbs, such as *tao ren* 桃仁 and *hong hua* 红花, listed the formula name as *Tao ren si wu tang* 桃仁四物汤. This is another well-known traditional formula that has a long history for use in gynaecological disorders. Addition of *tao ren* 桃仁 and *hong hua* 红花 to *Si wu tang* 四物汤 assists in resolving Blood stasis.[22]

Another, much smaller group of seven citations described formulas that were also named *Si wu tang* 四乌汤, but with different Chinese characters; however, the formulas in this group had different actions to those of the herbs listed above. Three herbs were common to all seven citations: *wu yao* 乌药, *dang gui* 当归, and *xiang fu* 香附. Both *xiang fu* 香附 and *wu yao* 乌药 regulate Liver *qi* and menstruation and alleviate pain. These actions were considered to be sufficiently different from those of the four-ingredient formula described above, so they were kept separate for analysis. This highlights the variation in formula names and herb ingredients in past eras.

Similar situations were encountered with other formulas, such as *Ba wu tang* 八物汤/*Ba zhen tang* 八珍汤, *Wen jing tang* 温经汤, and *Hu po san* 琥珀散. Analysis of formulas named *Ba wu tang* 八物汤 revealed two distinctly different formulas: those with actions to resolve *qi* stagnation and Blood stasis (*Ba wu tang* 八物汤 1) and those with actions to tonify *qi* and Blood (*Ba wu tang* 八物汤 2, also named *Ba zhen tang* 八珍汤). Due to these different actions, the formulas were separated for analysis. Both types of formulas were found in more than 10 citations each; *Ba wu tang* 八物汤 2, with its actions to tonify *qi* and Blood, was the more common of the two (Table 3.5).

The formula *Wen jing tang* 温经汤 was mentioned in 18 citations, but again, differences were evident in the actions of the herb ingredients. One variant included herbs for empty cold (*Wen jing tang* 温经汤 1), another included herbs for full cold (*Wen jing tang* 温经汤 2), while the third included herbs for resolving damp, with no obvious actions on cold at all (*Wen jin tang* 温经汤 3). Formulas with actions to alleviate empty cold (*Wen jing tang* 温经汤 1) were the most common of these three types. *Hu po san* 琥珀散 was also named as *Tong jing hu po san* 痛经琥珀散 and *Yan shi hu po san* 严氏琥珀散, although all had similar actions to invigorate Blood and expel cold.

For some formulas with the same name but highly variable herb ingredients, there was no 'core' formula on which to base any judgements of similarity. An example of this is the formula named *Mu dan tang/san*牡丹汤/散, which appeared in four citations. Two distinct actions were seen among the formulas: warming the meridians and relieving pain, and clearing *qi* and Blood stagnation. As there was no core formula on which to base an assessment of similarity, it was considered appropriate to separate the formulas with these different actions.

The earliest citation of the formula *Jue jin jian* 决津煎 was in the book *Fu Ren Gui* 妇人规 (c. 1624). In fact, this book provided five citations that described *Jue jin jian* 决津煎 for endometriosis-like symptoms. In three of the five citations, the formula was modified and named accordingly (*Jue jin jian jia jian* 决津煎加减; *jia jian* 加减 meaning modified). The other two citations of *Jue jin jian* 决津煎 contained the ingredients listed in Table 3.5, with one also including the herb *wu zhu yu* 吴茱萸. Another formula, *Tiao jing yin* 调经饮, found in 12 citations, described five different modifications in the earliest citation. Four of the five citations described modification of the core formula, which has been included in Table 3.5.

Many citations described modification of the CHM formula according to the stage of the menstrual cycle. Modification ranged from relatively minor changes, such as addition, removal, or substitution of one or more herbs from a formula, to using different formulas during different stages of the menstrual cycle as the CM syndrome changed. Two hundred and seven citations (30.2%) that mentioned oral CHM modified the treatment prior to menstruation, 241 citations (35.2%) modified treatment during menstruation, and 68 citations (9.9%) described modification of the formula after menstruation. Information about treatment modification was not reported in the 181 remaining citations.

Most frequent oral use herbs in possible endometriosis citations

Among the oral CHM citations that were possibly related to endometriosis, 293 different herbs were mentioned. Herbs prepared using different methods were merged for analysis, as were herbs from the same source. For example, *zhi gan cao* 炙甘草 is prepared by roasting *gan cao* 甘草, and both were counted as one herb for analysis. When different parts of the same herb were described, for example the roots or leaves from the same plant, analysis was conducted for the herb overall and additional types were noted.

The number of herb ingredients in included formulas ranged from one to 32, and the median number of herbs was eight. The most frequently used herb in citations judged as possible cases of endometriosis was *dang gui* 当归 (560 citations). As shown in Table 3.6, other parts from the same plant were also mentioned: *jiu dang gui*

Table 3.6. Most Frequent Oral Use Herbs in Possible Endometriosis Citations

Herb Name	Scientific Name	No. of Citations
Dang gui 当归 (dang gui shen 当归身, dang gui wei 当归尾, jiu dang gui 酒当归)	*Angelica sinensis* (Oliv.) Diels	560 (31, 26, 34)
Bai shao 白芍	*Paeonia lactiflora* Pall.	348
Chuan xiong 川芎	*Ligusticum chuangxiong* Hort.	336
Shu di huang 熟地黄	*Rehmannia glutinosa* Libosch.	247
Gan cao 甘草	*Glycyrrhiza* spp	229
Rou gui 肉桂	*Cinnamomum cassia* Presl	202
Xiang fu 香附	*Cyperus rotundus* L.	201

Table 3.6. (Continued)

Herb Name	Scientific Name	No. of Citations
Yan hu suo 延胡索	Corydalis yanhusuo W.T. Wang	188
Mu dan pi 牡丹皮	Paeonia suffruticosa Andr.	155
Fu ling 茯苓	Poria cocos (Schw.) Wolf	135
Tao ren 桃仁	Prunus spp	124
Ren shen 人参	Panax ginseng C. A. Mey.	122
Mu xiang 木香	Aucklandia lappa Decne.	119
Sheng di huang 生地黄	Rehmannia glutinosa Libosch.	114
Bai zhu 白术 (tu chao bai zhu 土炒白术, chao bai zhu 炒白术)	Atractylodes macrocephala Koidz.	108 (7, 4)
Sheng jiang 生姜	Zingiber officinale Rosc.	104
Niu xi 牛膝	Achyranthes bidentata Bl.	93
Chen pi 陈皮	Citrus reticulata Blanco	82
E zhu 莪术	Curcuma spp	81
Gan jiang 干姜	Zingiber officinale Rosc.	76

Note: The use of some herbs may be restricted in some countries. Readers are advised to comply with relevant regulations.

酒当归 was found in 34 citations, *dang gui shen* 当归身 was found in 31 citations, and *dang gui wei* 当归尾 was found in 26 citations. Other variants of *dang gui* 当归 that were found less frequently were *jiu dang gui shen* 酒当归身 (seven citations), *dang gui tan* 当归炭 (three citations), and *dang gui xu* 当归须 (one citation). Similarly, different variants of *bai zhu* 白术 were found; seven citations mentioned *tu chao bai zhu* 土炒白术 and four citations described *chao bai zhu* 炒白术.

Other herbs found in more than 200 citations included *bai shao* 白芍, *chuan xiong* 川芎, *shu di huang* 熟地黄, *gan cao* 甘草, *rou gui* 肉桂, and *xiang fu* 香附. These herbs have actions that nourish and invigorate Blood and *yin*, dispel cold, promote circulation of *qi* and Blood, and regulate menstruation. Many of these herbs continue to be used today and can be found in formulas recommended in textbooks and guidelines described in Chapter 2.

Most frequent oral use formulas in most likely endometriosis citations

Of the 44 citations judged most likely to be endometriosis, 22 citations described unnamed formulas. Due to the small number of citations in this subset, only three CHM formulas were found in multiple citations: *Si wu tang/Si wu tang jia jian* 四物汤/四物汤加减 (five citations), *Shun jing tang* 顺经汤 (five citations), and *Gui jing liang an tang* 归经两安汤 (two citations) (Table 3.7). Both *Shun jing tang* 顺经汤 and *Gui jing liang an tang* 归经两安汤 were found in two different books by the same author (Chen Shiduo 陈士铎). The two instances of *Gui jing liang an tang* 归经两安汤 came from the two books by Chen Shiduo 陈士铎 — *Bian Zheng Qi Wen* 辨证奇闻 and *Bian Zheng Lu* 辨证录 (both c. 1687).

Table 3.7. Most Frequent Formulas in Most Likely Endometriosis Citations

Formula Name	Herb Ingredients	No. of Citations
Si wu tang/Si wu tang jia jian 四物汤/四物汤加减	*Dang gui* 当归, *chuan xiong* 川芎, *bai shao* 白芍, *shu di huang* 熟地黄, *san leng* 三棱, *e zhu* 莪术, *hong hua* 红花, *wu yao* 乌药, *ren shen* 人参, *rou gui* 肉桂, *bai zhi* 白芷, *jing jie* 荆芥 (*Zheng Shi Jia Chuan Nv Ke Wan Jin Fang* 郑氏家传女科万金方 c. 1697).	5
Shun jing tang 顺经汤	*Dang gui* 当归, *shu di huang* 熟地黄, *mu dan pi* 牡丹皮, *bai shao* 白芍, *fu ling* 茯苓, *niu xi* 牛膝, *jing jie* 荆芥, *sha shen* 沙参 (*Bian Zheng Qi Wen* 辨证奇闻 and *Bian Zheng Lu* 辨证录, both c. 1687).	5
Gui jing liang an tang 归经两安汤	*Ren shen* 人参, *shan zhu yu* 山茱萸, *dang gui* 当归, *bai zhu* 白术, *bai shao* 白芍, *shu di huang* 熟地黄, *mai men dong* 麦门冬, *ba ji tian* 巴戟天, *jing jie* 荆芥, *sheng ma* 升麻 (*Bian Zheng Qi Wen* 辨证奇闻 and *Bian Zheng Lu* 辨证录, both c. 1687).	2

Note: The use of some herbs may be restricted in some countries. Readers are advised to comply with relevant regulations.

Most frequent oral use herbs in most likely endometriosis citations

One hundred and twelve different herbs were used in the 44 citations judged most likely to be endometriosis. Descriptive statistics of the number of herb ingredients showed the same result as was seen for possible endometriosis citations: the number of herb ingredients ranged from one to 32, and the median number of herbs was eight. The herb most often used was *dang gui* 当归, which was also the most frequently used herb in the total pool of citations. Other herbs used in most likely endometriosis citations included *bai shao* 白芍, *chuan xiong* 川芎, and *shu di huang* 熟地黄 (Table 3.8). These herbs appeared in the same rank as in the total pool.

Table 3.8. Most Frequent Herbs in Most Likely Endometriosis Citations

Herb Name	Scientific Name	No. of Citations
Dang gui 当归 (*dang gui shen* 当归身, *dang gui wei* 当归尾, *jiu dang gui* 酒当归)	*Angelica sinensis* (Oliv.) Diels	31 (5, 4, 4)
Bai shao 白芍	*Paeonia lactiflora* Pall.	23
Chuan xiong 川芎	*Ligusticum chuangxiong* Hort.	17
Shu di huang 熟地黄	*Rehmannia glutinosa* Libosch.	16
Mu dan pi 牡丹皮	*Paeonia suffruticosa* Andr.	14
Fu ling 茯苓	*Poria cocos* (Schw.) Wolf	13
Bai zhu 白术 (*tu chao bai zhu* 土炒白术)	*Atractylodes macrocephala* Koidz.	12 (1)
Ren shen 人参	*Panax ginseng* C. A. Mey.	10
Jing jie 荆芥 (*jing jie tan* 荆芥炭)	*Schizonepeta tenuifolia* Briq.	9 (3)
Gan cao 甘草	*Glycyrrhiza* spp	7
Zhi zi 栀子	*Gardenia jasminoides* Ellis	7
Niu xi 牛膝	*Achyranthes bidentata* Bl.	6
Sheng di huang 生地黄	*Rehmannia glutinosa* Libosch.	6

Note: The use of some herbs may be restricted in some countries. Readers are advised to comply with relevant regulations.

Of interest, *gan cao* 甘草 was mentioned less frequently (proportionally) in citations that were most likely to be endometriosis compared to the total pool of citations that were possibly related to endometriosis. *Gan cao* 甘草 is often used in formulas to harmonise the actions of other ingredients, but also has other actions that may be beneficial for endometriosis, such as to tonify the Spleen and *qi* and alleviate pain.[23] Such actions are related, although they may not be directly beneficial. In the total pool, *gan cao* 甘草 was the fifth-most frequently used herb, while in citations most likely to be endometriosis, *gan cao* 甘草 was the tenth-most frequently used herb. This may be due to the smaller number of citations in the 'most likely' group, more focused actions of formulas in the 'most likely' group, and greater variation in herbs in the total pool.

Treatment with Topical Chinese Herbal Medicine

Six citations described the use of topical CHM for endometriosis-like symptoms. All six were considered possible cases of endometriosis. The earliest of these citations was found in the book *Pu Ji Fang* 普济方 (c. 1406). This citation used *Long yan gao* 龙盐膏, consisting of the herbs *ding xiang* 丁香, *quan xie* 全蝎, *mu xiang* 木香, *liang jiang* 良姜, *wu tou* 乌头, *bai fan* 白矾, *long gu* 龙骨, *xiao hui xiang* 小茴香, *dang gui wei* 当归尾, *yan hu suo* 延胡索, *chao yan* 炒盐, *fang ji* 防己, *hou po* 厚朴, *chi xiao dou* 赤小豆, *rou gui* 肉桂, and *mu tong* 木通 as a vaginal pessary.

There was no overlap in formulas, with three named and three unnamed formulas described in the six citations. In addition to *Long yan gao* 龙盐膏, the other named formulas were *Jing feng xiang zhu* 金凤衔珠 and *San yin gao fu qi* 散阴膏敷脐 plus *Yao wu wai fu* 药物外敷. The combination of *San yin gao fu qi* 散阴膏敷脐 and *Yao wu wai fu* 药物外敷 was applied as a paste on the umbilicus. Two unnamed formulas, both consisting of the single ingredient *zi su* 紫苏, were used to steam the perineum, while the third unnamed formula included a variety of herb ingredients.

Table 3.9. Most Frequent Topical Use Herbs in Possible Endometriosis Citations

Herb Name	Scientific Name	No. of Citations
Rou gui 肉桂	Cinnamomum cassia Presl	3
Ding xiang 丁香	Eugenia caryophyllata Thunb.	2
Wu zhu yu 吴茱萸	Euodia rutaecarpa (Juss.) Benth. and variants	2
Yan hu suo 延胡索	Corydalis yanhusuo W.T. Wang	2
Zi su 紫苏	Perilla frutescens (L.) Britt.	2
Hu jiao 胡椒	Piper nigrum L.	2
She xiang 麝香	Moschus spp	2

Note: The use of some herbs may be restricted in some countries. Readers are advised to comply with relevant regulations.

Forty-three different herbs were described in the six topical CHM citations. The most frequently used herb was *rou gui* 肉桂, which was described in three citations. Other herbs used in two citations are described in Table 3.9.

Discussion of Chinese Herbal Medicine for Endometriosis

Chinese herbal medicine was commonly used to treat symptoms of endometriosis in past eras. The majority of citations described orally administered formulations, with many suggesting modifications according to the time of the menstrual cycle. Diversity was seen in the treatments used; 195 named formulas and many more unnamed formulas were described in the included citations. This diversity was also evident among herb ingredients, with more than 290 different herbs named in the citations.

Si wu tang 四物汤 was the most frequently described formula among citations judged as possible cases of endometriosis. *Si wu tang* 四物汤 is commonly used in gynaecology disorders due to its actions of nourishing Blood and promoting Blood circulation, regulating the Liver and therefore menstruation. While *Si wu tang* 四物汤 was not named in the textbooks and guidelines described in

Chapter 2, another formula, *Tao hong si wu tang* 桃红四物汤, is recommended in combination with other orally used formulas (see Chapter 2). *Tao hong si wu tang* 桃红四物汤 is a modification of *Si wu tang* 四物汤 with two herbs added: *tao ren* 桃仁 and *hong hua* 红花. Both herbs have actions that regulate Blood and resolve Blood stasis.[23]

Si wu tang 四物汤 is also one of the most frequently cited formulas among the citations considered most likely to relate to endometriosis. Only two other formulas were found in multiple citations: *Shun jing tang* 顺经汤 and *Gui jing liang an tang* 归经两安汤. *Shun jing tang* 顺经汤 is used to nourish *yin*, clear heat, and cool the Blood, while *Gui jing liang an tang* 归经两安汤 nourishes *qi* and Blood and regulates menstruation. The finding that only three formulas were found in multiple citations is likely to be due to the small number of citations that were judged most likely to be endometriosis.

Aside from *Tao hong si wu tang* 桃红四物汤, only one other formula that was found frequently in the classical literature was also recommended in the contemporary literature in Chapter 2: *Shi xiao san* 失笑散. This formula was described in one passage from *Lei Zheng Zhi Cai* 类证治裁 (c. 1839). While the actions of *Shi xiao san* 失笑散, invigorating Blood and dispelling Blood stasis, appear highly relevant to endometriosis, it is not clear why this formula was only found in one citation from past eras. One possible explanation is that this formula, which was first introduced in *Tai Ping Hui Min He Ji Ju Fang* 太平惠民和剂局方 (c. 992), was traditionally used for postpartum abdominal pain and pain diseases of the Liver meridian. The use of *Shi xiao san* 失笑散 for dysmenorrhoea was not documented until the publication of *Lei Zheng Zhi Cai* 类证治裁 (c. 1839).

The top four herb ingredients in possible endometriosis and most likely endometriosis are the same: *dang gui* 当归, *bai shao* 白芍, *chuan xiong* 川芎, and *shu di huang* 熟地黄. These four ingredients are the core ingredients of *Si wu tang* 四物汤. Although *Si wu tang* 四物汤 was the most frequently cited formula in the total pool of citations (found in 88 citations), this does not fully explain the high frequency of use of these herbs. Even the lowest ranked herb of these four (*shu di huang* 熟地黄, 247 citations) was found in many other formulas that were not *Si wu tang* 四物汤. The high frequency of use appears to be more related to their actions on tonifying Blood and promoting Blood circulation, which fits with the contemporary understanding of endometriosis being a disease primarily related to Blood stasis.

Topical CHM treatments were used far less frequently than oral CHM. Such treatments were used as vaginal pessaries, as a paste applied to the umbilicus, or as a steam wash for the genital area. Herbs used for topical application have actions that dispel cold (*hu jiao* 胡椒, *rou gui* 肉桂, and *wu zhu yu* 吴茱萸), invigorate Blood, and promote *qi* and Blood circulation (*rou gui* 肉桂, *she xiang* 麝香, and *yan hu suo* 延胡索). Topical treatments continue to be recommended in clinical guidelines and textbooks included in Chapter 2; for example, *yan hu suo* 延胡索 can be used as an enema for women with endometriosis.

Acupuncture and Other Chinese Medicine Therapies

Seven citations described acupuncture therapies and two described other CM therapies for endometriosis-like symptoms. All were considered as possible cases of endometriosis. Two citations from the Qing dynasty suggested that the abdomen could be massaged before menstruation. Among acupuncture therapy citations, treatment during the menstrual cycle was suggested in four of the seven citations; one suggested treatment administered prior to menstruation, while remaining citations did not specify this information.

Acupuncture was used as early as the pre-Tang dynasty, with one citation from *Zhen Jiu Jia Yi Jing* 针灸甲乙经 (c. 282 CE) describing acupuncture to ST25 *Tianshu* 天枢. This was the only citation that described the use of acupuncture alone. Three citations discussed using moxibustion for endometriosis-like symptoms, which was applied to single points: SP6 *Sanyinjiao* 三阴交, CV3 *Zhongji* 中极, and CV8 *Shenque* 神阙.

Two citations described the use of acupuncture and moxibustion together. Both citations applied the combination to ST28 *Shuidao*

水道. One additional citation mentioned acupuncture points without specifying the technique to be used. This citation suggested that points BL23 *Shenshu* 肾俞, CV4 *Guanyuan* 关元, and SP6 *Sanyinjiao* 三阴交 could be used.

Classical Literature in Perspective

The information contained in classical CM textbooks is the foundation for contemporary practice and continues to guide clinicians with an interest in endometriosis. Locating information about possible cases of endometriosis in these texts is reliant on searching for the characteristic symptoms, such as dysmenorrhoea, abdominal mass, abdominal pain, and menstruation. Cases of infertility in the context of the aforementioned symptoms may also provide insight into the understanding and treatment of endometriosis in past eras. This systematic analysis used terms for signs and symptoms of endometriosis to search a representative sample of classical CM books.

Contrary to what was expected, relatively few citations were identified by the various terms for dysmenorrhoea (388 hits). Far more citations were found when terms for mass were combined with terms for 'woman' (more than 15,000 hits). However, many of these citations were considered to be due to causes other than endometriosis and were excluded. Terms for mass and woman identified almost one-third of all included citations, while dysmenorrhoea identified fewer than 3% of included citations. Over half of the citations that were included were identified by terms for menstruation combined with *fu tong* 腹痛 (abdominal pain, 415 citations, 58.6%). This may reflect a different view of pain associated with endometriosis (as opposed to primary dysmenorrhoea), or it may simply be due to differences in terminology used in past eras.

Treatment of endometriosis-like symptoms was described as early as 282 CE in the well-known acupuncture text *Zhen Jiu Jia Yi Jing* 针灸甲乙经. This passage suggested that the acupuncture point ST25 *Tianshu* 天枢 should be used to alleviate symptoms. The earliest citation of CHM was found in later books from the Tang and Five dynasties (*Hua Tuo Shen Fang* 华佗神方 and *Qian Jin Yi Fang* 千金翼方, both dated c. 682 CE); both books described unnamed CHM formulas for menstrual pain or abdominal mass.

Oral CHM was the most common treatment described in included citations; *Si wu tang* 四物汤 was the most frequently cited formula overall as well as in citations most likely to be endometriosis. Modification of formulas to address each individual's signs and symptoms is typical of clinical practice and was seen in descriptions from classical texts. As highlighted, many citations made modifications to the four core ingredients of *Si wu tang* 四物汤, with *Tao ren si wu tang* 桃仁四物汤 being one of the most notable examples. *Tao ren si wu tang* 桃仁四物汤 continues to be a key formula in CM clinical practice and is recommended in contemporary clinical textbooks and guidelines included in Chapter 2.

The most frequently cited herbs in citations most likely to relate to endometriosis were generally reflective of the herbs found in all included citations, which is somewhat surprising given the much smaller numbers of citations judged most likely to relate to endometriosis (707 possible endometriosis citations versus 44 most likely endometriosis citations). This may reflect overlap in the herbs used for abdominal pain due to endometriosis and abdominal pain due to other gynaecological diseases, such as primary dysmenorrhoea. Herbs with a high frequency of use have actions that tonify and regulate Blood and dispel Blood stasis.

Three herbs that were among the most frequently described herbs in citations considered most likely to relate to endometriosis were *jing jie* 荆芥 (*jing jie tan* 荆芥炭) and *zhi zi* 栀子. As the citations most likely to be endometriosis are a subset of the overall group, these herbs naturally also appeared in the overall group, but with much lower frequency. For example, *jing jie* 荆芥 was found in 12 of the 707 included citations, compared with nine of the 44 citations most likely to be endometriosis, and *zhi zi* 栀子 was found in 13 of the 707 included citations, compared with 13 of the 44 citations most likely to be endometriosis. While *jing jie* 荆芥 is typically used to release the exterior, it also has actions that stop uterine bleeding or bleeding from the bowel.[23] *Zhi zi* 栀子 is traditionally used to drain heat and can also cool the Blood,[23] so it may be beneficial for the CM syndromes of dampness-heat and stasis obstructing the uterus. Neither herb was included in formulas recommended in Chapter 2, but this may relate to the fact that Chapter 2 describes the herbs for the more common endometriosis of the pelvic cavity, while most classical literature citations judged most likely to be endometriosis (32 of 44) described symptoms suggestive of endometriosis outside the pelvic cavity, such as haemoptysis and haematochezia.

Topical CHM and acupuncture therapies were infrequently described in classical CM texts for endometriosis-like symptoms. Despite this, both treatments continue to be used in contemporary clinical practice and are included in clinical textbooks and guidelines included in Chapter 2. Clinicians can consider these as adjunct treatments to oral CHM.

This systematic review of the classical CM literature was designed to capture key information about endometriosis-like signs and symptoms in past eras. The criteria for selecting citations was developed according to the typical symptoms of endometriosis. Of course, laparoscopic confirmation of diagnosis was not possible in ancient China. As such, the findings presented in this chapter should be considered only as examples most likely to be endometriosis, not definite cases of endometriosis.

Further, a search of the ZHYD was conducted using terms for some of the most common symptoms and complications of endometriosis. Not all women with endometriosis will have symptoms,[24] and it is unlikely that cases or descriptions of asymptomatic endometriosis will have been identified in this search.

In order to identify the most frequently used formulas described in classical CM texts, decisions were made to group some formulas with the same or similar names together, while others were separated according to actions of the formula. The findings of analyses would be different if other approaches were used to categorise treatments. Nevertheless, it seems clear that the formula *Si wu tang* 四物汤 and herbs *dang gui* 当归, *shu di huang* 熟地黄, *bai shao* 白芍, and *chuan xiong* 川芎 were important treatments for endometriosis-like symptoms in past eras.

References

1. Needham J, Lu G, Sivin N. (2000) *Science and civilisation in China. Vol 5, Part VI: Medicine.* Cambridge University Press; Cambridge.
2. Hu R. (2000) *Encyclopedia of Traditional Chinese Medicine.* Hunan Electronic and Audio-Visual Publishing House, Changsha.
3. May B, Lu Y, Lu C, *et al.* (2013) Systematic assessment of the representativeness of published collections of the traditional literature on Chinese medicine. *J Altern Complement Med* **19**(5): 403–409.
4. May B, Lu C, Xue C. (2012) Collections of traditional Chinese medical litearture as resources for systematic searches. *J Altern Complement Med* **18**(12): 1101–1107.
5. Benagiano G, Brosens I, Lippi D. (2014) The history of endometriosis. *Gynecologic and Obstetric Investigation* **78**(1): 1–9.
6. 欧阳慧卿. (2002) 中医妇科学. 北京: 人民卫生出版社.
7. 中华中医药学会. (2012) 中医妇科常见病诊疗指南. 北京: 中国中医药出版社.
8. 司徒仪. (2008) 中西医结合妇科学(第二版). 北京: 科学出版社.
9. 王小云. (2017) 中西医结合妇科学研究新进展. 北京: 人民卫生出版社.
10. 王小云, 黄建玲. (2013) 妇科专病中医临床诊治 (第三版). 北京: 人民卫生出版社.
11. 梁雪芳. (2015) 子宫内膜异位症. 北京: 人民卫生出版社.
12. 司徒仪. (2004) 子宫内膜异位症中西医结合治疗. 北京: 人民卫生出版社.
13. 罗云坚, 张英哲. (2003) 常见病中西医结合诊疗常规. 北京: 广东科技出版社.
14. 张玉珍. (2002) 中医妇科学 北京: 中国中医药出版社.
15. 罗颂平, 刘雁峰. (2016) 中医妇科学(第三版). 北京: 人民卫生出版社.
16. 欧阳慧卿. (2012) 中西医结合妇产科学(新世纪第二版). 北京: 中国中医药出版社.
17. 罗云坚, 孙塑伦. (2007) 中医临床治疗特色与优势指南. 北京: 人民卫生出版社.
18. 林昭庚. (2002) 中西医病名对照大词典. 北京: 人民卫生出版社.
19. World Health Organization. Regional Office for the Western Pacific. (2007) *WHO international standard terminologies on traditional medi-*

cine in the Western Pacific Region. WHO Regional Office for the Western Pacific; Manila.
20. 梁雪芳, 曹立幸, 王小云. (2015) 痛经. 北京: 中国中医药出版社.
21. 郑玮琳. (2016) 痛经文献分析及益气化瘀法治疗子宫内膜异位症痛经临床研究: 广州中医药大学, 中医妇科学 (专业学位), 硕士.
22. Lyttleton J. (2004) *Treatment of Infertility with Chinese Medicine.* Churchill Livingstone; Edinburgh, UK.
23. Bensky D, Clavey S, Stoger E. (2004) *Chinese herbal medicine Materia Medica.* 3rd ed. Eastland Press, Inc; Seattle, US.
24. Rawson JM. (1991) Prevalence of endometriosis in asymptomatic women. *J Reprod Med* **36**(7): 513–515.

4

Methods for Evaluating Clinical Evidence

OVERVIEW

Clinical studies that evaluated Chinese medicine interventions for women with endometriosis were identified through searches of electronic biomedical databases. Studies were reviewed against eligibility criteria and a review was conducted using internationally accepted methods. This chapter describes the methods used to evaluate the efficacy and safety of Chinese medicine treatment for endometriosis and endometriosis-related infertility.

Introduction

Chinese medicine (CM) treatments for endometriosis have been described in the contemporary literature (Chapter 2) and classical CM texts (Chapter 3). The efficacy, effectiveness, and safety of several CM treatments have been tested in clinical studies and published in scientific journals. Systematic reviews of a selection of these studies have been conducted and are presented for Chinese herbal medicine (CHM; see Chapter 5), acupuncture and related therapies (see Chapter 7), and combinations of CM therapies (see Chapter 8).

This chapter describes the methods used to evaluate the evidence from clinical studies. References to clinical studies were obtained and assessed by an expert group. The characteristics of randomised controlled trials (RCTs) and non-randomised controlled clinical trials (CCTs) were described, as were details of the interventions tested. Results for selected outcome measures were evaluated with meta-analysis using the approach outlined below. This approach was not possible for non-controlled studies. Instead, a summary of the characteristics of the studies, CM treatments, and any adverse events were reported.

References for studies that evaluated CHM are indicated by an 'H' followed by a number (e.g., H1), studies of acupuncture therapies are indicated by an 'A' (e.g., A1), and studies that tested a combination of CHM and acupuncture therapies are indicated by a 'C' (e.g., C1). No studies that evaluated other CM therapies met the inclusion criteria, and the evidence for such interventions is uncertain.

Search Strategy

A comprehensive search was conducted in English and Chinese language databases following the methods of the Cochrane Handbook of Systematic Reviews.[1] English language databases included PubMed, Excerpta Medica Database (Embase), Cumulative Index of Nursing and Allied Health Literature (CINAHL), Cochrane Central Register of Controlled Trials (CENTRAL) including the Cochrane Library, and Allied and Complementary Medicine Database (AMED). Chinese language databases included China BioMedical Literature (CBM), China National Knowledge Infrastructure (CNKI), Chongqing VIP (CQVIP), and Wanfang. Chinese and English language databases were searched from inception to November 2018. No restrictions were applied. Search terms were mapped to controlled vocabulary (where applicable) in addition to being searched as keywords.

To conduct a comprehensive search of the literature, searches were run according to study design (reviews, controlled trials, non-controlled studies). This was done for each of the three intervention types (CHM, acupuncture and related therapies, and other CM therapies), resulting in nine searches in each of the nine databases:

1. CHM reviews;
2. CHM controlled trials (randomised and non-randomised);
3. CHM non-controlled studies;
4. Acupuncture and related therapies reviews;
5. Acupuncture and related therapies controlled trials (randomised and non-randomised);

6. Acupuncture and related therapies non-controlled studies;
7. Other CM therapies reviews;
8. Other CM therapies controlled trials (randomised and non-randomised);
9. Other CM therapies non-controlled studies.

Studies of combination CM therapies were identified through the above searches. In addition to electronic databases, reference lists of systematic reviews and included studies were searched for additional publications. Clinical trial registries were searched on December 2018 to identify clinical trials that were ongoing or completed, and where required, trial investigators were contacted to obtain data. The searched trial registries included the Australian New Zealand Clinical Trial Registry (ANZCTR), the Chinese Clinical Trial Registry (ChiCTR), the European Union Clinical Trials Register (EU-CTR), and the United States National Institutes of Health register (ClinicalTrials.gov).

If required, trial investigators were contacted to obtain further information. Trial investigators were contacted by email or telephone and were followed up after two weeks if no reply was received. When no response was received after one month, any unknown information was marked as not available.

Inclusion Criteria

Inclusion criteria were developed in consultation with clinical experts. Studies that met eligibility criteria for participants, interventions, comparators, and outcomes were included. Studies were included when:

- Participants were adolescent girls or adult women with 1) endometriosis diagnosed based on symptoms, examination, biochemical results, imaging, or laparoscopy/laparotomy/visualisation (with or without histological confirmation), or 2) adenomyosis.
- Interventions were CHM, acupuncture and related therapies, or combinations of CM therapies (Table 4.1).

Table 4.1. Chinese Medicine Interventions Included in Clinical Evidence Evaluation

Category	Intervention
CHM	CHM for oral or topical use, CHM enema.
Acupuncture and related therapies	Acupuncture, moxibustion, electroacupuncture.
Combination CM therapies	Combination therapies are defined as two or more CM interventions from different categories administered together (e.g., CHM plus acupuncture, CHM plus *qigong* 气功).

- Comparators included no treatment or waitlist control, placebo or sham, and interventions recommended in clinical practice guidelines for treatment of endometriosis or endometriosis-related infertility.
- One or more of the pre-specified outcome measures were reported (Table 4.2).

Laparoscopy with histological confirmation is considered the gold standard for diagnosis of endometriosis, although robust evidence is lacking.[2] As stated in the European Society of Human Reproduction and Embryology,[2] a diagnosis of endometriosis is suspected based on history, signs, and symptoms, is further supported by pelvic examination, and is confirmed by laparoscopy. Not all women will undergo laparoscopy to confirm diagnosis of endometriosis and, in many cases, diagnosis is made according to history, signs, symptoms, and examination. Such studies were included in this review.

Studies that tested the effectiveness of CM therapies in treating endometriosis symptoms were included, as were studies that examined the effects of CM therapies on fertility outcomes and menopausal symptoms induced by gonadotropin-releasing hormone agonists (GnRHa). Guideline-recommended treatments included surgery, analgesics, hormonal treatment such as oral contraceptives or progestogen treatment, danazol (a synthetic steroid), GnRHa, mifepristone, and combinations of these or other treatments, such as assisted reproductive treatments. Studies that combined a CM therapy with a guideline-recommended treatment were included if the same guideline-recommended treatment was used as the comparator.

Methods for Evaluating Clinical Evidence

Table 4.2. Pre-specified Outcomes

Outcome Categories	Outcome Measures	Scoring
Pain	1. VAS	Score
	2. VRS/NRS	Score
	3. CMSS[3]	0–90, lower is better
	4. CPGQ[4]	Variable, see text
	5. 1993 Guideline[5]	Variable, see text
	6. Number of people with pain	Lower is better
Recurrence	1. Recurrence	Various, lower is better
Uterine or cyst volume	1. Volume (see text)	Various, lower is better
Menstrual volume	1. Number of sanitary napkins	Lower is better
	2. Weight of sanitary napkins	Lower is better
Pregnancy outcomes	1. Pregnancy rate	Higher is better
	2. Live birth rate	Higher is better
	3. Miscarriage rate	Lower is better
Health-related quality of life	1. EHP-30[6]	0–100 points, lower is better
	2. EHP-5[7]	0–100 points, lower is better
	3. WHOQOL-BREF[8]	0–20 or 0–100 points per domain, higher is better
	4. SF-36[9]	0–100 points per domain, higher is better
	5. NHP[10]	0–1 point for each domain, lower is better
Other outcomes	1. Kupperman Index[11]	0–51 points, lower is better
	2. Bone density	See text
Adverse events	Number and type of adverse events	

Abbreviations: CMSS, Cox Menstrual Symptom Scale; CPGQ, Chronic Pain Grade Questionnaire; EHP, Endometriosis Health Profile; NHP, Nottingham Health Profile; NRS, numerical rating scale; SF-36, Medical Outcome Study 36-Item Short-Form Health Survey; VAS, visual analogue scale; VRS, verbal rating scale; WHOQOL-BREF, World Health Organization Quality of Life instrument (brief version).

Exclusion Criteria

Studies were excluded when participants:

- Were diagnosed with primary dysmenorrhoea;
- Were post-menopausal women;
- Reported dysmenorrhoea, pelvic pain, or dyspareunia (pain on sexual intercourse) due to inflammation, tumour, uterine myoma, or other causes;
- Had previously undergone hysterectomy and/or unilateral or bilateral salpingo-ovariectomy due to endometriosis; or
- Had previously undergone bilateral salpingo-ovariectomy.

Outcomes

Outcomes were selected in consultation with clinical experts. Outcomes included signs and symptoms of endometriosis, fertility outcomes, side effects of treatment, and health-related quality of life. Outcomes were grouped into the following categories: pain, recurrence, uterine or cyst volume, menstrual volume, pregnancy outcomes, health-related quality of life, and other outcomes that were not related to clinical presentation but were important for endometriosis management (Table 4.2). The nature and quantity of adverse events were documented.

These outcomes were selected in the review planning stages in 2018. Since then, a core outcome set for endometriosis research has been published.[12] Three core outcomes were selected for studies evaluating treatments for pain and other endometriosis symptoms: overall pain, improvement in the most bothersome symptom, and health-related quality of life. Eight outcomes were selected for trials evaluating interventions for infertility: intrauterine pregnancy confirmed by ultrasound, pregnancy loss (including miscarriage, ectopic pregnancy, termination, and stillbirth), live birth, time to pregnancy resulting in live birth, gestational age at birth, birth weight, neonatal mortality, and congenital abnormalities. Two outcomes were relevant to all trials: adverse events and patient satisfaction. The

Methods for Evaluating Clinical Evidence

outcomes selected for this review (Table 4.2) include pain and the most bothersome symptoms of endometriosis. Pregnancy outcomes were limited to pregnancy rate, live birth rate, and miscarriage rate. Future research may investigate the effects of CM interventions on other pregnancy outcomes, such as those included in the core outcome set.

Pain

Women with endometriosis may report dysmenorrhoea, pelvic pain, or dyspareunia. Many scales are used to assess pain. The visual analogue scale (VAS) is commonly used to assess pain due to various causes. Patients indicate their level of pain on the 10 cm line, where zero refers to no pain and 10 refers to the worst imaginable pain. Results may be reported as a score in centimetres (0–10 cm) or millimetres (0–100 mm). The verbal rating scale (VRS) assesses pain on a four- or five-point scale, where higher scores indicate worse pain. The numerical rating scale (NRS) measures pain on an 11-point scale from zero (no pain) to 10 (worst imaginable pain).

The Cox Menstrual Symptom Scale (CMSS)[3] assesses the severity of 18 menstrual symptoms. Severity is rated on a five-point scale where higher scores indicate worse severity. The sum of individual item scores provides a total score ranging from zero to 90. Two additional questions relate to time spent in bed due to menstrual problems and use of medication for menstrual symptoms, and results for these are reported separately. The original version of the CMSS included assessments of both severity and duration of each item, but the developers of the instrument found that assessing only severity was sufficient. The Chinese version of the CMSS includes assessments for both severity and duration.

The Chronic Pain Grade Questionnaire is a seven-item scale that assesses chronic pain in the previous six months.[4] Six of the items are scored on an 11-point scale where a score of zero means 'no pain' and a score of 10 means 'pain as bad as it could be'. The final item records the number of days that pain has affected usual activities. Scores are reported for three subscales: pain intensity (range 0–100), disability score (range 0–100), and the disability points score (derived from a combination of the number of disability days and the disability score; range 0–3). Subscale scores are used to classify one of five pain severity grades: grade 0 (no pain), grade I (low disability–low intensity), grade II (low disability–high intensity), grade III (high disability–moderately limiting), and grade IV (high disability–severely limiting). Studies conducted in China frequently use a different score range for the disability points score (range 0–6).

The 1993 *Guideline for Clinical Research on New Chinese Herbal Medicine Drugs* (中药新药临床研究指导原则)[5] includes a scale to assess the severity of dysmenorrhoea. The scale includes 17 items. A score of five points is allocated for the presence of dysmenorrhoea, and scores of 0.5, one, or two are allocated for additional symptoms and for the duration of pain. The lowest possible score is five points while the upper score (excluding points for additional days of pain) is 18 points.

Finally, studies that reported the number of people with pain were also included.

Recurrence

Recurrence of endometriosis is common. Assessment of recurrence can be based on several features; for example, recurrence of dysmenorrhoea, pelvic pain, mass, or cyst. Recurrence may be diagnosed based on clinical examination, biomarkers such as the cancer antigen 125, imaging, or laparoscopy. Details relating to the criteria for recurrence were extracted from studies that reported this information. Results were analysed for studies that reported women who underwent surgery prior to receiving the intervention, and for those that reported the number of women who achieved a cure at the end of treatment.

Uterine and Cyst Volume

The uterine and cyst volume were included when calculated using formulas for an ellipsoid (volume = $4/3\pi abc$ when using the radius or volume = 1/6πabc when using the diameter) or when calculated through ultrasound measurement. Volume is typically reported in either cubic centimetres (cm³) or millimetres (mm³). Data were excluded for studies that did not describe the method used to calculate uterine or cyst volume.

Menstrual Volume

Menstrual volume can be measured in several ways. The number of sanitary napkins used can be recorded for each menstrual period. Volume can be calculated by measuring the weight of each sanitary napkin, assuming that one gram is equivalent to one millilitre. Other approaches to measure menstrual volume were also included, such as the pictorial blood loss assessment chart (PBAC), which provides visual guides for assessing menstrual volume.

Pregnancy Outcomes

Pregnancy outcomes were extracted for studies that described the number of women with endometriosis-related infertility, regardless of whether pregnancy was conceived naturally or with assisted reproductive technologies. Outcomes included the pregnancy rate (number of pregnancies), live birth rate (number of live births), and miscarriage rate (number of miscarriages). Data were extracted where pregnancy was confirmed by presence of gestational sac with or without foetal heartbeat. Data for biochemical pregnancy were not extracted.

Health-related Quality of Life

Disease-specific health-related quality of life scales were included, as were generic wellbeing scales. The Endometriosis Health Profile questionnaire (EHP-30)[6] includes 53 items; 30 core items are grouped into five scales and 23 additional items are included in six supplementary modules. The core scales are for pain, control and powerlessness, emotional wellbeing, social support, and self-image.

Supplementary modules include work, sexual relationship, relationship with child/children, feelings about infertility, feelings about treatment, and feelings about the medical profession. Supplementary modules may not be applicable to every woman. Each item is scored from zero to four, and the raw scores are transformed to provide a score between zero and 100, where a lower score indicates less impact on health-related quality of life. A short version of the questionnaire (EHP-5) includes 11 items, one core item for each of the five scales, and one question for each of the supplementary modules.[7]

The abbreviated version of the World Health Organization Quality of Life Instruments (WHOQOL-BREF) is a generic quality of life scale.[8] The WHOQOL-BREF includes 26 items; 24 items are grouped into four domains (physical health, psychological health, social relationships, and environment), one question assesses the individual's overall perception of their quality of life and the final question assesses their overall perception of their health. Each item is rated on a five-point scale. Domain scores are calculated as the mean score of items within each domain. The raw scores can be transformed to provide a score from four to 24 that is comparable with the longer version (WHOQOL-100), and a second transformation converts the domain score to a scale from zero to 100.

The Medical Outcome Study 36-Item Short-Form Health Survey (SF-36) contains 36 items on eight domains: physical functioning, role functioning due to health problems, role functioning due to emotional problems, bodily pain, general health perceptions, vitality, social function, and mental health.[9] The scores are weighted for each domain and transformed into a score that ranges from zero to 100. Higher scores indicate better outcomes.

The Nottingham Health Profile (NHP) is a generic quality of life scale that evaluates perceived physical mobility, pain, sleep, emotional reactions, social isolation, and energy.[10] The scale is divided into two parts. The first part includes 38 questions relating to the six sections. The second part includes seven questions about the life areas affected; for example, work, home life, and vacations. Responses to all questions are either yes or no, and responses are

Methods for Evaluating Clinical Evidence

weighted to provide a score between zero and one for each domain. Higher scores indicate greater perceived dysfunction.

Other Outcomes

Patients who use GnRHa can experience menopause-like symptoms and decreased bone density due to lower levels of oestrogen. The severity of these symptoms can be reduced when GnRHa is combined with low dose oestrogens, tibolone (a synthetic steroid), or low dose progestin ('add-back therapy'). Two outcome measures were included that assessed these side effects of GnRHa: the Kupperman Index (KI) and bone density.

The original KI (also known as the Kupperman Menopause Index and the Blatt-Kuperman Menopausal Index) assesses the severity of 11 common symptoms associated with menopause: vasomotor symptoms, paraesthesia, insomnia, nervousness, melancholia, vertigo, weakness/fatigue, arthralgia and myalgia, headaches, palpitation, and formication (a type of paraesthesia or a tactile hallucination where a physical sensation is felt where there is no physical cause).[11] Each item is scored from zero (no symptoms) to three (severe symptoms). The severity is multiplied by a conversion factor, and the total score is the sum of individual scores. The Chinese version of the KI typically includes two extra items related to dyspareunia and urinary tract infections.

Bone density decreases during GnRHa treatment, but usually recovers within 18–24 months. Bone mineral density can be measured using a central dual-energy X-ray absorptiometry (DXA). This test is typically used to assess bone mineral density in the hip and lumbar vertebra. Results are usually reported as standard deviations (SD) from the normal result for a healthy young adult. A result between −1 and 1 SD indicates a normal result. A result between 1 and 2.5 SD lower than the healthy young adult norm is considered as having low bone mass, a result of 2.5 SD lower than the healthy young adult norm indicates osteoroposis, and a result of more than 2.5 SD lower than the healthy young adult norm indicates severe osteoporosis.[13]

Evaluating the safety of CHM is important to inform patient choice. For controlled studies, the nature and type of adverse events were extracted when adverse events were reported for each group.

Risk of Bias Assessment

Risk of bias was assessed for RCTs using the Cochrane Collaboration's tool.[1] In clinical trials, bias can be categorised as selection bias, performance bias, detection bias, attrition bias, and reporting bias. Each domain is assessed to determine whether the bias poses low, high, or unclear risk. Low risk of bias indicates that bias is unlikely, high risk indicates plausible bias that seriously weakens confidence in the results, and unclear bias indicates lack of information or uncertainty over potential bias and raises some doubt about the results. Risk of bias assessment was verified by two researchers and disagreement was resolved by discussion or consultation with a third person.

Risk of bias is categorised using the following six domains:

- Sequence generation: the method used to generate the allocation sequence is given in sufficient detail to allow an assessment of whether it should produce comparable groups. Low risk of bias refers to a random number table or computerised random generator. High risk of bias includes studies that describe a non-random sequence generation such as odd or even date of birth or date of admission.
- Allocation concealment: the method used to conceal the allocation sequence is given in enough detail to determine whether intervention allocations could have been foreseen before or during enrolment. Low risk of bias includes central randomisation or sealed envelopes while high risk of bias includes open random sequence etc.
- Blinding of participants and personnel: the measures used to describe if the study participants and personnel are blind to the intervention received. In addition, information relating to whether the blinding was effective is also assessed. Studies that

ensure blinding of participants and personnel are at low risk of bias. If the study is not blind or incompletely blind, it is at high risk of bias.
- Blinding of outcome assessors: the measures used to describe if the outcome assessors are blind to knowledge of which intervention a participant received. In addition, information relating to whether the blinding was effective is also assessed. Studies that ensure blinding of outcome assessors are at low risk of bias. If the study is not blind or incompletely blind, it is at high risk of bias.
- Incomplete outcome data: completeness of outcome data for each main outcome, including dropouts, exclusions from the analysis with numbers missing in each group, and reasons for dropping out or exclusions. Studies with low risk of bias would include all outcome data, or if there is missing data, it is unlikely to relate to the true outcome or is balanced between groups. Studies at high risk of bias would have unexplained missing data.
- Selective reporting: the study protocol is available and the pre-specified outcomes are included in the report. Studies with a published protocol and that include all pre-specified outcomes in their report would be at low risk of bias. Studies at high risk of bias would not include all pre-specified outcomes or the outcome data may be reported incompletely.

Statistical Analyses

Studies that included people with adenomyosis or endometriosis outside the pelvic cavity were reported separately from those that included women with endometriosis in the pelvic cavity. Descriptive statistics were used to summarise the frequency of CM syndromes, CHM formulas, herbs, and acupuncture reported in included studies. Chinese medicine syndromes reported in two or more studies were presented. The 10 most frequently reported CHM formulas and 20 most frequently reported herbs are presented when used in at least two studies. The top 10 acupuncture points used in two or more studies are presented, or as available. Where data were limited, reports of single CM syndromes or acupuncture points were provided as a guide for the reader.

Definitions of statistical tests and results are described in the glossary. Dichotomous data are reported as a risk ratio (RR) with 95% confidence intervals (CI), and continuous data are reported as a mean difference (MD) or standardised mean difference (SMD) with 95% CI. For dichotomous data, when the RR is greater than one and the upper and lower values of the 95% CI are both greater than one, this indicates that we can be 95% certain that there is a difference between groups and that the true effect lies within these CIs. The same is true for values less than one. In such cases, we can say that there is a 'significant difference' between the groups. For continuous data, when the MD is greater than zero and both the upper and lower values of the 95% CI are greater than zero, we can say that there is a 'significant difference' between the groups. The same is true on the negative side of the scale.[1] For all analyses, RR or MD and 95% CI were reported, together with a formal test for heterogeneity using the I^2 statistic. An I^2 score greater than 50% was considered to indicate substantial heterogeneity.[1]

Sensitivity analyses were undertaken to explore potential sources of heterogeneity. This included studies judged as posing low risk of bias for the risk of bias domain 'sequence generation'. Planned subgroup analyses included participant age (adolescents, adults, both adolescents and adults), diagnosis (laparoscopy), CM formulas, duration of treatment, and comparator type. Available cases analysis with a random effects model was used in all analyses. The random effects model was used to account for possible clinical heterogeneity within and between included studies, as well as the variation in treatment effects between included studies.

Assessment Using Grading of Recommendations Assessment, Development and Evaluation

The Grading of Recommendations Assessment, Development, and Evaluation (GRADE) approach was used.[14,15] The GRADE approach summarises and rates the strength and quality ('certainty') of evidence in systematic reviews using a structured process for the presentation of evidence summaries. The results are presented in summary of findings tables and provide an important overview for endometriosis outcomes.

A panel of experts was established to evaluate the certainty of evidence. The panel included the systematic review team, CM practitioners, integrative medicine experts, research methodologists, and conventional medicine physicians. The experts were asked to rate the clinical importance of key interventions from CHM and acupuncture therapies, as well as comparators and outcomes. Results were collated and, based on the rating scores and subsequent discussion, a consensus on the content for the summary of findings tables was achieved.

The quality of evidence for each outcome was rated according to five factors outlined in the GRADE approach. The certainty of evidence may be rated based on:

- Limitations in study design (risk of bias);
- Inconsistency of results (unexplained heterogeneity);
- Indirectness of evidence (interventions, populations, and outcomes important to the patients with the condition);
- Imprecision (uncertainty about the results);
- Publication bias (selective publication of studies).

These five factors are additive, and a reduction in one factor or more will reduce the certainty of the evidence for that outcome. The GRADE approach also includes methods for assessing observational studies. In this monograph, GRADE summaries only include RCTs.

Treatment recommendations can also be assessed using the GRADE approach, but due to the diverse nature of CM practice, treatment recommendations were not included with the summary of findings. Therefore, the reader should interpret the evidence with reference to the local practice environment. It should also be noted that the GRADE approach requires judgements about the strength and quality of evidence and some subjective assessment. However, the experience of the panel members suggests that the judgements are reliable and transparent representations of the certainty of evidence. The GRADE levels of evidence are grouped into four categories:

1) High certainty evidence: We are very confident that the true effect lies close to that of the estimate of the effect.
2) Moderate certainty evidence: We are moderately confident in the effect estimate — the true effect is likely to be close to the estimate of the effect, but there is also a possibility that it is substantially different.
3) Low certainty evidence: Our confidence in the effect estimate is limited — the true effect may be substantially different from the estimate of the effect.
4) Very low certainty evidence: We have very little confidence in the effect estimate — the true effect is likely to be substantially different from the estimate of the effect.

References

1. Higgins JPT, Green S, eds. Cochrane Handbook for Systematic Reviews of Interventions Version 5.1.0 [updated March 2011]. The Cochrane Collaboration. Available from www.cochrane-handbook.org2011.
2. Dunselman GA, Vermeulen N, Becker C, *et al.* (2014) ESHRE guideline: Management of women with endometriosis. *Hum Reprod* **29**(3): 400–412.
3. Cox DJ, Meyer RG. (1978) Behavioral treatment parameters with primary dysmenorrhea. *J Behav Med* **1**(3): 297–310.
4. Von Korff M, Dworkin SF, Le Resche L. (1990) Graded chronic pain status: An epidemiologic evaluation. *Pain* **40**(3): 279–291.
5. 郑筱萸. (1993) 中药新药临床指导原则. 北京: 中国医药科技出版社.
6. Jones G, Kennedy S, Barnard A, *et al.* (2001) Development of an endometriosis quality-of-life instrument: The Endometriosis Health Profile-30. *Obstet Gynecol* **98**(2): 258–264.
7. Jones G, Jenkinson C, Kennedy S. (2004) Development of the Short Form Endometriosis Health Profile Questionnaire: The EHP-5. *Qual Life Res* **13**(3): 695–704.

8. World Health Organization. Division of Mental Health. (1996) WHOQOL-BREF: Introduction, administration, scoring and generic version of the assessment: Field trial version. World Health Organization. https://apps.who.int/iris/handle/10665/63529.
9. Ware JJ, Sherbourne C. (1992) The MOS 36-item Short-form Health Survey (SF-36). I. Conceptual framework and item selection. *Med Care* **30:** 473–483.
10. Hunt SM, McEwen J. (1980) The development of a subjective health indicator. *Sociol Health Illn* **2**(3): 231–246.
11. Kupperman HS, Wetchler BB, Blatt MH. (1959) Contemporary therapy of the menopausal syndrome. *J Am Med Assoc* **171:** 1627–1637.
12. Duffy J, Hirsch M, Vercoe M, *et al.* (2020) A core outcome set for future endometriosis research: An international consensus development study. *BJOG* **127**(8): 967–974.
13. National Institue of Health Osteoporosis and Related Bone Diseases National Resouce Centre. (2018) Bone mass measure: What the numbers mean. National Institue of Health Osteoporosis and Related Bone Diseases National Resouce Centre, [updated October 2018; cited 2019 13th October]. Available from: https://www.bones.nih.gov/health-info/bone/bone-health/bone-mass-measure.
14. Schunemann H, Brozek J, Guyatt G, Oxman, A, eds. (2013) *GRADE Handbook for Grading Quality of Evidence and Strength of Recommendations.* The GRADE Working Group (ed.). Available from: http://www.guidelinedevelopment.org/handbook.
15. Schünemann H, Higgins J, Vist G, *et al.*, eds. Chapter 14: Completing 'Summary of findings' tables and grading the certainty of the evidence. In: Higgins JPT, Thomas J, Chandler J, Cumpston M, Li T, Page MJ, Welch VA, eds. (2019) Cochrane Handbook for Systematic Reviews of Interventions version 6.0 (updated July 2019). Available from: http://www.training.cochrane.org/handbook.

5
Clinical Evidence for Chinese Herbal Medicine

OVERVIEW

Chinese herbal medicines have been tested in clinical studies and results have been published in scientific journals. A selection of 434 such studies that met the inclusion criteria was subject to systematic review and meta-analysis. This chapter presents an overview of the Chinese medicine syndromes described in studies, the herbal medicines investigated, and the efficacy and safety of these products for women with endometriosis and adenomyosis.

Introduction

Chinese herbal medicine (CHM) is used for many gynaecological disorders, including endometriosis and adenomyosis. The formulas described in contemporary clinical textbooks and guidelines in Chapter 2 can be considered according to each woman's Chinese medicine (CM) syndrome differentiation. The classical literature (Chapter 3) provides insight into the treatments that were used for endometriosis-like symptoms in past eras. Clinical studies, including randomised controlled trials (RCTs), controlled clinical trials (CCTs), and non-controlled studies, provide evidence of the effects of such interventions.

Chapter Structure

This chapter reviews the evidence from clinical studies of CHM for women with endometriosis and adenomyosis. Studies have been grouped according to the primary diagnosis of study participants and according to subtypes of studies, such as those that focused on the role of CHM in alleviating side effects of hormone therapy (HT). The findings from reviews are presented in five parts:

- Part 1: Endometriosis.
- Part 2: Adenomyosis.
- Part 3: Endometriosis and adenomyosis.
- Part 4: Side effects of gonadotropin-releasing hormone agonists (GnRHa).
- Part 5: Endometriosis outside the pelvic cavity.

Within parts 1–5, results are presented according to the route of administration: oral CHM, topical CHM, and both oral and topical CHM. Studies are indicated by the letter 'H' followed by a number, and the references for studies can be found at the end of the chapter.

Previous Systematic Reviews

The literature search identified 27 published systematic reviews (SRs) of CHM for endometriosis[1-25] and adenomyosis.[26,27] Three were published in English,[1-3] and the remainder were published in Chinese. Many SRs have evaluated the potential role of CHM for women with endometriosis or adenomyosis, with some showing that CHM may be beneficial for women with endometriosis. However, many review authors have noted that the quality of the literature was generally low, so confidence in the results is limited. Systematic reviews of CHM for endometriosis and adenomyosis, and SRs of specific formulas, are summarised below.

Systematic Reviews of Chinese Herbal Medicine for Endometriosis

One Cochrane SR by Flower *et al.* (2012) examined the role of CHM in alleviating endometriosis-related pain and infertility.[1] Analysis of results from each of the two studies included in the Cochrane SR showed that the effects of CHM were comparable to gestrinone for symptom severity after surgery and the total pregnancy rate. Chinese herbal medicine administered orally and as an enema resulted in a greater reduction in dysmenorrhoea scores than the conventional medicine danazol.

Among the Chinese SRs, three included studies of women with endometriosis-related infertility,[9,17,18] two assessed the efficacy of CHM for endometrioma,[8,19] and one examined the effect of CHM on endometriosis-related pain.[12] Ten SRs focused on women post-surgery,[5,8,10,11,15–18,21,24] nine SRs included studies of women who had not undergone surgery,[6,9,12–14,20,22,26,27] and five SRs included studies of all women, regardless of previous surgery.[4,7,19,23,25] Systematic reviews evaluated CHM used alone[5–7,9–18,21,22,25] or in combination with pharmacotherapy,[20,24,26,27] while others included both studies of CHM alone and as integrative medicine with conventional medicine.

Six SRs evaluated the effect of CHM alone in post-operative women.[5,8,10,11,19,21] Three SRs found a higher pregnancy rate among women who received CHM,[5,11,19] while one study showed a negative result compared with pharmacotherapy.[8] One SR found a higher effective rate with CHM than with pharmacotherapy.[8] Three SRs compared CHM with no treatment in post-operative women[5,8,19]; all three found CHM to be more effective in increasing the pregnancy rate and reducing the recurrence rate than no treatment. Two SRs showed that women who received CHM had a higher effective rate.[8,19] Xiao et al. (2016)[21] focused on quality of life in post-operative women; results from the seven included RCTs and case-control studies showed improved quality of life, measured using the World Health Organization Quality of Life Instruments (WHOQOL-BREF), with CHM compared to HT.

Three SRs found the combination of CHM and pharmacotherapy to be more effective than pharmacotherapy alone in increasing the effective rate and reducing recurrence rate in post-operative women.[8,19,24] Only one SR examined the role of CHM in relation to fertility and found the pregnancy rate to be higher when CHM and pharmacotherapy were used together.[24]

Five SRs focused on endometriosis in women who had not undergone surgery.[9,13,14,19,22] Two SRs found that CHM improved the effective rate compared with pharmacotherapy,[14,19] while a third showed CHM to be more effective than gestrinone and danazol, but equally as effective as mifepristone/Nemestran®.[22] Four SRs evaluated the effect of CHM on dysmenorrhoea in women with endometriosis[13,14,19,22]; two showed that CHM could reduce dysmenorrhoea compared with pharmacotherapy,[14,22] while the other two found no significant difference between CHM and pharmacotherapy.[13,19] Results were mixed in SRs that examined outcomes relating to ovarian cysts,[14,19,22] recurrence rate,[14,19,22] and pregnancy rate;[9,19,22] some studies suggested that CHM led to improved outcomes while others showed a similar result to pharmacotherapy.

One network meta-analysis focused on recurrence of endometriosis after surgery.[15] The result showed that formulas designed to nourish the Kidneys and remove stasis, promote Blood and remove stasis, and regulate *qi* and promote Blood could reduce the recurrence rate after surgery compared with no treatment.

Fifteen SRs reported the safety of CHM. Generally, there were fewer side effects in the CHM groups than in the pharmacotherapy groups[19,20] and fewer cases of abnormal liver function.[6,7] The nature of side effects differed between CHM and pharmacotherapy — the most frequent side effects of CHM were gastrointestinal symptoms and allergies,[11-14,18,22,25] while the side effects of pharmacotherapy were specific to the biological actions of the drugs and were generally known side effects.

Systematic Reviews of Chinese Herbal Medicine Formulas for Endometriosis

Several SRs evaluated the efficacy and safety of specific formulas. Two English language SRs reviewed the evidence for CHM formulas: *Bu shen huo xue* 补肾活血 prescriptions[3] and *Dan e fu kang jian gao* 丹莪妇康煎膏.[2] In a review of 13 RCTs, *Bu shen huo xue* 补肾活血 prescriptions were more effective than conventional medicine in improving the total effective rate (a global assessment of symptom severity) and pregnancy rate, but was not different from conventional medicine in reducing the number of women with dysmenorrhoea at the end of treatment.[3] Li et al. (2017)[2] included 39 RCTs that compared *Dan e fu kang jian gao* 丹莪妇康煎膏 with HT. The authors found that *Dan e fu kang jian gao* 丹莪妇康煎膏 had a higher effective rate than gestrinone, but was comparable with danazol, mifepristone, Marvelon®, and levonorgestrel-releasing intrauterine systems (LNG-IUS). The rate of recurrence was lower with *Dan e fu kang jian gao* 丹莪妇康煎膏 than gestrinone, but similar to that of mifepristone. Levels of cancer antigen 125 (CA125) were also lower among women who received *Dan e fu kang jian gao* 丹莪妇康煎膏, and fewer women who received *Dan e fu kang jian gao* 丹莪妇康煎膏 reported adverse events.

Two meta-analyses compared the effectiveness of a commercially manufactured product, *San jie zhen tong jiao nang* 散结镇痛胶囊, with HT. Results from one SR of nine RCTs that included women with endometriosis who did not undergo surgery[6] showed that CHM had a higher effective rate and pregnancy rate compared with HT, but CHM was not superior to HT in improving dyspareunia. The second SR included 13 studies: five studies included women with previous surgery while eight included women without previous surgery.[7] *San jie zhen tong jiao nang* 散结镇痛胶囊 was superior to HT in increasing the effective rate and pregnancy rate in women without previous surgery, but was not statistically different from HT in terms of the effective rate and pregnancy outcomes in women with previous laparoscopic surgery. Abnormal liver function was less frequent in women who received *San jie zhen tong jiao nang* 散结镇痛胶囊, regardless of previous surgical history.

Two reviews evaluated the effectiveness and safety of *Gui zhi fu ling jiao nang* 桂枝茯苓胶囊.[20,23] Lian et al. (2016)[20] reviewed 11 RCTs and documented the effectiveness and safety of *Gui zhi fu ling jiao nang* 桂枝茯苓胶囊 as integrative medicine compared with mifepristone alone. The effective rate and pregnancy rate with *Gui zhi fu ling jiao nang* 桂枝茯苓胶囊 were higher than in the control group, the recurrence rate was lower, and there were fewer side effects. This SR also evaluated hormone levels; the levels of oestrogen and progestin were lower in the treatment group than in the control group, while the levels of follicle-stimulating hormone and luteinising hormone were similar in both groups. Han *et al.* (2016)[23] included nine RCTs and reached conclusions similar to those of Lian *et al.* (2016).[20] Analysis of four of the nine included RCTs showed a higher effective rate for women who received *Gui zhi fu ling jiao nang* 桂枝茯苓胶囊 plus mifepristone compared with mifepristone only. The effective rate was not statistically different between *Gui zhi fu ling jiao nang* 桂枝茯苓胶囊 and HT.

A SR by He *et al.* (2012)[4] evaluated *Dan leng fu kang jian gao* 丹棱妇康煎膏 for endometriosis. Twenty-one studies were included and meta-analysis showed that *Dan leng fu kang jian gao* 丹棱妇康煎膏 had a similar effective rate, pregnancy rate, and recurrence rate to no treatment and to HT. Wang *et al.* (2016)[17] reviewed three articles that evaluated the effect of *Luo shi nei yi fang* 罗氏内异方 in improving pregnancy outcomes for post-operative women and found that *Luo shi nei yi fang* 罗氏内异方 after laparoscopy could improve the pregnancy rate and reduce the miscarriage rate compared to waitlist control groups. Another SR of four studies[16] that evaluated the formula *Dan zhu xiao yi fang* 丹术消异方 showed similar pregnancy and miscarriage results to Wang *et al.* (2016),[17] but a lower rate of recurrence than waitlist controls.

Three SRs assessed the effectiveness of herbs with actions to promote Blood circulation and remove stasis, while Huang *et al.* (2012)[25] reviewed 16 studies of herbs to nourish the Kidneys and remove stasis. The results showed that CHM was more effective than HT in increasing the pregnancy rate, but was equally effective in reducing dysmenorrhoea. Zhang (2010)[12] found similar results for pregnancy outcomes when CHM was compared with HT. In addition, Zhang (2010) found CHM to be more effective than HT in reducing dysmenorrhoea, pelvic pain, and anal pain, improving the effective rate, and reducing the chance of recurrence, but was similar to HT in reducing dyspareunia, cyst size, nodule tenderness, and hormone levels.

Wang *et al.* (2017)[18] reviewed 18 studies and found that CHM plus laparoscopy could improve the pregnancy rate when compared with laparoscopy alone. Further, the authors found that fewer women who received CHM plus laparoscopy had a miscarriage, and fewer cases of endometriosis recurrence were reported.

Systematic Reviews of Chinese Herbal Medicine for Adenomyosis

Two SRs evaluated the effectiveness and safety of CHM for adenomyosis. Feng et al. (2016)[26] reviewed 14 studies that compared the combination of CHM plus pharmacotherapy to pharmacotherapy alone and concluded that the combination was more effective than pharmacotherapy alone, but the SR did not describe the results for selected outcomes. The second SR assessed the effect of combining *San jie zhen tong jiao nang* 散结镇痛胶囊 with LNG-IUS against LNG-IUS alone.[27] Among the six included studies, the effective rate was higher in the combination group, there was a greater reduction in adenomyoma and dysmenorrhoea, the endometrium was thinner, and CA125 was lower compared with LNG-IUS alone.

Identification of Clinical Studies

Search of English and Chinese language databases identified 37,518 potentially relevant studies. Search results were exported to reference management software for further assessment. Many of these citations were duplicates, which were removed prior to screening the title and abstract of each citation (Figure 5.1). In total, 23,997 citations were reviewed, of which 20,989 were excluded after reviewing the titles and abstracts. The full-text article was retrieved for more than 3,000 citations and 436 studies met the inclusion criteria. Two articles described treatment approaches that are not commonly used outside China and were not included in the review. The CHM treatments used and treatment effects are presented for the 434 included studies. Among these, 279 studies were RCTs, 44 were CCTs, and 111 were non-controlled studies.

Part 1. Endometriosis

Among the 434 included studies, 305 studies focused on women with endometriosis. Oral CHM was the main form of treatment investigated (268 studies), with other studies testing topical CHM (15 studies) and the

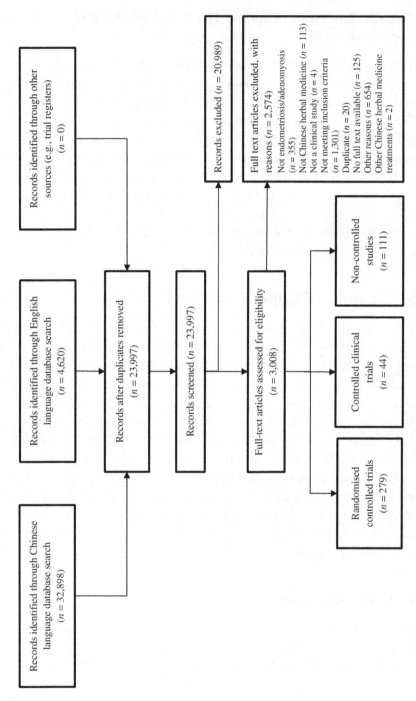

Figure 5.1. Flowchart of study selection process: Chinese herbal medicine.

combination of oral plus topical CHM (22 studies). Analyses of these studies are presented according to the route of administration and grouped by study type, for example, RCTs, CCTs and non-controlled studies.

Oral Chinese Herbal Medicine for Endometriosis

Oral CHM was tested in 175 RCTs (H1–H175), 27 CCTs (H176–H202) and 53 non-controlled studies (H203–H255). The findings from the evaluation of these studies are presented.

Randomised Controlled Trials of Oral Chinese Herbal Medicine for Endometriosis

In total, 16,106 women with endometriosis participated in the 175 RCTs of oral CHM (H1–H175). All studies were conducted in China except for one, which was conducted in the United Kingdom (H1). Twenty-six studies included three groups (H1–H26); these studies either included two treatment groups (CHM alone and as integrative medicine with pharmacotherapy) or two control groups (typically one group that received no treatment and another that received pharmacotherapy). One RCT included four arms (H27); the results for the groups that received acupuncture therapy or combined CM therapies are presented in Chapter 7 and Chapter 9, respectively.

One study included both women and adolescents (H28), while all other RCTs included adult women. Women were recruited from a range of settings, including hospital inpatient and outpatient departments and community clinics. More than half of all included studies (101 of 175 RCTs, 57.7%) reported that women received surgery prior to the study, and 26 focused on women with endometriosis-related infertility (H15, H18, H21, H26, H29–H50).

Over half of all included studies confirmed endometriosis via laparoscopy (98 RCTs, 56%); diagnosis in other studies was either based on other criteria, such as signs and symptoms (71 RCTs, 40.6%), or was not reported (six RCTs, 3.4%). Eighty-four studies (48%) reported the revised American Society for Reproductive Medicine (rASRM) stage: 10 RCTs included women with stage I or II endometriosis, 3 RCTs included women with stage II or III endometriosis, 28 RCTs included women with stage III or IV endometriosis, 13 RCTs included women with stage II–IV endometriosis, 29 RCTs included women with any of the four stages, and one RCT included only women with stage III endometriosis. The duration of endometriosis ranged from as little as two months (H51) to as many as 22 years (H28), and some studies reported a mean duration of close to 10 years (H52, H53).

Eighty RCTs described using CM syndrome differentiation as an inclusion criterion or to guide treatment, with many RCTs describing multiple syndromes. The most frequently documented syndromes were Kidney deficiency with Blood stasis (24 studies; H3, H4, H27, H31, H34, H44, H50, H53–H69) and *qi* stagnation and Blood stasis (23 studies; H7, H17, H38, H46, H54, H68, H70–H86). Other CM syndromes found three or more times among included studies were cold coagulation and Blood stasis (12 studies; H6, H42, H54, H68, H74, H81, H82, H87–H91), *qi* deficiency and Blood stasis (eight studies; H5, H20, H27, H54, H81, H82, H92, H93), damp-heat stasis (four studies; H94–H97), Liver *qi* stagnation (four studies; H5, H48, H98, H99), damp-heat (three studies; H13, H98, H100), and phlegm-dampness (three studies; H5, H48, H101).

One hundred and twelve RCTs tested oral CHM alone, while 63 RCTs tested the combination of oral CHM with pharmacotherapy. Treatment with oral CHM ranged from one month (H21) to 56 menstrual cycles (H37). Most studies provided treatment for three (100 RCTs) or six months (52 RCTs). Follow-up assessment was reported in 110 RCTs (62.8%); women were followed for between one month (H13) and three years (H100, H102, H103). Twenty-eight RCTs reported loss to follow-up.

Many studies used CHM formulas developed by investigators or unspecified treatments that were tailored according to the time of the menstrual cycle. These studies were excluded from formula frequency analysis. Several formulas were used in multiple studies. One hundred and eight different formulas or combinations of formulas were reported in the 175 RCTs, and the most commonly tested oral formula was *San jie zhen tong jiao nang/tang* 散结镇痛胶囊/汤 (Table 5.1). The low number of formulas used in multiple studies,

Table 5.1. Frequently Reported Oral Formulas in Randomised Controlled Trials

Most Common Formulas	No. of Uses	Ingredients
San jie zhen tong jiao nang/tang 散结镇痛胶囊/汤*	10	*Long xue jie* 龙血竭, *san qi* 三七, *yi yi ren* 薏苡仁, *zhe bei mu* 浙贝母
Dan leng fu kang jian gao 丹棱妇康煎膏	9	Variant 1: *dan shen* 丹参, *e zhu* 莪术, *san leng* 三棱, *chai hu* 柴胡, *dang gui* 当归, *chi shao* 赤芍, *xiang fu* 香附, *xuan hu suo* 玄胡索, *gan cao* 甘草 (H150, H151, H175); plus *san qi* 三七 and *zhu ye* 竹叶 (H71, H112, H114, H115) Variant 2: *dan shen* 丹参, *e zhu* 莪术, *san leng* 三棱, *chai hu* 柴胡, *dang gui* 当归, *chi shao* 赤芍, *xiang fu* 香附, *yan hu suo* 延胡索, *gan cao* 甘草, *san qi* 三七 (H152) Variant 3: *zi dan shen* 紫丹参, *e zhu* 莪术, *san qi* 三七, *dang gui* 当归, *zhu ye* 竹叶, *chai hu* 柴胡, and 10 other herbs (H113)
Xue fu zhu yu jiao nang/tang 血府逐瘀胶囊/汤	7	*Dang gui* 当归, *sheng di huang* 生地黄, *tao ren* 桃仁, *hong hua* 红花, *zhi he* 枳壳, *chi shao* 赤芍, *chai hu* 柴胡, *gan cao* 甘草, *jie geng* 桔梗, *chuan xiong* 川芎, *niu xi* 牛膝
Wen jing tang 温经汤	5	Variant 1: *dang gui* 当归, *chuan xiong* 川芎, *shao yao* 芍药, *rou gui* 肉桂, *mu dan pi* 牡丹皮, *e zhu* 莪术, *ren shen* 人参, *gan cao* 甘草, *niu xi* 牛膝 Variant 2: *ren shen* 人参, *bai zhu* 白术, *dang gui* 当归, *bai shao* 白芍, *chuan xiong* 川芎, *shu di huang* 熟地黄, *sha ren* 砂仁, *xiao hui xiang* 小茴香, *fu ling* 茯苓, *gan cao* 甘草, *xiang fu* 香附, *chen pi* 陈皮, *chen xiang* 沉香, *wu zhu yu* 吴茱萸, *xuan hu suo* 玄胡索, *lu rong* 鹿茸

(Continued)

Table 5.1. (Continued)

Most Common Formulas	No. of Uses	Ingredients
Yi qi hua yu fang 益气化瘀方	5	Variant 1: *huang qi* 黄芪, *dang shen* 党参, *chuan xiong* 川芎, *dang gui* 当归, *zhe bei* 浙贝, *yi yi ren* 薏苡仁, *yan hu suo* 延胡索, *tu si zi* 菟丝子, *gui zhi* 桂枝, etc 等 (H136, H173) Variant 2: *huang qi* 黄芪, *dang shen* 党参, *bai zhu* 白术, *shan yao* 山药, *san leng* 三棱, *e zhu* 莪术, *ji nei jin* 鸡内金, *dan shen* 丹参, *dang gui* 当归, *tao ren* 桃仁, *hong hua* 红花, *yan hu suo* 延胡索, *xiang fu* 香附, *jiu gan cao* 灸甘草 (H19) Variant 3: *huang qi* 黄芪, *dang shen* 党参, *bai zhu* 白术, *chai hu* 柴胡, *bai shao* 白芍, *dang gui* 当归, *dan shen* 丹参, *yan hu* 延胡, *wu ling zhi* 五灵脂, *sheng pu huang* 生蒲黄, *liu ji nu* 刘寄奴 (H135) Variant 4: *san leng* 三棱, *e zhu* 莪术, *ru xiang* 乳香, *mo yao* 没药, *huang qi* 黄芪, *dang gui* 当归, *bai zhu* 白术, *fu ling* 茯苓 (H86)
Gui zhi fu ling jiao nang/wan 桂枝茯苓胶囊/丸	4	*Gui zhi* 桂枝, *fu ling* 茯苓, *mu dan pi* 牡丹皮, *tao ren* 桃仁, *shao yao* 芍药 (H14, H68, H92, H108)

Ingredients are referenced to the original studies where possible. If herb ingredients varied across studies, the herb ingredients were sourced from *Zhong Yi Fang Ji Da Ci Dian* 中医方剂大辞典. *Ingredients for *San jie zhen tong jiao nang/tang* 散结镇痛胶囊/汤 were sourced from the *Zhong Hua Ren Min Gong He Guo Yao Dian* 中华人民共和国药典 (*Pharmacopoeia of the People's Republic of China*). Note: the use of some herbs may be restricted in some countries. Readers are advised to comply with relevant regulations.

combined with the high number of formulas tested, highlights the diversity in treatments tested in the clinical studies included.

Diversity was also seen in the herb ingredients of tested formulas. In total, 189 different herb ingredients were reported in the included studies. The most frequently used herbs were *dang gui* 当归, *e zhu* 莪术, *yan hu suo* 延胡索, *dan shen* 丹参, and *chi shao* 赤芍 (Table 5.2).

Table 5.2. Frequently Reported Orally Used Herbs in Randomised Controlled Trials

Most Common Herbs	Scientific Name	Frequency of Use
Dang gui 当归	Angelica sinensis (Oliv.) Diels	108
E zhu 莪术	Curcuma spp.	98
Yan hu suo 延胡索	Corydalis yanhusuo W.T. Wang	84
Dan shen 丹参	Salvia miltiorrhiza Bge.	81
Chi shao 赤芍	Paeonia spp.	74
San leng 三棱	Sparganium stoloniferum Buch. -Ham.	71
Gan cao 甘草	Glycyrrhiza spp.	67
Xiang fu 香附	Cyperus rotundus L.	62
Tao ren 桃仁	Prunus spp.	60
Chuan xiong 川芎	Ligusticum chuanxiong Hort.	55
Huang qi 黄芪	Astragalus membranaceus (Fisch.) Bge.	50
Tu si zi 菟丝子	Cuscuta spp.	50
Wu ling zhi 五灵脂	Trogopterus xanthipes Milne-Edwards	48
Mu dan pi 牡丹皮	Paeonia suffruticosa Andr.	41
Pu huang 蒲黄	Typha spp.	41
Bai shao 白芍	Paeonia spp.	37
Chai hu 柴胡	Bupleurum spp.	37
Dang shen 党参	Codonopsis spp.	37
Hong hua 红花	Carthamus tinctorius L.	36
Shu di huang 熟地黄	Rehmannia glutinosa Libosch.	36

Note: the use of some herbs may be restricted in some countries. Readers are advised to comply with relevant regulations.

These herbs have actions that tonify, nourish, cool, and invigorate Blood, dispel Blood stasis, regulate *qi*, and clear heat.

Risk of bias assessment

All RCTs were described as randomised controlled trials but lacked critical detail on potential sources of bias (Table 5.3). Sixty-two studies

Table 5.3. Risk of Bias Assessment of Randomised Controlled Trials: Oral CHM

Risk of Bias Domain	Low Risk n (%)	Unclear Risk n (%)	High Risk n (%)
Sequence generation	62 (35.4)	96 (54.9)	17 (9.7)
Allocation concealment	4 (2.3)	166 (94.9)	5 (2.9)
Blinding of participants	14 (8.0)	0 (0)	161 (92.0)
Blinding of personnel	11 (6.3)	2 (1.1)	162 (92.8)
Blinding of outcome assessors	11 (6.3)	6 (3.4)	158 (90.3)
Incomplete outcome data	158 (90.3)	16 (9.1)	1 (0.6)
Selective outcome reporting	0 (0)	175 (100)	0 (0)

(35.4%) used appropriate methods to allocate women to groups, such as random number tables or central randomisation. Inappropriate methods, including allocation according to visit order or hospital number, resulted in a judgement of high risk for sequence generation (9.7%). Four RCTs adequately concealed group allocation using central randomisation or sealed, sequentially numbered envelopes.

Most studies did not report the details of allocation concealment. Fourteen studies were judged as having low risk of bias for blinding of participants, mainly through use of a placebo or objective outcome measures. Eleven studies were judged as having low risk of bias for blinding of personnel and outcome assessors, largely for the same reasons. Over 90% of studies were judged as having low risk of bias for incomplete outcome data. For these studies, there was either no missing data, a small amount of missing data, balanced data across groups, or low likelihood that the missing data would influence the outcomes. No trial protocols or trial registrations could be identified for any of the included RCTs, and all were judged as posing unclear risk of bias for selective outcome reporting.

Outcomes

Unsurprisingly, the most frequently documented clinical outcomes were those related to dysmenorrhoea (83 studies; H1, H2, H6, H7,

H13, H15, H17, H20, H28, H29, H36, H39, H42–H45, H54, H55, H57–H62, H64, H66, H69–H71, H73–H75, H77–H80, H83, H86, H87, H89, H90, H93–H97, H101, H109–H144) and recurrence (82 studies; H2, H3, H5, H8–H12, H14, H16, H17, H19, H20, H22–H24, H27, H30, H38, H40, H55–H57, H59, H60, H63, H66, H67, H69, H70, H75, H81, H82, H85, H87, H91, H92, H98, H100–H108, H110, H113, H118–H120, H125, H127, H128, H136, H140, H143, H145–H168).

Other outcomes were those related to pregnancy (34 studies; H12, H15, H18, H21, H25, H26, H29–H42, H44–H50, H90, H92, H105, H124, H160, H169, H170), ovarian cyst size (30 studies; H7, H20, H51–H53, H56, H58, H61, H62, H64, H65, H72, H74, H76, H88, H90, H94, H99, H111, H117, H130–H132, H134, H138, H144, H171–H174), dyspareunia (16 studies; H1, H15, H17, H39, H43, H45, H54, H59, H74, H90, H94, H110, H119, H120, H138, H142), pelvic pain (14 studies; H17, H25, H39, H43, H45, H54, H59, H77, H86, H94, H99, H119, H120, H157), health-related quality of life (14 studies; H4, H17, H27, H68, H69, H82, H84, H94, H95, H112, H126, H133, H142, H175), menopausal symptoms measured with the Kupperman Index (KI)[28] (five studies; H43, H133, H140, H143, H147), uterine volume (four studies; H43, H116, H138, H142), menstrual volume (two studies; H116, H142), fatigue (one study; H128), and bone density (one study; H147).

Ninety-six RCTs documented the safety of oral CHM (H1, H6–H14, H16, H22–H25, H27, H30, H33–H35, H37, H40, H43–H45, H49–H53, H55, H56, H58, H60, H61, H64–H66, H70, H75, H76, H81–H83, H85, H86, H90, H93, H94, H96–H99, H101, H102, H104–H107, H113–H115, H118, H119, H121, H128–H132, H136, H138–H140, H143, H145, H146, H148–H152, H154–H157, H162–H170, H173).

Some studies reported data in a way that did not allow for re-analysis; such data were excluded from further review. The results of analyses are described for each outcome according to the comparison made, for example, oral CHM versus no treatment.

Dysmenorrhoea

Dysmenorrhoea was measured in a variety of ways among included studies, including a 10 cm visual analogue scale (VAS), the scale described in the 1993 *Guidelines for Clinical Research in New Chinese Medicine Drugs* (中药新药临床研究指导原则; 'the 1993 Guideline'),[29] the Chronic Pain Grade Questionnaire (CPGQ),[30] the Cox Menstrual Symptom Scale (CMSS),[31] a verbal rating scale (VRS), and the number of people who reported dysmenorrhoea at the end of treatment. Meta-analyses were conducted where possible, with studies grouped according to the comparison.

Oral Chinese herbal medicine versus no treatment

Four RCTs compared oral CHM with no treatment (H2, H7, H17, H57). Oral CHM reduced the mean dysmenorrhoea VAS score at the end of treatment by 1.35 cm more than no treatment (124 women, [95% confidence intervals −2.54, −0.17], I^2 = 87%; H2, H17). Statistical heterogeneity was detected that could not be explored through planned subgroup analyses. Confidence in this result is low.

One study examined the long-term benefits of *Shao yao zhi tong he ji* 芍药止痛合剂 at a nine-month follow-up. The VAS score at follow-up was 0.37 cm lower with *Shao yao zhi tong he ji* 芍药止痛合剂 than with no treatment (64 women, [−0.65, −0.09]; H17). Despite this being a statistically significant result, the small magnitude of the change is unlikely to be clinically important.

When dysmenorrhoea was assessed using the 1993 Guideline, the mean score at follow-up within three months was not statistically different between women who received oral CHM and those who received no treatment (60 women, mean difference [MD] −0.23 points [−0.76, 0.30]; H57). Finally, results from one study of 50 women showed no difference between groups in the number of women with dysmenorrhoea at the end of treatment (risk ratio [RR] 0.67 [0.41, 1.07]; H7).

Oral Chinese herbal medicine versus placebo

One small RCT of 29 women used a VAS to measure dysmenorrhoea (H6). Treatment with *Chi pu ke li* 赤蒲颗粒 resulted in a mean decrease of 2.37 cm compared to placebo ([–3.40, –1.34]). Another study that assessed dysmenorrhoea using the 1993 Guideline found that women who received *Nei yi xiao jiao nang* 内异消胶囊 scored 3.8 points lower than women who received a placebo (42 women, [–4.83, –2.77]; H61).

Oral Chinese herbal medicine versus pharmacotherapy

Fourteen RCTs that compared oral CHM and pharmacotherapy used the VAS to measure dysmenorrhoea (H2, H28, H42, H54, H75, H80, H87, H89, H97, H122, H126, H129, H131, H143). Women who received oral CHM reported a lower mean VAS score at the end of treatment than women who received pharmacotherapy (1,062 women, MD –0.63 cm [–0.91, –0.36], $I^2 = 71\%$). Considerable statistical heterogeneity was detected, which was examined through planned sensitivity and subgroup analyses. All studies provided treatment for three months or greater, and this was considered unlikely to contribute to heterogeneity. Statistical heterogeneity was greater among studies assessed as having low risk of bias (Table 5.4), which is surprising given that sequence generation is considered one of the key elements for reducing bias in clinical studies. Studies in which women had not received surgery prior to enrolling in the study had much lower heterogeneity, which seems unusual as one would generally expect greater variation among women with endometriosis than those without (i.e., those who had undergone surgery). The reasons for statistical heterogeneity are unclear, so the results should be interpreted accordingly.

One study conducted follow-up assessments three and six months after the end of treatment (H75). Among the 60 participants, women who received *Mu da tang* 木达汤 reported VAS scores similar to women who received gestrinone at three months (MD –0.16 cm [–0.49, 0.17]) and at six months (MD –0.17 cm [–0.66, 0.32]).

Table 5.4. Oral Chinese Herbal Medicine versus Pharmacotherapy for Endometriosis: Dysmenorrhoea Visual Analogue Scale

VAS	No. of Studies (Participants)	Effect Size MD [95% CI], I^2	Included Studies
VAS – EoT	14 (1,062)	–0.63 [–0.91, –0.36]*, 71%	H2, H28, H42, H54, H75, H80, H87, H89, H97, H122, H126, H129, H131, H143
Subgroup: low risk of bias SG	6 (456)	–0.51 [–0.97, –0.06]*, 84%	H2, H54, H75, H97, H126, H143
Subgroup: prior surgery	6 (422)	–0.42 [–0.75, –0.10]*, 65%	H2, H75, H87, H126, H129, H143
Subgroup: no prior surgery	8 (640)	–0.96 [–1.20, –0.71]*, 13%	H28, H42, H54, H80, H89, H97, H122, H131

*Statistically significant, see Statistical Analysis in Chapter 4.
Abbreviations: CI, confidence intervals; EoT, end of treatment; MD, mean difference; SG, sequence generation; VAS, visual analogue scale.

The 1993 Guideline was used to measure dysmenorrhoea in 22 studies. At the end of treatment, women who received oral CHM had a mean score that was 1.59 points lower than women who received pharmacotherapy (1,730 women, MD –1.59 points [–2.32, –0.86], I^2 = 97%; Table 5.5). Substantial statistical heterogeneity highlighted variance among studies in the treatment effect. Heterogeneity was examined through sensitivity analysis with studies judged as having low risk of bias for sequence generation, and subgroup analysis according to surgical history. As these potential sources of bias did not explain the statistical heterogeneity detected, confidence in the results is limited.

Meta-analysis was also possible with studies that conducted follow-up assessments after the end of treatment. When measured with the 1993 Guideline, oral CHM showed benefits in reducing dysmenorrhoea for women followed up at six months (125 women, MD –1.65 points [–2.54, –0.76], I^2 = 20%; Table 5.6) and at one year (272 women, MD –3.22 points [–4.11, –2.32], I^2 = 61%). No such

Table 5.5. Oral Chinese Herbal Medicine versus Pharmacotherapy for Endometriosis: 1993 Guideline at End of Treatment

1993 Guideline	No. of Studies (Participants)	Effect Size MD [95% CI], I^2	Included Studies
1993 Guideline — EoT	20 (1,730)	−1.59 [−2.32, −0.86]*, 97%	H13, H20, H58, H69, H73, H90, H93, H95, H96, H101, H112, H114, H115, H118, H120, H123, H127, H130, H134, H135
Subgroup: low risk of bias SG	6 (811)	−2.20 [−3.36, −1.04]*, 98%	H13, H69, H101, H112, H115, H127
Subgroup: prior surgery	5 (442)	−1.11 [−1.57, −0.64]*, 52%	H69, H101, H118, H120, H127
Subgroup: no prior surgery	15 (1,288)	−1.78 [−2.80, −0.76]*, 97%	H13, H20, H58, H73, H90, H93, H96, H95, H112, H114, H115, H123, H130, H134, H135

*Statistically significant, see Statistical Analysis in Chapter 4.
Abbreviations: CI, confidence intervals; EoT, end of treatment; MD, mean difference; SG, sequence generation.

Table 5.6. Oral Chinese Herbal Medicine versus Pharmacotherapy for Endometriosis: 1993 Guideline at Follow-up Assessment

1993 Guideline	No. of Studies (Participants)	Effect Size MD [95% CI], I^2	Included Studies
Follow-up ≤ 3 m	2 (252)	−2.92 [−10.10, 4.27], 98%	H13, H95
Follow-up at 6 m	2 (125)	−1.65 [−2.54, −0.76]*, 20%	H57, H136
Follow-up at 1 y	2 (272)	−3.22 [−4.11, −2.32]*, 61%	H57, H69
Follow-up at 18 m	1 (212)	−3.30 [−3.89, −2.71]*, NA	H69
Follow-up at 2 y	1 (212)	−2.80 [−3.46, −2.14]*, NA	H69

*Statistically significant, see Statistical Analysis in Chapter 4.
Abbreviations: CI, confidence intervals; m, months; MD, mean difference; NA, not applicable; y, years.

benefit was seen when follow-up assessment occurred within three months. Results from individual studies showed long-term benefit with oral CHM at 18 months and two years (Table 5.6).

Two RCTs used the CPGQ to measure dysmenorrhoea (H15, H116), with both reporting the pain intensity component of the scale. Pain intensity at the end of treatment was not statistically different between women who received oral CHM and those who received HT (110 women, MD −5.19 points [−17.43, 7.05], I^2 = 90%). One RCT involving 60 women (H116) documented the other two components of the CPGQ: disability score and disability points score (a composite measure of disability score and disability days). Women who received *Wu wei san* 五味散 scored lower on both the disability score (MD −12.00 points [−18.41, −5.59]) and the disability points score (MD −0.90 points [−1.58, −0.22]) than women who received mifepristone.

The CMSS was used to measure dysmenorrhoea in one RCT (H117). Results of analysis showed that women who received *Fu fang e zhu san* 复方莪术散 scored 1.17 points lower than women who received gestrinone ([−1.74, −0.60]; H117).

Seven studies reported the number of women with dysmenorrhoea at the end of treatment (H7, H29, H39, H45, H74, H90, H138). Women who received oral CHM were no more or less likely to report dysmenorrhoea at the end of treatment than women who received pharmacotherapy (424 women, RR 0.88 [0.68, 1.15], I^2 = 8%).

Oral Chinese herbal medicine plus pharmacotherapy versus pharmacotherapy

Seventeen studies that tested the combination of oral CHM and pharmacotherapy used a 10 cm VAS to measure dysmenorrhoea. The combined treatment resulted in a mean VAS score of 1.26 points lower at the end of treatment than for pharmacotherapy alone (1,372 women, MD −1.26 [−1.56, −0.95], I^2 = 99%; Table 5.7). Statistical heterogeneity was examined through sensitivity and subgroup analyses and was only reduced in the subgroup of studies with women who had not undergone surgery prior to enrolling in the study. This

Table 5.7. Oral Chinese Herbal Medicine plus Pharmacotherapy versus Pharmacotherapy for Endometriosis: Dysmenorrhoea Visual Analogue Scale

VAS	No. of Studies (Participants)	Effect Size MD [95% CI], I^2	Included Studies
VAS – EoT	17 (1,372)	−1.26 [−1.56, −0.95]*, 99%	H43, H55, H64, H66, H70, H71, H77–H79, H86, H110, H113, H124, H128, H137, H140, H141
Subgroup: low risk of bias SG	9 (786)	−1.08 [−1.39, −0.76]*, 99%	H43, H55, H71, H77–H79, H86, H113, H141
Subgroup: no previous surgery	4 (341)	−1.46 [−1.55, −1.37]*, 0%	H64, H78, H79, H141
Subgroup: previous surgery	13 (1,028)	−1.18 [−1.49, −0.87]*, 99%	H43, H55, H66, H70, H71, H77, H86, H110, H113, H124, H128, H137, H140
Subgroup: stage III or IV	4 (274)	−1.68 [−1.95, −1.41]*, 91%	H79, H110, H128, H140
Subgroup: stage II or III	1 (68)	−0.07 [−0.08, −0.06]*, NA	H43
Subgroup: all stages	2 (183)	−1.95 [−5.68, 1.77], 99%	H55, H71
Subgroup: stage NS	10 (844)	−1.05 [−1.61, −0.49]*, 98%	H64, H66, H70, H77, H78, H86, H113, H124, H137, H141

*Statistically significant, see Statistical Analysis in Chapter 4.
Abbreviations: CI, confidence intervals; EoT, end of treatment; MD, mean difference; NA, not applicable; NS, not specified; SG, sequence generation, VAS, visual analogue scale.

finding seems counter-intuitive; women who had previous surgery to remove endometriosis should, in theory, be a more homogenous group. The reasons for the large variation in the treatment effect among studies remain unclear, which reduces our confidence in the results.

Several studies assessed the long-term effects of oral CHM as integrative medicine with pharmacotherapy. Meta-analysis showed no difference between women who received oral CHM plus pharmacotherapy and those who received pharmacotherapy alone in VAS scores when follow-up was conducted within six months (120 women, MD −0.60 cm [−1.52, 0.32], I² = 74%; H59, H70). However, when follow-up assessment was conducted at one year, women who received oral CHM plus pharmacotherapy scored lower on the VAS than those who received pharmacotherapy alone (170 women, −1.13 cm [−2.19, −0.07], I² = 73%; H59, H128).

One RCT followed up participants until two years after the end of treatment (H128). In this study, women who received *Yi shen xiao zheng tang* 益肾消癥汤 plus triptorelin, oestrogen, and medroxyprogesterone acetate reported lower VAS scores than women who received HT alone (110 women, MD −0.72 cm [−0.91, −0.53]; H128). Another RCT that followed women until their first menstrual period also found that women who received oral CHM in combination with HT had lower dysmenorrhoea VAS scores than women who received HT alone (86 women, MD −0.10 [−0.16, −0.04]; H77).

One study reported using a VAS to measure dysmenorrhoea, but the scale was scored from zero to nine with lower scores indicating better outcomes (H133). This study was kept separate for analysis. Results favoured *Xue jie an yi fang* 血竭安异方 plus goserelin over goserelin alone (90 women, MD −1.86 points [−2.06, −1.66]).

Six RCTs used the 1993 Guideline to assess dysmenorrhoea (H20, H62, H83, H109, H111, H139). Women who received oral CHM plus HT scored an average of 2.20 points lower than women who received HT alone (498 women, [−3.58, −0.83], I² = 94%). Sensitivity analysis including three RCTs judged as having low risk of bias also showed benefit, but with no statistical heterogeneity (255 women, MD −2.95 points [−3.37, −2.52], I² = 0%). This result may provide the best evidence for the potential role of oral CHM plus HT in reducing dysmenorrhoea as measured using the 1993 Guideline.

Results from single studies showed that *Bu shen huo xue tang* 补肾活血汤 plus gestrinone lowered dysmenorrhoea scores more than gestrinone alone as measured using the VRS (52 women, MD

−0.39 points [−0.65, −0.13]; H60). Another study, which reported CPGQ pain intensity, found no benefit of adding *Kang yi zhong yu tang* 抗异种玉汤 to goserelin over goserelin alone (50 women, MD −0.90 points [−5.19, 3.39]; H15).

Finally, there was no difference between the combination of oral CHM and HT and HT alone in reducing the chance of dysmenorrhoea. This result was found at the end of treatment (198 women, RR 0.47 [0.09, 2.35], I^2 = 90%; H44, H70) and at follow-up (198 women, RR 0.84 [0.65, 1.08], I^2 = 0%; H70, H119).

Oral Chinese herbal medicine plus hormone therapy versus placebo plus hormone therapy

When *Zhi tong hua zheng jiao nang* 止痛化癥胶囊 was combined with triptorelin, women received a lower dysmenorrhoea score as measured using the 1993 Guideline compared to women who received placebo plus triptorelin (44 women, MD −2.61 points [−3.53, −1.69]; H142).

Pelvic pain

Pelvic pain was measured in several ways: using a VAS, a four-point scale (0–3 points, lower is better), and by determining the number of women with pelvic pain.

Oral Chinese herbal medicine versus no treatment

One RCT with 64 women (H17) assessed pelvic pain at the end of treatment and at nine-month follow-up. *Shao yao zhi tong he ji* 芍药止痛合剂 resulted in a greater reduction in VAS pain scores, both at the end of treatment (MD −0.42 cm [−0.74, −0.10]) and at follow-up (MD −0.21 cm [−0.38, −0.04]). A second study found that the number of women with pelvic pain at the end of treatment was not statistically different between women who received *Dan zhu xiao yi fang* 丹术消异方 plus *Zhu yun san hao wan* 助孕三号丸 and those who received no treatment (50 women, RR 0.50 [0.24, 1.03]; H45).

Oral Chinese herbal medicine versus pharmacotherapy

Two RCTs assessed pelvic pain severity using a VAS (H17, H157). Meta-analysis showed no difference in the mean VAS score at the end of treatment between women who received oral CHM and those who received triptorelin (107 women, MD −0.07 cm [−0.26, 0.11], $I^2 = 0\%$). Both studies also documented pelvic pain scores at follow-up; however, the small standard deviation reported in one study (H17) meant that statistical analysis of results could not be calculated. Results from 45 women included in the other study also showed no difference between groups during follow-up assessment (MD −0.04 cm [−0.65, 0.57]; H157).

Three RCTs reported the number of women with pelvic pain at the end of treatment (H39, H99, H120). Results of meta-analysis indicated that there was no difference between oral CHM and pharmacotherapy in reducing the number of women with pelvic pain (RR 0.62 [0.31, 1.25], $I^2 = 31\%$).

In another study (H54), pelvic pain was measured on a four-point scale (0–3, lower is better). Results showed that pelvic pain was less severe at the end of treatment in women who received modified *Hu po san* 琥珀散 compared to women who received mifepristone (129 women, MD −0.32 points [−0.43, −0.21]).

Oral Chinese herbal medicine plus hormone therapy versus hormone therapy

Five RCTs that tested oral CHM in combination with HT assessed pelvic pain at the end of treatment and/or at follow-up assessment (H43, H59, H77, H86, H119). Three RCTs that measured pelvic pain using a 10 cm VAS were pooled for analysis (H43, H77, H86). Results showed that adding oral CHM to HT did not result in a greater improvement in pelvic pain than HT alone (272 women, MD −1.16 [−2.37, 0.04], $I^2 = 99\%$). Substantial statistical heterogeneity was identified. All three studies were judged as having low risk of bias for sequence generation, provided treatment for three months or more, and included women who had previously undergone surgery.

As such, these factors were not likely to be contributing to the statistical heterogeneity seen. The reasons for diversity in the results are unclear, which lowers confidence in these results.

Results from individual studies showed mixed conclusions. One RCT of 60 women (H59) found no benefit of treatment with *Bu shen qu yu fang* 补肾祛瘀方 and leuprolide (and the rice bran oil oryzanol, where necessary) over leuprolide alone at six-month follow-up (MD −0.37 cm [−0.80, 0.06]), while the combination was superior at 12-month follow-up (MD −1.14 cm [−1.79, −0.49]). Another study that followed up women until their first menstrual period showed that the combination of *San jie zhen tong tang* 散结镇痛汤 and leuprolide resulted in a greater improvement in VAS pain score compared to women who received leuprolide alone (86 women, MD −0.19 cm [−0.25, −0.13]; H77). While this was a statistically significant improvement, the magnitude of the change (0.19 cm) is small and may not be clinically important.

One RCT assessed the number of women with pelvic pain (H119). The number of women with pelvic pain at follow-up was not statistically different between the two groups (138 women, RR 0.50 [0.13, 1.92]).

Dyspareunia

Fourteen studies that reported re-analysable results for dyspareunia were included (H15, H17, H39, H43, H45, H54, H59, H74, H90, H110, H119, H120, H138, H142). Dyspareunia was measured using 10 cm VAS or CPGQ, with some studies reporting the number of women with dyspareunia. Results are reported according to the comparison.

Oral Chinese herbal medicine versus no treatment

One study, comparing *Shao yao zhi tong he ji* 芍药止痛合剂 with no treatment, assessed dyspareunia using a 10 cm VAS (H17). At the end of treatment, women who received *Shao yao zhi tong he ji* 芍药止痛合剂 had similar VAS scores to women who received no treatment

(64 women, MD −0.52 cm [−1.13, 0.09]). This study also documented VAS scores at nine-month follow-up; however, as the mean score and standard deviation for the oral CHM group were zero, no statistical analysis was conducted.

The number of women with dyspareunia at the end of treatment was reported in another study (H45). Among the 50 women, those who received *Dan zhu xiao yi fang* 丹术消异方 plus *Zhu yun san hao wan* 助孕三号丸 were no more likely to have dyspareunia at the end of treatment (RR 0.64 [0.34, 1.20]).

Oral Chinese herbal medicine versus pharmacotherapy

Studies that compared oral CHM with pharmacotherapy assessed dyspareunia in different ways. When dyspareunia was assessed using VAS, there was no difference at the end of treatment between women who received *Shao yao zhi tong he ji* 芍药止痛合剂 and those who received triptorelin (64 women, MD −0.05 cm [−0.47, 0.37]; H17). At nine-month follow-up, the mean VAS score and the standard deviation in the intervention group were zero, indicating no dyspareunia.

In another study (H54), a four-point scale (0–3 points, where lower scores indicate less dyspareunia) was used to measure dyspareunia. Women who received modified *Hu po san* 琥珀散 scored lower than women who received mifepristone (129 women, MD −0.36 points [−0.45, −0.27]).

Five RCTs reported the number of women with dyspareunia (H39, H74, H90, H120, H138). Among the 324 participants, women who received oral CHM were as likely to have dyspareunia at the end of treatment as women who received pharmacotherapy (RR 0.74 [0.42, 1.29], $I^2 = 0\%$).

Oral Chinese herbal medicine plus hormone therapy versus hormone therapy

Five RCTs that tested the combination of oral CHM and HT did so in different ways (H43, H59, H110, H119). When dyspareunia was measured using a 10 cm VAS, the combination of oral CHM plus HT was not statistically different from HT alone at the end of treatment in reducing dyspareunia scores (116 women, MD −0.68 cm [−1.94, 0.59], I^2 = 97%; H43, H110). There was considerable statistical heterogeneity that could not be explored due to the small number of studies; this lowers confidence in these results.

One study conducted follow-up assessments of dyspareunia, both six and 12 months after the end of treatment (H59). This study showed that the benefits of Bu shen qu yu fang 补肾祛瘀方 combined with leuprolide acetate (and a rice bran oil, oryzanol, if necessary) were long lasting. VAS scores at six months were 0.63 cm lower (60 women, [−1.24, −0.02]), and scores at 12 months were one centimetre lower in the treatment group (60 women, [−1.65, −0.35]). The absence of an agreed minimal clinically important difference makes it difficult to determine the clinical relevance of these results.

In another study, the number of women with dyspareunia at the end of treatment was reported (H119). There was no statistical difference between women who received oral CHM plus mifepristone and those who received mifepristone alone in the chances of having dyspareunia at the end of treatment (138 women, RR 0.67 [0.11, 3.87]). One final study reported dyspareunia pain intensity as measured with the CPGQ (H15). Among the 50 participants, women who received Kang yi zhong yu tang 抗异种玉汤 had CPGQ scores that were 12.40 points lower at the end of treatment compared to women who received goserelin (50 women, [−18.09, −6.71]).

Oral Chinese herbal medicine plus hormone therapy versus placebo plus hormone therapy

One study that compared Zhi tong hua zheng jiao nang 止痛化癥胶囊 plus triptorelin with placebo plus triptorelin (H142) found that the mean dyspareunia score was 1.28 cm lower among women who received oral CHM than those who received placebo (44 women, [−1.63, −0.93]).

Recurrence

Recurrence was one of the most frequently reported outcomes. The lack of consistency in criteria for assessing recurrence and the various time points at which recurrence was assessed meant that many studies were separated for analysis. Results are reported according to the comparison.

Oral Chinese herbal medicine versus no treatment

Ten RCTs that compared oral CHM with no treatment reported on recurrence (H8, H11, H14, H19, H24, H38, H57, H152, H158, H168). Several studies reported the same criteria and/or time at which recurrence was assessed and were pooled for meta-analysis. Results showed that oral CHM did not reduce the recurrence of signs and symptoms at the end of treatment (240 women, RR 0.25 [0.03, 2.24], $I^2 = 0\%$; Table 5.8), nor did it reduce recurrence between six and 30 months after treatment (73 women, RR 0.27 [0.06, 1.26], $I^2 = 0\%$).

Table 5.8. Oral Chinese Herbal Medicine versus No Treatment for Endometriosis: Recurrence

Recurrence	No. of Studies (Participants)	Effect Size RR [95% CI], I^2	Included Studies
Signs and symptoms — EoT	4 (240)	0.25 [0.03, 2.24], 0%	H8, H14, H57, H152
Signs and symptoms 6 m after surgery	3 (240)	0.28 [0.12, 0.67]*, 0%	H8, H14, H159
Signs and symptoms at 1 y	5 (304)	0.53 [0.33, 0.86]*, 0%	H2, H8, H17, H57, H152
Signs and symptoms at 2 y	3 (234)	0.30 [0.16, 0.54]*, 0%	H12, H16, H22
Criteria NS, 6–30 m after EoT	2 (73)	0.27 [0.06, 1.26], 0%	H24, H38

*Statistically significant, see Statistical Analysis in Chapter 4.
Abbreviations: CI, confidence intervals; EoT, end of treatment; m, months; NS, not specified; RR, risk ratio; y, year.

Clinical Evidence for Chinese Herbal Medicine

Of note, two of the four studies that assessed recurrence of signs and symptoms at the end of treatment reported no recurrence in either group (H8, H57).

When recurrence of signs and symptoms was assessed six months after surgery, women who received oral CHM had a lower chance of recurrence than women who received no treatment (240 women, RR 0.28 [0.12, 0.67], $I^2 = 0\%$; Table 5.8). Similar findings were seen when recurrence was assessed at 12 months (304 women, RR 0.53 [0.33, 0.86], $I^2 = 0\%$) and at 24 months (234 women, RR 0.30 [0.16, 0.54], $I^2 = 0\%$).

Results from individual studies showed that oral CHM resulted in a lower chance of recurrence when compared to no treatment for:

- Recurrence of cysts one year after treatment (60 women, RR 0.30 [0.09, 0.98]; H19);
- Recurrence of signs and symptoms 21 months after treatment (64 women, RR 0.18 [0.04, 0.74]; H11);
- Recurrence of signs and symptoms between three and 12 months after treatment (86 women, RR 0.19 [0.04, 0.84]; H168).

No such benefit was seen in one study (H158) for reducing recurrence of pain (138 women, RR 0.50 [0.13, 1.92]) or recurrence of cysts at follow-up (138 women, RR 0.25 [0.03, 2.18]).

Oral Chinese herbal medicine versus hormone therapy

Recurrence was reported in 48 RCTs that used various criteria for assessment. Results were grouped according to signs, symptoms, or physiological features (e.g., cysts) and the time at which recurrence was assessed. Results of meta-analyses are presented in Table 5.9. Oral CHM was superior to HT in reducing recurrence of:

- Signs and symptoms after two years (589 women, RR 0.50 [0.26, 0.97], $I^2 = 56\%$);
- Pain one year after surgery (216 women, RR 0.32 [0.17, 0.58], $I^2 = 0\%$).

Table 5.9. Oral Chinese Herbal Medicine versus Hormone Therapy for Endometriosis: Recurrence

Recurrence	No. of Studies (Participants)	Effect Size RR [95% CI], I^2	Included Studies
Signs and symptoms — EoT	7 (622)	0.99 [0.22, 4.53], 0%	H8, H14, H69, H75, H82, H118, H136
Signs and symptoms at 3–6 m	10 (685)	0.75 [0.51, 1.12], 0%	H8, H14, H23, H40, H67, H75, H107, H136, H151, H157
Signs and symptoms at 1 y	11 (1,092)	0.74 [0.51, 1.05], 0%	H2, H8, H17, H30, H63, H69, H81, H104, H106, H120, H143
Signs and symptoms at 2 y	5 (589)	0.50 [0.26, 0.97]*, 56%	H12, H16, H22, H69, H166
Signs and symptoms at 3 y	2 (308)	0.95 [0.66, 1.36], 0%	H3, H102
Pain at 1 y after surgery	3 (216)	0.32 [0.17, 0.58]*, 0%	H101, H127, H155
Cyst at 1 y	7 (499)	1.13 [0.75, 1.70], 0%	H19, H127, H146, H148, H150, H155, H156
Recurrence NS at 6–30 m	2 (135)	0.38 [0.14, 1.03], 0%	H24, H87

*Statistically significant, see Statistical Analysis in Chapter 4.
Abbreviations: CI, confidence intervals; EoT, end of treatment; m, months; NS, not specified; RR, risk ratio; y, year.

Oral CHM was not superior to HT in reducing recurrence of:

- Signs and symptoms at the end of treatment (622 women, RR 0.99 [0.22, 4.53], I^2 = 0%);
- Signs and symptoms between three and six months after treatment (685 women, RR 0.75 [0.51, 1.12], I^2 = 0%);
- Signs and symptoms one year after treatment (1,092 women, RR 0.74 [0.51, 1.05], I^2 = 0%);

- Signs and symptoms three years after treatment (308 women, RR 0.95 [0.66, 1.36], $I^2 = 0\%$);
- Cysts one year after treatment (499 women, RR 1.13 [0.75, 1.70], $I^2 = 0\%$).

Among the seven studies that documented recurrence of signs and symptoms at the end of treatment, five studies reported no recurrence in either group (H8, H14, H75, H136, H69). Meta-analysis of two studies that did not specify the criteria for assessment showed no difference between groups when recurrence was assessed between six and 30 months (135 women, RR 0.38 [0.14, 1.03], $I^2 = 0\%$).

As other studies that reported on recurrence could not be included in meta-analyses, results were analysed for individual studies. None of these studies showed any benefit of oral CHM over HT for recurrence of:

- Endometriosis one year after surgery (60 women, RR 2.17 [0.09, 51.10]; H155);
- Signs and symptoms between three and 12 months (112 women, RR 0.50 [0.05, 5.36]; H154);
- Signs and symptoms eight months after surgery (68 women, RR 1.18 [0.35, 4.02]; H165);
- Signs and symptoms within nine months (66 women, RR 0.80 [0.14, 4.48]; H67);
- Signs and symptoms 18 months after surgery (212 women, RR 0.75 [0.33, 1.71]; H69);
- Signs and symptoms at 21 months (64 women, RR 0.44 [0.09, 2.24]; H11);
- Signs and symptoms at an unspecified time point (66 women, RR 1.13 [0.12, 10.13]; H105);
- Cysts at the end of treatment (85 women, RR 0.95 [0.26, 3.55]; H148);
- Cysts six months after treatment (40 women, RR 1.50 [0.28, 8.04]; H5);
- Cysts at an unspecified time point (60 women, RR 0.67 [0.21, 2.13]; H160).

Oral Chinese herbal medicine plus hormone therapy versus hormone therapy

Twenty-eight studies tested the combination of oral CHM and HT. While diversity was seen in the criteria for assessing recurrence, there was sufficient overlap among studies such that most RCTs could be included in the meta-analysis. Benefits were seen with adding oral CHM to HT in reducing recurrence of signs and symptoms across a range of time points (Table 5.10) and in reducing recurrence of cysts up to one year. For most analyses, statistical heterogeneity was low or non-existent, suggesting that studies were showing similar effects.

Two studies reported different criteria for recurrence and were analysed individually. Among 90 participants, the combination of

Table 5.10. Oral Chinese Herbal Medicine versus Hormone Therapy for Endometriosis: Recurrence

Recurrence	No. of Studies (Participants)	Effect Size RR [95% CI], I^2	Included Studies
Signs and symptoms — EoT	3 (461)	0.17 [0.05, 0.52]*, 6%	H66, H128, H164
Signs and symptoms at ≤ 6 m	6 (414)	0.57 [0.35, 0.95]*, 0%	H55, H66, H70, H110, H147, H153
Signs and symptoms at 1 y	3 (447)	0.68 [0.49, 0.93]*, 0%	H128, H145, H167
Signs and symptoms at 2 y	7 (563)	0.48 [0.32, 0.72]*, 0%	H10, H91, H108, H128, H149, H161, H163
Signs and symptoms at 3 y	3 (355)	0.55 [0.38, 0.81]*, 0%	H3, H100, H103
Cysts at ≤ 6 m	3 (140)	0.20 [0.05, 0.75]*, 0%	H5, H27, H140
Cysts at 1 y	2 (144)	0.37 [0.15, 0.89]*, 0%	H59, H92

*Statistically significant, see Statistical Analysis in Chapter 4.
Abbreviations: CI, confidence intervals; EoT, end of treatment; m, months; RR, risk ratio; y, years.

Dan leng fu kang jian gao 丹棱妇康煎膏 and triptorelin did not result in a lower chance of endometriosis at six months compared to triptorelin alone (RR 0.30 [0.09, 1.02]; H113). The second study found no difference between oral CHM plus mifepristone and mifepristone alone in the chance of recurrence of signs and symptoms at an unspecified time point (126 women, RR 0.45 [0.17, 1.23]; H98).

Ovarian cyst size

Studies that assessed ovarian cyst size did so in various ways, including measuring the cyst diameter, area, and volume.

Oral Chinese herbal medicine versus no treatment

One RCT that compared *E ling jiao nang* 莪棱胶囊 with no treatment found ovarian cyst diameter to be 0.97 cm lower among women who received *E ling jiao nang* 莪棱胶囊 (50 women, [−1.66, −0.28]; H7).

Oral Chinese herbal medicine versus placebo

Meta-analysis of two RCTs showed that the ovarian cyst diameter was 0.85 cm smaller in women who received oral CHM than in women who received a placebo (103 women, [−1.59, −0.12], $I^2 = 51\%$; H61, H132).

Oral Chinese herbal medicine versus hormone therapy

Studies that compared oral CHM with HT measured ovarian cyst diameter, area, and volume. Findings from meta-analyses showed that oral CHM was not superior to HT in reducing ovarian cyst diameter (872 women, MD −0.22 cm [−0.64, 0.21], $I^2 = 91\%$) or area (252 women, MD −0.04 cm^2 [−0.89, 0.81], $I^2 = 0\%$) (Table 5.11). Statistical heterogeneity among studies that assessed ovarian cyst diameter was explored in sensitivity analyses. Among three studies assessed as having low risk of bias for sequence generation (H56, H88, H99), there was no statistical difference between groups (189

Table 5.11. Oral Chinese Herbal Medicine versus Hormone Therapy for Endometriosis: Ovarian Cyst Size

Cyst Measurement	No. of Studies (Participants)	Effect Size MD [95% CI], I^2	Included Studies
Diameter (cm)	13 (872)	−0.22 [−0.64, 0.21], 91%	H7, H20, H51, H56, H76, H88, H90, H94, H99, H117, H130, H131, H173
Area (cm^2)	4 (252)	−0.04 [−0.89, 0.81], 0%	H52, H58, H134, H138

Abbreviations: CI, confidence intervals; MD, mean difference.

women, MD −0.70 cm [−1.48, 0.08], I^2 = 88%) and statistical heterogeneity remained considerable. As such, the certainty of findings is unclear.

One study that assessed ovarian cyst size by measuring volume (H53) found that cyst volume was smaller among women who received oral CHM than in those who received mifepristone (60 women, MD −3.74 [−6.84, −0.64]).

Oral Chinese herbal medicine plus hormone therapy versus hormone therapy

Meta-analysis was conducted with six studies that tested the effect of a combination of oral CHM and HT on ovarian cyst diameter (H20, H65, H144, H171, H172, H174). Cyst diameter was 0.72 cm smaller in women who received oral CHM plus HT than in women who received HT alone ([−0.95, −0.48], I^2 = 71%). Substantial statistical heterogeneity lowers confidence in the result; in addition, the clinical importance of such a change is uncertain.

In individual studies, the combination of *Tong jing ke li* 痛经颗粒 and mifepristone produced a greater reduction in ovarian cyst volume compared to mifepristone alone (100 women, MD −1.21 cm^3 [−1.81, −0.61]; H64). A second study found that *Huo xue san yu tang* 活血散瘀汤 used in combination with mifepristone was not superior to mifepristone alone in reducing the ovarian cyst area (120 women, MD 0.04 cm^2 [−1.18, 1.26]; H62).

Uterine volume

Results from one RCT that reported uterine volume measured by ultrasound could be analysed (H116), and women who received *Wu wei san* 五味散 had lower uterine volume than women who received mifepristone (MD −12.60 cm^3 [−18.69, −6.51]).

Menstrual volume

Two RCTs measured menstrual volume at the end of treatment (H116, H142). Studies tested different comparisons and measured menstrual volume in different ways, and were separated for analysis.

Oral Chinese herbal medicine versus hormone therapy

One RCT measured menstrual volume by weighing sanitary napkins (H116); one milligram was considered equal to one millilitre. Menstrual volume was lower in women who received *Wu wei san* 五味散 than in women who received mifepristone (MD −19.70 [−29.55, −9.85]).

Oral Chinese herbal medicine plus hormone therapy versus placebo plus hormone therapy

Menstrual volume was assessed in one small RCT with 44 women (H142). Women who received *Zhi tong hua zheng jiao nang* 止痛化癥胶囊 plus triptorelin used fewer sanitary napkins than women who received triptorelin alone (MD −5.09 [−6.31, −3.87]).

Pregnancy outcomes

Pregnancy outcomes were examined in studies that reported the number of women with endometriosis-related infertility. Some studies reported pregnancy outcomes only for women with endometriosis-related infertility, while others reported pregnancy outcomes for all women. Studies in the latter category were included where the number of women with endometriosis-related infertility was clearly specified; this approach was taken to ensure that at least some of the women for which pregnancy outcomes were documented were intending to become pregnant. Outcomes included pregnancy rate (confirmed by the presence of the gestational sac through ultrasound), miscarriage rate, and live birth rate.

Oral Chinese herbal medicine versus no treatment

Meta-analysis of two studies that reported pregnancy rate at the end of treatment showed that the chance of achieving a pregnancy was greater among women who received oral CHM than in those who received no treatment (90 women, RR 3.80 [1.02, 14.16], $I^2 = 0\%$). The pregnancy rate at follow-up was also greater in women who received oral CHM (Table 5.12). Reassuringly, there was no difference in the miscarriage rate between oral CHM and no treatment (57 women, RR 1.09 [0.31, 3.92], $I^2 = 0\%$), although the number of women included in this analysis was small.

Table 5.12. Oral Chinese Herbal Medicine versus No Treatment for Endometriosis: Pregnancy Outcomes

Pregnancy Outcome	No. of Studies (Participants)	Effect Size RR [95% CI], I^2	Included Studies
Pregnancy rate — EoT	2 (90)	3.80 [1.02, 14.16]*, 0%	H38, H45
Pregnancy rate — follow-up	4 (522)	2.13 [1.47, 3.07]*, 0%	H12, H21, H38, H45
Miscarriage rate — follow-up	2 (57)	1.09 [0.31, 3.92], 0%	H25, H45

*Statistically significant, see Statistical Analysis in Chapter 4.
Abbreviations: CI, confidence intervals; EoT, end of treatment; RR, risk ratio.

Oral Chinese herbal medicine versus pharmacotherapy

Among the studies that compared oral CHM with pharmacotherapy, most used HT as the treatment; however, two stated that conventional therapy was used in the control group without specifying the details (H39, H124). In analyses of pregnancy outcomes, the comparison is referred to as 'oral CHM versus pharmacotherapy', although it is likely that this is actually a comparison of oral CHM and HT. All results were for women with endometriosis-related infertility.

While oral CHM did not result in a higher pregnancy rate at the end of treatment than pharmacotherapy (187 women, RR 1.61 [0.89, 2.92], $I^2 = 26\%$; Table 5.13), the pregnancy rate was higher at follow-up assessment (1,062 women, RR 1.73 [1.45, 2.06], $I^2 = 0\%$). In addition, the miscarriage rate among women who achieved a pregnancy was lower with oral CHM (RR 0.49 [0.30, 0.81], $I^2 = 0\%$). Oral

Table 5.13. Oral Chinese Herbal Medicine versus Pharmacotherapy for Endometriosis: Pregnancy Outcomes

Pregnancy Outcome	No. of Studies (Participants)	Effect Size RR [95% CI], I^2	Included Studies
Pregnancy rate — EoT	4 (187)	1.61 [0.89, 2.92], 26%	H15, H30, H90, H160
Pregnancy rate — follow-up	12 (1,062)	1.73 [1.45, 2.06]*, 0%	H12, H18, H21, H29, H30, H39, H40, H42, H46, H49, H105, H169
Miscarriage rate — follow-up	10 (305)	0.49 [0.30, 0.81]*, 0%	H18, H25, H29, H30, H39, H40, H42, H46, H49, H169
Live birth rate	3 (79)	1.17 [0.90, 1.54], 0%	H25, H46, H169

*Statistically significant, see Statistical Analysis in Chapter 4.
Abbreviations: CI, confidence intervals; EoT, end of treatment; RR, risk ratio.

CHM did not increase the chance of a live birth (79 women, RR 1.17 [0.90, 1.54], I^2 = 0%), although this analysis was based on a small number of women.

One study assessed pregnancy rate at a second follow-up visit after two years (H46). Among the 33 women, the pregnancy rate was higher in women who received *Dan chi yin* 丹赤饮 than in those who received GnRHa (RR 1.97 [1.07, 3.65]). Results from another small study showed that the miscarriage rate at the end of treatment was not statistically different between women who received *Kang yi zhong yu tang* 抗异种玉汤 and those who received goserelin (15 women, RR 0.57 [0.06, 5.03]; H15).

Oral Chinese herbal medicine plus pharmacotherapy versus pharmacotherapy

Fourteen studies that tested the combination of oral CHM and pharmacotherapy reported on pregnancy outcomes, including rates of pregnancy, miscarriage, and live births. Differences were noted in participants among the studies; for example, some studies included women undergoing assisted reproductive techniques (ART), including *in vitro* fertilisation (IVF). Such studies were considered sufficiently different to be separated for meta-analysis.

At the end of treatment, the pregnancy rate among women with endometriosis-related infertility was higher in those who received oral CHM plus pharmacotherapy compared to those who received pharmacotherapy alone; this result was seen irrespective of whether they were receiving HT treatment (208 women, RR 2.10 [1.31, 3.37], I^2 = 0%) or ART (175 women, RR 2.08 [1.28, 3.38], I^2 = 0%; Table 5.14). The benefits of oral CHM plus pharmacotherapy persisted until follow-up assessment in studies that used pharmacotherapy as the comparator (774 women, RR 1.39 [1.18, 1.64], I^2 = 17%). Not surprisingly, there was no difference between groups at follow-up in one study of women undergoing IVF (53 women, RR 1.49 [0.76, 2.93]); women who are undergoing IVF treatment are unlikely to have conceived naturally during the follow-up period.

Table 5.14. Oral Chinese Herbal Medicine plus Pharmacotherapy versus Pharmacotherapy for Endometriosis: Pregnancy Rate

Assessment Time; Comparator	No. of Studies (Participants)	Effect Size RR [95% CI], I^2	Included Studies
Women with endometriosis-related infertility			
EoT; ART	3 (175)	2.08 [1.28, 3.38]*, 0%	H36, H37, H41
EoT; HT	3 (208)	2.10 [1.31, 3.37]*, 0%	H15, H35, H48
Follow-up; IVF	1 (53)	1.49 [0.76, 2.93], NA	H47
Follow-up; Pharmacotherapy	9 (774)	1.39 [1.18, 1.64]*, 17%	H26, H32–H34, H44, H48, H50, H92, H124
All women			
Follow-up; Pharmacotherapy	8 (754)	1.39 [1.17, 1.64]*, 23%	H32–H34, H44, H48, H50, H92, H124
Follow-up; IVF	2 (73)	1.60 [0.84, 3.03], 0%	H26, H47

*Statistically significant, see Statistical Analysis in Chapter 4.
Abbreviations: ART, assisted reproductive techniques; CI, confidence intervals; EoT, end of treatment; HT, hormone therapy; IVF, in vitro fertilisation; NA, not applicable; RR, risk ratio.

In studies that reported the pregnancy rate for all women, the chances of achieving a pregnancy at follow-up were greater with the combination of oral CHM and pharmacotherapy than with pharmacotherapy alone (754 women, RR 1.39 [1.17, 1.64], I^2 = 23%). No such benefit at follow-up was seen in women undergoing IVF (73 women, RR 1.60 [0.84, 3.03], I^2 = 0%).

The miscarriage rate among women who achieved a pregnancy was not statistically different between groups at the end of treatment (78 women, RR 0.34 [0.08, 1.50], I^2 = 0%), but was lower among women who received the combination of oral CHM plus pharmacotherapy at follow-up (418 women, RR 1.39 [1.18, 1.63], I^2 = 0%; Table 5.15).

Table 5.15. Oral Chinese Herbal Medicine plus Pharmacotherapy versus Pharmacotherapy for Endometriosis: Miscarriage Rate

Assessment Time	No. of Studies (Participants)	Effect Size RR [95% CI], I²	Included Studies
EoT	3 (78)	0.34 [0.08, 1.50], 0%	H15, H31, H35
Follow-up	4 (418)	0.51 [0.31, 0.83]*, 0%	H32, H34, H44, H124

*Statistically significant, see Statistical Analysis in Chapter 4.
Abbreviations: CI, confidence intervals; EoT, end of treatment; RR, risk ratio.

One study that assessed the live birth rate of 48 participants (H124) found no statistical difference between women who received oral CHM plus pharmacotherapy and those who received pharmacotherapy alone (RR 1.13 [0.79, 1.61]).

Fatigue

The number of women with fatigue was measured in one RCT (H128). Among the 110 women, the chance of having fatigue at the end of treatment was lower in women who received *Yi shen xiao zheng tang* 益肾消癥汤 plus triptorelin, oestrogen, and medroxyprogesterone acetate than in women who received HT alone (MD 0.40 [0.19, 0.83]).

Health-related quality of life

Three different measures of health-related quality of life were used in included studies: the Medical Outcome Study 36-Item Short-Form Health Survey (SF-36),[32] the World Health Organization Quality of Life Instruments (WHOQOL-BREF),[33] and the 30- and five-item versions of the Endometriosis Health Profile (EHP) questionnaire.[34,35] Results were analysed according to comparisons.

Oral Chinese herbal medicine versus no treatment

Two studies examined health-related quality of life using the SF-36 (H95, H126); however, only one RCT reported results for all eight

Table 5.16. Oral Chinese Herbal Medicine versus No Treatment for Endometriosis: SF-36

Domain	No. of Studies (Participants)	Effect Size MD [95% CI], I^2	Included Studies
Physical function	2 (150)	1.57 [−8.17, 11.31], 92%	H17, H68
Emotional role function	2 (150)	7.86 [4.11, 11.61]*, 0%	H17, H68
Social function	2 (150)	6.20 [0.30, 12.10]*, 78%	H17, H68
Mental health	2 (150)	3.73 [−3.76, 11.21], 81%	H17, H68
Physical role function	1 (64)	−5.42 [−19.79, 8.95]	H17
Bodily pain	1 (64)	1.75 [−6.86, 10.36]	H17
General health	1 (64)	−21.00 [−28.24, −13.76]*	H17
Vitality	1 (64)	2.25 [−5.03, 9.53]	H17

*Statistically significant, see Statistical Analysis in Chapter 4.
Abbreviations: CI, confidence intervals; MD, mean difference.

domains. Meta-analysis showed higher scores with oral CHM — indicating better outcomes — on the emotional role function (150 women, MD 7.86 points [4.11, 11.61], I^2 = 0%; H17, H68) and social function domains (150 women, MD 6.20 points [0.30, 12.10], I^2 = 78%; H17, H68) (Table 5.16). No such benefits were seen on the physical function and mental function domains.

Results from one study of 64 women (H17) showed no difference between *Shao yao zhi tong he ji* 芍药止痛合剂 and no treatment in improving scores on the physical role function, bodily pain, and vitality domains of the SF-36 (Table 5.15); however, women who received no treatment reported better outcomes on the general health domain. The same study also reported SF-36 scores at follow-up after nine months. Women who received *Shao yao zhi tong he ji* 芍药止痛合剂 had better scores on the bodily pain domain (MD 5.27 [0.55, 9.99]), while women who received no treatment had better scores on the physical function domain (MD −4.83 [−8.62, −1.04]). No differences were seen between groups for physical role function (MD −5.08 [−15.19, 5.03]), emotional role function (MD −1.39 [−18.41, 15.63]), general health (MD 4.75 [−1.46, 10.96]), vitality (MD 2.58 [−3.74, 8.90]), social function (MD 1.92 [−1.77, 5.61]), and mental health (MD −4.33 [−9.45, 0.79]).

Another small study that compared oral CHM with no treatment assessed health-related quality of life using the WHOQOL-BREF (H4). Women who received oral CHM scored higher — indicating better quality of life — on the questions relating to overall quality of life (MD 0.80 points [0.35, 1.25]) and general health (MD 0.42 points [0.10, 0.74]) than women who received no treatment. In terms of the WHOQOL-BREF domain scores, women who received oral CHM had higher scores on the physical domain (MD 1.53 points [0.75, 2.31]), yet scores were not statistically different between the two groups on the psychological (MD 0.39 [−0.29, 1.07]), social (MD −0.46 [−1.53, 0.61]), or environmental domains (MD −0.36 [−1.04, 0.32]).

Oral Chinese herbal medicine versus hormone therapy

Studies that compared oral CHM with HT measured health-related quality of life using different scales. Two studies that used the WHOQOL-BREF were pooled for meta-analysis (H4, H82). Results showed that women who received oral CHM scored higher — indicating better outcomes — on the general health (243 women, MD 0.21 points [0.02, 0.40], $I^2 = 0\%$) and physical domains (243 women, MD 0.50 points [0.01, 0.98], $I^2 = 32\%$) compared to women who received HT. There was no difference between groups for the questions relating to overall quality of life or the psychological, social, or environmental domains (Table 5.17).

The SF-36 was used to assess health-related quality of life in one RCT (H17). This study included two control arms: one that received no treatment (described previously) and another that received triptorelin. Among the 62 women in these two groups, scores at the end

Table 5.17. Oral Chinese Herbal Medicine versus Hormone Therapy for Endometriosis: WHOQOL-BREF

Domain	No. of Studies (Participants)	Effect Size MD [95% CI], I^2	Included Studies
Overall quality of life	2 (243)	0.06 [−0.10, 0.22], 0%	H4, H82
General health	2 (243)	0.21 [0.02, 0.40]*, 0%	H4, H82
Physical	2 (243)	0.50 [0.01, 0.98]*, 32%	H4, H82
Psychological	2 (243)	0.16 [−0.24, 0.57], 13%	H4, H82
Social	2 (243)	0.30 [−0.27, 0.87], 31%	H4, H82
Environmental	2 (243)	0.01 [−0.49, 0.51], 17%	H4, H82

*Statistically significant, see Statistical Analysis in Chapter 4.
Abbreviations: CI, confidence intervals; MD, mean difference.

of treatment were lower for women who received *Shao yao zhi tong he ji* 芍药止痛合剂 — indicating worse outcomes — on the emotional role function domain than for women who received triptorelin (MD −29.86 points [−43.34, −16.38]). *Shao yao zhi tong he ji* 芍药止痛合剂 was not statistically different from triptorelin in terms of SF-36 scores for the physical function (MD 2.67 points [−3.37, 8.71]), physical role function (MD 6.89 points [−9.38, 23.16]), bodily pain (MD −0.06 points [−5.84, 5.72]), general health (MD −4.15 points [−10.40, 2.10]), vitality (MD −0.10 points [−6.78, 6.58]), social function (MD −1.29 points [−5.85, 3.27]), and mental health domains (MD −2.41 points [−15.72, 10.90]).

This study also assessed SF-36 scores nine months after treatment and similar findings were seen. People who received *Shao yao zhi tong he ji* 芍药止痛合剂 fared worse than people who received triptorelin on the emotional role function domain (MD −21.06 points [−33.82, −8.30]). In comparison, there was no difference between groups for physical function (MD 2.25 points [−4.08, 8.58]), physical role function (MD 3.88 points [−7.93, 15.69]), bodily pain (MD 1.82 points [−3.45, 7.09]), general health (MD −3.17 points [−10.20, 3.86]), vitality (MD −1.15 points [−7.15, 4.85]), social function (MD −2.46 points [−5.94, 1.02]), and mental health (MD −1.04 points [−14.00, 11.92]).

Different versions of the EHP were used to assess health-related quality of life in other studies. Two studies that tested the formula *Qing re hua yu fang* 清热化瘀方 reported the total score for the EHP-30 (H95, H126). Meta-analysis showed that the EHP-30 total score at the end of treatment was 4.39 points lower with *Qing re hua yu fang* 清热化瘀方 than with HT (131 women, [−5.27, −3.51], I^2 = 0%). Another RCT documented the five core scales of the EHP-30 (H126). This study of 60 women found lower scores at the end of treatment — indicating better health outcomes — on the control and powerlessness (MD −1.04 points [−1.69, −0.39]), social support (MD −1.56 points [−2.13, −0.99]), emotional wellbeing (MD −1.43 points [−2.09, −0.77]), and self-image (MD −0.85 points [−1.61, −0.09]) scales with *Qing re hua yu fang* 清热化瘀方 than with triptorelin. Despite these results, no benefit was seen between groups based on the pain scale of the EHP-30 (MD 0.41 points [−0.26, 1.08]).

Two studies used the shorter version of the EHP, the EHP-5 (H94, H112). One study found that women who received *Dan leng fu kang jian gao* 丹棱妇康煎膏 had higher scores at the end of treatment — indicating worse quality of life — than women who received mifepristone (H112). The second study (H94), involving 70 women, reported both the five core scales and the six supplementary modules of the EHP-5. Women who received *Nei yi kang fu pian* 内异康复片 scored lower than women who received gestrinone for four of the five core scales: control and powerlessness (MD −8.17 [−15.84, −0.51]), social support (MD −10.89 [−15.72, −6.05]), emotional wellbeing (MD −16.46 [−23.48, −9.43]), and self-image (MD −17.57 [−21.35, −13.79]). No difference was seen between the two groups on the pain scale (MD −7.86 [−16.01, 0.30]). Among the supplementary modules, benefits of *Nei yi kang fu pian* 内异康复片 over gestrinone were found based on feelings about the medical profession (MD −18.57 [−21.85, −15.30]), work (MD −13.73 [−18.73, −8.73]), feelings about treatment (MD −10.45 [−18.96, −1.95]), feelings about infertility (MD −7.71 [−10.48, −4.95]), and relationship with children (MD −8.00 [−14.04, −1.96]). There was no difference between groups in the sexual relationship module (MD 2.29 [−3.55, 8.13]).

Kupperman Index

Four studies measured menopausal symptoms using the KI (H43, H133, H140, H147). As some RCTs modified the KI, results were analysed using the standardised mean difference (SMD). Women who received oral CHM plus HT reported similar KI scores at the end of treatment compared with women who received HT alone (SMD −1.67 [−3.64, 0.30], I² = 98%). Considerable statistical heterogeneity was detected. Planned subgroup analyses according to CHM formulas and previous surgery could not be conducted as all studies used different formulas and all women had had previous surgery. Subgroup analysis of three RCTs that provided treatment for three months or longer also exhibited statistical heterogeneity (SMD −1.96 [−5.10, 1.19], I² = 98%; H43, H133, H140). As such, confidence in this result is low.

Bone density

One RCT tested the effectiveness of adding *Yu yin qian yang fang* 育阴潜阳方 to tibolone as add-back therapy on bone density (H147). Bone density of the L1–L4 vertebra was measured in 84 women. Women who received oral CHM plus tibolone had a statistically higher bone density — indicating poorer outcomes — than women who received tibolone as add-back therapy (MD 0.02 standard deviations [0.01, 0.03]), although it is important to note that the end of treatment results for both groups were within the normal range. Further, while the result shows a statistically significant difference, it is not clear whether this is clinically important in the absence of an agreed minimal clinically important difference for osteoporosis.[36]

Assessment using Grading of Recommendations Assessment, Development and Evaluation

The Grading of Recommendations Assessment, Development, and Evaluation (GRADE) framework was used to summarise the strength and quality ('certainty') of clinically important questions. Group consensus, involving experts in endometriosis and members of the research team, on the items for inclusion in summary-of-findings tables was reached after following the process described in Chapter 4. The group considered endometriosis to be the most important disease subtype to focus on, and the comparisons of oral CHM versus placebo, oral CHM versus HT, and oral CHM plus HT versus HT alone to be critically important.

In addition, three formulas were considered important for clinical practice: *Shao fu zhu yu tang* 少腹逐瘀汤, *Xue fu zhu yu tang* 血府逐瘀汤, and *Gui zhi fu ling jiao nang/wan* 桂枝茯苓胶囊/丸. We planned to prepare summary-of-findings tables for each of these formulas compared to HT and to placebo. None of the RCTs compared:

- *Shao fu zhu yu tang* 少腹逐瘀汤 versus placebo;
- *Shao fu zhu yu tang* 少腹逐瘀汤 verus HT;
- *Shao fu zhu yu tang* 少腹逐瘀汤 plus placebo versus placebo;
- *Xue fu zhu yu tang* 血府逐瘀汤 versus placebo;
- *Xue fu zhu yu tang* 血府逐瘀汤 plus placebo versus placebo;
- *Gui zhi fu ling jiao nang/wan* 桂枝茯苓胶囊/丸 versus placebo;
- *Gui zhi fu ling jiao nang/wan* 桂枝茯苓胶囊/丸 plus placebo versus placebo.

As such, we were unable to prepare summary-of-findings tables for these comparisons. The certainty of the evidence for these important clinical questions remains unclear.

The most important outcomes, determined by group consensus, included VAS pain scores (dysmenorrhoea, pelvic pain, and dyspareunia), recurrence, live birth rate, health-related quality of life measured with the EHP-30, and adverse events. Some studies reported outcome data in ways that differed from conventional use (e.g., VAS score from 0–9) or reported results incompletely (e.g., missing mean and/or standard deviation at the end of treatment); such data were not used in the preparation of summary-of-findings tables.

Studies documented recurrence in different ways, including recurrence at varying time points from baseline or surgery. A pragmatic decision was made to include all results for comparisons where there were few studies and to focus on studies that reported endometriosis for comparisons involving a large number of studies.

Three summary-of-findings tables were prepared for oral CHM:

- Oral CHM versus placebo;
- Oral CHM versus HT;
- Oral CHM plus HT versus HT.

Five summary-of-findings tables were prepared for specific formulas:

- *Shao fu zhu yu tang* 少腹逐瘀汤 plus HT versus HT;
- *Xue fu zhu yu tang* 血府逐瘀汤 versus HT;
- *Xue fu zhu yu tang/jiao nang* 血府逐瘀汤/胶囊 plus HT versus HT;
- *Gui zhi fu ling jiao nang/wan* 桂枝茯苓胶囊/丸 versus HT;
- *Gui zhi fu ling jiao nang/wan* 桂枝茯苓胶囊/丸 plus HT versus HT.

Oral Chinese herbal medicine versus placebo

Four RCTs that compared oral CHM with placebo reported on dysmenorrhea VAS as the outcome measure (H1, H6, H61, H132). Moderate certainty evidence from one study showed that oral CHM resulted in a lower dysmenorrhoea VAS score at the end of treatment than placebo did (Table 5.18).

Table 5.18. GRADE: Oral Chinese Herbal Medicine versus Placebo

Outcome	Absolute Effect		Relative Effect (95% CI) No. of Participants & Studies	Certainty of the Evidence (GRADE)
	With Oral CHM	With Placebo		
Dysmenorrhoea VAS Treatment duration: 12 w	1.94 cm Average difference: 2.37 cm (95% CI: 3.4 to 1.34 cm lower)	4.31 cm	MD −2.37 (−3.40 to −1.34) Based on data from 29 patients in 1 study	⊕⊕⊕⊝ MODERATE[a]

Abbreviations: CHM, Chinese herbal medicine; CI, confidence intervals; MD, mean difference; VAS, visual analogue scale; w, weeks.
[a]Small sample size; downgraded one level.

References
Dysmenorrhoea VAS: H6.

All four studies reported on the safety of oral CHM. Adverse events (AEs) among women who received oral CHM included one case of abnormal liver function and an unspecified number of cases of nausea and vomiting. Adverse events among women who received placebo included two cases of abnormal liver function associated with paracetamol-based analgesia use and one case of elevated creatinine at baseline.

Oral Chinese herbal medicine versus hormone therapy

Of the 96 studies that compared oral CHM with HT, 20 RCTs reported on the clinical outcomes selected for summary-of-findings tables (H2, H17, H25, H28, H42, H46, H54, H75, H80, H87, H95, H97, H122, H126, H129, H131, H143, H155, H157, H169). The certainty of the evidence was low in studies that assessed patient-reported outcomes and moderate in studies that reported objective outcomes, such as recurrence of endometriosis and live birth rate (Table 5.19). Low certainty evidence showed that oral CHM lowered dysmenorrhoea VAS scores and EHP-30 scores at the end of treatment, indicating better outcomes. No such benefit of oral CHM over HT was seen for pelvic pain and dyspareunia as measured using the VAS (low certainty evidence). Women who received oral CHM were no more likely to experience recurrence or give birth to a live baby than women who received HT (moderate certainty evidence). In the one study that documented recurrence of endometriosis (H155), there was one recurrence in the treatment group and no recurrence in the control group.

Sixty of the 96 RCTs that compared oral CHM with HT reported on AEs (H5, H7–H9, H11, H12, H14, H16, H22–H25, H30, H40, H49, H51–H53, H56, H58, H75, H76, H81, H82, H85, H90, H93, H94, H96, H97, H99, H101, H102, H104–H107, H114, H115, H118, H129–H131, H136, H138, H143, H146, H148, H150, H151, H154–H157, H165, H166, H169, H170, H173). Studies that reported the nature of the event but not the number were not included in the description of AEs below. The number of AEs among women who received oral CHM was much lower than among women who received HT (132 versus 1,148).

Table 5.19. GRADE: Oral Chinese Herbal Medicine versus Hormone Therapy

Outcome	Absolute Effect		Relative Effect (95% CI) No. of Participants & Studies	Certainty of the Evidence (GRADE)
	With Oral CHM	With HT		
Dysmenorrhoea VAS Treatment duration: 3 to 6 m	2.18 cm Average difference: 0.62 cm lower (95% CI: 0.91 to 0.34 cm lower)	2.8 cm	MD −0.62 (−0.91 to −0.34) Based on data from 1,002 patients in 13 studies	⊕⊕☐☐ LOW[a,b]
Pelvic pain VAS Treatment duration: 3 m	1.23 cm Average difference: 0.07 cm lower (95% CI: 0.26 lower to 0.11 cm higher)	1.3 cm	MD −0.07 (−0.26 to 0.11) Based on data from 107 patients in 2 studies	⊕⊕☐☐ LOW[a,c]
Dyspareunia VAS Treatment duration: 3 m	0.33 cm Average difference: 0.05 cm lower (95% CI: 0.47 lower to 0.37 cm higher)	0.38 cm	MD −0.05 (−0.47 to 0.37) Based on data from 64 patients in 1 study	⊕⊕☐☐ LOW[a,c]
Recurrence of endometriosis 1 y after surgery Treatment duration: 3 m	0 per 100 Difference: 0 fewer per 100 patients (95% CI: 0 to 0 fewer per 100 patients)	0 per 100	RR 2.17 (0.09 to 51.1) Based on data from 60 patients in 1 study	⊕⊕⊕☐ MODERATE[c]
Live birth rate Treatment duration: 63 d to 6 m	80 per 100 Difference: 12 more per 100 patients (95% CI: 7 fewer to 36 more per 100 patients)	68 per 100	RR 1.17 (0.90 to 1.54) Based on data from 79 patients in 3 studies	⊕⊕⊕☐ MODERATE[c]

(Continued)

Table 5.19. (*Continued*)

Outcome	Absolute Effect		Relative Effect (95% CI) No. of Participants & Studies	Certainty of the Evidence (GRADE)
	With Oral CHM	With HT		
EHP-30 (total score) Treatment duration: 3 to 4 m	25.56 points Average difference: 4.39 points lower (95% CI: 5.27 to 3.51 points lower)	29.95 points	MD −4.39 (−5.27 to −3.51) Based on data from 131 patients in 2 studies	⊕⊕⊡⊡ LOW[a,c]

Abbreviations: CHM, Chinese herbal medicine; CI, confidence intervals; d, days; EHP-30, Endometriosis Health Profile-30; HT, hormone therapy; m, months; MD, mean difference; RR, risk ratio; VAS, visual analogue scale; y, years.
[a]High risk of bias due to lack of blinding; downgraded one level.
[b]Considerable differences in magnitude of effect and substantial statistical heterogeneity; downgraded one level.
[c]Small sample size; downgraded one level.

References
Dysmenorrhoea VAS: H2, H28, H42, H54, H75, H80, H87, H97, H122, H126, H129, H131, H143.
Pelvic pain VAS: H17, H157.
Dyspareunia VAS: H17.
Recurrence of endometriosis: H155.
Live birth rate: H25, H46, H169.
EHP-30: H95, H126.

Adverse events reported in the oral CHM groups included 35 cases of gastrointestinal discomfort or reactions, 26 cases of irregular vaginal bleeding, 13 cases of nausea and bowel symptoms such as diarrhoea and constipation, 10 cases of breast discomfort, nine cases of hot flushes and sweating, seven cases of nausea and gastrointestinal discomfort, seven cases of weight gain, seven cases of abnormal liver function, five cases of diarrhoea, four cases of amenorrhoea, three cases of rashes, two cases of dry mouth, two cases of acne, and one case each of constipation and dizziness.

The number of AEs was higher among women who received HT, with 1,148 AEs reported. These included 225 cases of irregular vaginal bleeding, 185 cases of abnormal liver function, 172 cases of amenorrhoea,

Clinical Evidence for Chinese Herbal Medicine

136 cases of menopausal symptoms such as hot flushes, insomnia, and loss of libido, 66 cases of weight gain, 40 cases of gastrointestinal symptoms such as discomfort, nausea, vomiting, and diarrhoea, 26 cases of vaginal dryness, 23 cases of haemorrhoids, 22 cases of acne and weight gain, 14 cases of mood changes, 12 cases of abnormal liver and kidney function, 11 cases of elevated androgen levels, 11 cases of acne, 10 cases of loss of libido, eight cases of bone pain, seven cases of elevated white blood cell count, two cases of emotional changes, two cases of headache, two cases of malignant vomiting, two cases of hyperhidrosis, two cases of menstrual disorders, and one case each of treatment interruptions, rash, voice changes, and allergic reaction. Several studies reported the overall number of cases for a diverse range of AEs — a total of 166 cases were of this nature.

Oral Chinese herbal medicine plus hormone therapy versus hormone therapy

Among the 63 RCTs that tested the combination of oral CHM and HT, 18 reported on the selected clinical outcomes (H43, H48, H55, H64, H66, H70, H71, H77–H79, H86, H110, H113, H128, H133, H137, H140, H141). Evidence from these studies ranged from very low to moderate certainty. Very low certainty evidence suggests that oral CHM plus HT may reduce VAS scores for dysmenorrhoea (Table 5.20). There was no evidence that the combination of oral CHM and HT was better than HT alone in reducing pelvic pain or dyspareunia (very low certainty evidence). Further, there was neither evidence that oral CHM plus HT reduced the chance of recurrence of endometriosis when assessed one year after surgery (low certainty evidence) nor evidence that the combination increased the live birth rate (moderate certainty evidence).

Thirty RCTs reported on safety (H10, H15, H27, H33–H35, H37, H43, H44, H50, H55, H60, H64–H66, H70, H83, H86, H98, H113, H119, H128, H139, H140, H145, H149, H162–H164, H167). Studies that did not report the number of AEs were not included in the counts below. Fewer AEs were seen in women who received the combination of oral CHM plus HT (244 versus 560).

Table 5.20. GRADE: Oral Chinese Herbal Medicine plus Hormone Therapy versus Hormone Therapy

Outcome	Absolute Effect		Relative Effect (95% CI) No. of Participants & Studies	Certainty of the Evidence (GRADE)
	With Oral CHM plus HT	With HT		
Dysmenorrhoea VAS Treatment duration: 3 to 6 m	1.89 cm Average difference: 1.25 cm lower (95% CI: 1.56 to 0.94 cm lower)	3.14 cm	MD −1.25 (−1.56 to −0.94) Based on data from 1,299 patients in 17 studies	⊕☐☐☐ VERY LOW[a,b]
Pelvic pain VAS Treatment duration: 3 to 6 m	0.93 cm Average difference: 1.16 cm lower (95% CI: 2.37 cm lower to 0.04 cm higher)	2.09 cm	MD −1.16 (−2.37 to 0.04) Based on data from 272 patients in 3 studies	⊕☐☐☐ VERY LOW[a,c,d]
Dyspareunia VAS Treatment duration: 5 m to 24 w	1.11 cm Average difference: 0.68 cm lower (95% CI: 1.94 cm lower to 0.59 cm higher)	1.79 cm	MD −0.68 (−1.94 to 0.59) Based on data from 116 patients in 2 studies	⊕☐☐☐ VERY LOW[a,c,d]
Recurrence of endometriosis 1 y after surgery Treatment duration: 6 m	7 per 100 Difference: 15 fewer per 100 patients (95% CI: 20 to 0 fewer per 100 patients)	22 per 100	RR 0.30 (0.09 to 1.02) Based on data from 90 patients in 1 study	⊕⊕☐☐ LOW[a,d]

Table 5.20. (*Continued*)

Outcome	Absolute Effect		Relative Effect (95% CI) No. of Participants & Studies	Certainty of the Evidence (GRADE)
	With Oral CHM plus HT	With HT		
Live birth rate Treatment duration: 3 m	**77 per 100** Difference: 9 more per 100 patients (95% CI: 14 fewer to 42 more per 100 patients)	**68 per 100**	RR 1.13 (0.79 to 1.61) Based on data from 48 patients in 1 study	⊕⊕⊕⊘ MODERATE[d]

Abbreviations: CHM, Chinese herbal medicine; CI, confidence intervals; HT, hormone therapy; m, months; MD, mean difference; RR, risk ratio; VAS, visual analogue scale; w, weeks; y year.
[a]High risk of bias due to lack of blinding; downgraded one level.
[b]High statistical heterogeneity in many studies; downgraded two levels.
[c]Statistical heterogeneity; downgraded one level.
[d]Small sample size; downgraded one level.

References
Dysmenorrhoea VAS: H43, H55, H64, H66, H70, H71, H77–H79, H86, H110, H113, H128, H137, H140, H141.
Pelvic pain VAS: H43, H77, H86.
Dyspareunia VAS: H43, H110.
Recurrence of endometriosis: H113.
Live birth rate: H48.

Adverse events with the combination of oral CHM and HT included 73 cases of menstrual disorders, 45 cases of menopausal symptoms such as hot flushes and night sweats, 20 cases of gastrointestinal discomfort, 19 cases of vaginal dryness, 15 cases of irregular vaginal bleeding, 12 cases of abnormal liver function, 10 cases of joint or bone pain, nine cases of sleep disorders such as insomnia, eight cases of fatigue, seven cases of nausea, four cases of mood changes, three cases of fatigue, three cases of weakness and insomnia, three cases of pruritis, two cases of acne, two cases of diarrhoea, two cases of weight gain and liver function abnormality, two cases of weight gain, two cases of loss of libido, and one case each of breast pain, dizziness, and amenorrhoea. In addition, one study reported five unspecified AEs (H149) while another reported four cases of a wide range of events (H98).

Adverse events with HT included 115 cases of menopausal symptoms such as hot flushes and night sweats, 81 cases of abnormal liver function, 81 cases of menstrual disorders, 56 cases of irregular vaginal bleeding, 37 cases of bone or joint pain, 36 cases of weight gain, 31 cases of fatigue, 27 cases of sleep disturbance, 23 cases of vaginal dryness, 12 cases of acne, 12 cases of mood changes, seven cases of gastrointestinal discomfort, six cases of loss of libido, five cases of nausea, five cases of weakness and insomnia, three cases of dizziness, three cases of weight gain and abnormal liver function, and one case each of breast pain and seborrheic dermatitis. One study documented 18 cases of unspecified AEs (H149).

Shao fu zhu yu tang 少腹逐瘀汤 plus hormone therapy versus hormone therapy

Two RCTs tested the combination of Shao fu zhu yu tang 少腹逐瘀汤 with HT (H162, H172), but neither reported usable data for the selected outcome measures. Safety was reported in one of the two studies (H162). Adverse events in the CHM plus HT group included two cases each of pruritis, hot flushes, and night sweats and one case each of vaginal bleeding, vaginal dryness, and amenorrhoea. Adverse events in the HT group were similar: two cases of night sweats, two cases of hot flushes, two cases of irregular vaginal bleeding, and one case each of vaginal dryness and gastrointestinal reactions.

Xue fu zhu yu tang 血府逐瘀汤 versus hormone therapy

One RCT that compared Xue fu zhu yu tang 血府逐瘀汤 and HT provided low certainty evidence (H160). Results showed no difference between groups in terms of the chance of cyst recurrence at an

Clinical Evidence for Chinese Herbal Medicine

Table 5.21. GRADE: *Xue fu zhu yu tang* 血府逐瘀汤 versus Hormone Therapy

Outcome	Absolute Effect		Relative Effect (95% CI) No. of Participants & Studies	Certainty of the Evidence (GRADE)
	With *Xue Fu Zhu Yu Tang* 血府逐瘀汤	With HT		
Recurrence of cyst (time NS) Treatment duration: 6 m	13 per 100 Difference: 7 fewer per 100 patients (95% CI: 16 fewer to 23 more per 100 patients)	20 per 100	RR 0.67 (0.21 to 2.13) Based on data from 60 patients in 1 study	⊕⊕☐☐ LOW[a,b]

Abbreviations: CI, confidence intervals; HT, hormone therapy; m, months; NS, not specified; RR, risk ratio.
[a]High risk of bias due to lack of blinding; downgraded one level.
[b]Small sample size; downgraded one level.

References
Recurrence of cyst: H160.

unspecified time point (Table 5.21). The study did not report on the safety of *Xue fu zhu yu tang* 血府逐瘀汤.

Xue fu zhu yu tang 血府逐瘀汤 plus hormone therapy versus hormone therapy

The combination of *Xue fu zhu yu tang* 血府逐瘀汤 plus HT was compared with HT alone in five RCTs that reported the selected outcomes (H43, H110, H137, H163, H164). Low certainty evidence showed that the combination of *Xue fu zhu yu tang* 血府逐瘀汤 plus HT resulted in a greater reduction in pelvic pain VAS score than did HT alone (low certainty evidence; Table 5.22) and reduced the likelihood of signs and symptoms recurring at the end of treatment (low certainty evidence). Results showed no benefit for the combination of CHM and HT over HT alone in reducing VAS scores for dysmenorrhoea (very low certainty evidence) and dyspareunia (very low certainty evidence) or reduction in the recurrence of signs and symptoms two years after surgery (low certainty evidence).

Table 5.22. GRADE: Xue fu zhu yu tang 血府逐瘀汤 plus Hormone Therapy versus Hormone Therapy

Outcome	Absolute Effect		Relative Effect (95% CI) No. of Participants & Studies	Certainty of the Evidence (GRADE)
	With Xue Fu Zhu Yu Tang/ Jiao Nang Plus HT	With HT		
Dysmenorrhoea VAS Treatment duration: range 3 m to 24 w	1.26 cm Average difference: 1.25 cm lower (95% CI: 2.57 cm lower to 0.08 cm higher)	2.51 cm	MD −1.25 (−2.57 to 0.08) Based on data from 206 patients in 3 studies	⊕⊝⊝⊝ VERY LOW[a,b,c]
Pelvic pain VAS Treatment duration: 24 w	0.22 cm Average difference: 0.14 cm lower (95% CI: 0.16 to 0.12 cm lower)	0.36 cm	MD −0.14 (−0.16 to −0.12) Based on data from 68 patients in 1 study	⊕⊕⊝⊝ LOW[a,c]
Dyspareunia VAS Treatment duration: 5 m to 24 w	1.11 cm Average difference: 0.68 cm lower (95% CI: 1.94 cm lower to 0.59 cm higher)	1.79 cm	MD −0.68 (−1.94 to 0.59) Based on data from 116 patients in 2 studies	⊕⊝⊝⊝ VERY LOW[a,b,c]
Recurrence of signs and symptoms at EoT Treatment duration: 3–5 m	2 per 100 Difference: 15 fewer per 100 patients (95% CI: 16 to 11 fewer per 100 patients)	17 per 100	RR 0.14 (0.05 to 0.39) Based on data from 334 patients in 2 studies	⊕⊕⊝⊝ LOW[a,c]

Recurrence of signs and symptoms 2 y after surgery	17 per 100	21 per 100	RR 0.81 (0.41 to 1.61)	⊕⊕⊟⊟ LOW[a,c]
Treatment duration: 3 m	Difference: 4 fewer per 100 patients (95% CI: 13 fewer to 13 more per 100 patients)		Based on data from 139 patients in 1 study	

Abbreviations: CI, confidence intervals; EoT, end of treatment; HT, hormone therapy; m, months; MD, mean difference; RR, risk ratio; VAS, visual analogue scale; w, weeks; y, years.
[a]High risk of bias due to lack of blinding of participants and personnel; downgraded one level.
[b]Substantial statistical heterogeneity; downgraded one level.
[c]Small sample size; downgraded one level.

References
Dysmenorrhoea VAS: H43, H110, H137.
Pelvic pain VAS: H43.
Dyspareunia VAS: H43, H110.
Recurrence of signs and symptoms at EoT: H110, H164.
Recurrence of signs and symptoms 2 y after surgery: H163.

Three of the five RCTs evaluated the safety of *Xue fu zhu yu tang* 血府逐瘀汤 plus HT (H43, H163, H164). Women who received the combination of oral CHM and HT reported fewer AEs (21 versus 96). Adverse events documented in women who received oral CHM included seven cases of abnormal liver function, seven cases of irregular vaginal bleeding, five cases of menopausal symptoms, and two cases of weight gain and abnormal liver function. Adverse events in women who received HT included 32 cases of irregular vaginal bleeding, 28 cases of hot flushes, 28 cases of abnormal liver function, five cases of menopausal symptoms, and three cases of weight gain and abnormal liver function.

Gui zhi fu ling jiao nang 桂枝茯苓胶囊 versus hormone therapy

One RCT compared *Gui zhi fu ling jiao nang* 桂枝茯苓胶囊 and HT (H14). Low certainty evidence showed that *Gui zhi fu ling jiao nang* 桂枝茯苓胶囊 did not reduce the chance of recurrence of signs and symptoms six months after surgery (Table 5.23). None of the women

Table 5.23. GRADE: *Gui zhi fu ling jiao nang* 桂枝茯苓胶囊 versus Hormone Therapy

Outcome	Absolute Effect		Relative Effect (95% CI) No. of Participants & Studies	Certainty of the Evidence (GRADE)
	With *Gui Zhi Fu Ling Jiao Nang* 桂枝茯苓胶囊	With HT		
Recurrence of signs and symptoms 6 m after surgery Treatment duration: 3 m	0 per 100 Difference: 0 more per 100 patients (95% CI: 0 to 0 fewer per 100 patients)	0 per 100	RR 3.00 (0.13 to 70.83) Based on data from 60 patients in 1 study	⊕⊕□□ LOW[a,b]

Abbreviations: CI, confidence intervals; HT, hormone therapy; m, months; RR, risk ratio.
[a]High risk of bias due to lack of blinding of participants and personnel; downgraded one level.
[b]Small sample size; downgraded one level.

References
Recurrence of signs and symptoms 6 m after surgery: H14.

in the HT group reported recurrence of signs and symptoms, and one woman in the *Gui zhi fu ling jiao nang* 桂枝茯苓胶囊 group reported recurrence. Adverse events in the treatment group were eight cases of hot flushes, seven cases of irregular vaginal bleeding, and four cases each of abnormal liver function and amenorrhoea. Adverse events in the HT group were 16 cases of irregular vaginal bleeding, 15 cases of hot flushes, 11 cases of amenorrhoea, and five cases of abnormal liver function.

Gui zhi fu ling jiao nang 桂枝茯苓胶囊 *plus hormone therapy versus hormone therapy*

Two RCTs that tested the combination of *Gui zhi fu ling jiao nang* 桂枝茯苓胶囊 plus HT reported on important clinical outcomes (H92, H108). Low certainty evidence showed that the combination of *Gui zhi fu ling jiao nang* 桂枝茯苓胶囊 plus HT reduced the chance of signs and symptoms recurring two years after treatment (Table 5.24), but did not reduce the chance of cyst recurrence one year after surgery. Neither study reported on safety.

Randomised controlled trial evidence for individual oral formulas

For several outcomes, meta-analysis could be conducted to determine the effectiveness of specific oral CHM formulas: *Dan leng fu kang jian gao* 丹棱妇康煎膏, *Xue fu zhu yu jiao nang/tang* 血府逐瘀胶囊/汤, *San jie zhen tong jiao nang* 散结镇痛胶囊, and *Luo shi nei yi fang* 罗氏内异方. Neither *Dan leng fu kang jian gao* 丹棱妇康煎膏 nor *Xue fu zhu yu jiao nang/tang* 血府逐瘀胶囊/汤 reduced the mean dysmenorrhoea VAS score when combined with pharmacotherapy, compared with pharmacotherapy alone (Table 5.25).

When dysmenorrhoea was measured using the 1993 Guideline, the combination of *Dan leng fu kang jian gao* 丹棱妇康煎膏 and pharmacotherapy resulted in a mean score that was 3.36 points lower than that of pharmacotherapy alone (3 RCTs, 406 women, MD −3.36 [−4.52, −2.20], $I^2 = 93\%$; H112, H114, H115).

Table 5.24. GRADE: *Gui zhi fu ling jiao nang* 桂枝茯苓胶囊 plus Hormone Therapy versus Hormone Therapy

Outcome	Absolute Effect		Relative Effect (95% CI) No. of Participants & Studies	Certainty of the Evidence (GRADE)
	With *Gui Zhi Fu Ling Jiao Nang* plus HT	With HT		
Recurrence of cyst 1 y after surgery Treatment duration: 6 m	10 per 100 Difference: 9 fewer per 100 patients (95% CI: 16 fewer to 10 more per 100 patients)	19 per 100	RR 0.50 (0.16 to 1.53) Based on data from 84 patients in 1 study	⊕⊕?? LOW[a,b]
Recurrence of signs and symptoms 2 y after treatment Treatment duration: 4 m	7 per 100 Difference: 17 fewer per 100 patients (95% CI: 22 to 2 fewer per 100 patients)	24 per 100	RR 0.28 (0.08 to 0.93) Based on data from 76 patients in 1 study	⊕⊕?? LOW[a,b]

Abbreviations: CI, confidence intervals; HT, hormone therapy; m, months; RR, risk ratio; y, years.
[a]High risk of bias due to lack of blinding of participants and personnel; downgraded one level.
[b]Small sample size; downgraded one level.

References
Recurrence of cyst: H92.
Recurrence of signs and symptoms: H108.

Table 5.25. Oral CHM Formulas plus Pharmacotherapy versus Pharmacotherapy for Endometriosis: Dysmenorrhoea Visual Analogue Scale

Formula	No. of Studies (Participants)	Effect Size MD [95% CI], I^2	Included Studies
Dan leng fu kang jian gao 丹棱妇康煎膏	2 (210)	−2.28 [−5.35, 0.78], 100%	H71, H113
Xue fu zhu yu jiao nang/ tang 血府逐瘀胶囊/汤	3 (206)	−1.25 [−2.57, 0.08], 100%	H43, H110, H137

*Statistically significant, see Statistical Analysis in Chapter 4.
Abbreviations: CI, confidence intervals; MD, mean difference.

San jie zhen tong jiao nang 散结镇痛胶囊 appeared beneficial in preventing recurrence of signs and symptoms two years after treatment when compared with:

- No treatment (2 RCTs, 139 women, RR 0.35 [0.18, 0.66], $I^2 = 0\%$; H12, H16);
- HT (2 RCTs, 144 women, RR 1.03 [0.44, 2.37], $I^2 = 0\%$; H12, H16).

Meta-analyses of individual formulas were also possible for pregnancy outcomes. *San jie zhen tong jiao nang* 散结镇痛胶囊 was equally as effective as gestrinone in terms of the number of confirmed pregnancies (2 RCTs, 70 women, RR 1.34 [0.83, 2.14], $I^2 = 0\%$; H12, H105). *Luo shi nei yi fang* 罗氏内异方 was not statistically different from pharmacotherapy in reducing the chance of miscarriage (2 RCTs, 29 women, RR 0.39 [0.08, 1.98], $I^2 = 0\%$; H39, H40).

Frequently reported orally used herbs in meta-analyses showing favourable effect

For several outcomes, meta-analyses showed positive effects of oral CHM, both when alone or combined with pharmacotherapy. To identify the herbs that may contribute to these positive treatment effects, we calculated the most frequently used herbs in studies that were included in the meta-analyses.

Analyses were conducted according to outcome category; for example, meta-analyses that showed benefits with oral CHM for dysmenorrhoea as assessed with the VAS, 1993 Guideline, or any other outcome measure were grouped in the category 'dysmenorrhoea'. Categories were: dysmenorrhoea, pelvic pain, dyspareunia, recurrence, pregnancy outcomes, sonographic outcome measurements (ovarian cyst size and uterine volume), menstrual changes, health-related quality of life, and HT side effects (including the KI and bone density).

For most outcomes, calculations were based on results for between-group comparisons at the end of treatment; however, exceptions were made for recurrence and pregnancy outcomes. Many studies tested the effectiveness of oral CHM in preventing recurrence which, by necessity, required follow-up beyond the end of treatment. The rate of miscarriage and live births could only be feasibly assessed at follow-up. As meta-analyses did not show superiority of oral CHM for pelvic pain, dyspareunia, menstrual changes, and HT side effects, analyses of herbs were not undertaken for these categories.

Five meta-analyses, including 57 RCTs, showed greater benefits with oral CHM than with comparators for dysmenorrhoea. Herbs that were frequently used included *dang gui* 当归, *e zhu* 莪术, *gan cao* 甘草, and *yan hu suo* 延胡索 (Table 5.26). With the exception of *yan hu suo* 延胡索, the most frequently used herbs in positive meta-analyses for dysmenorrhoea were also found in the overall pool (see Table 5.2), suggesting that the treatments used for dysmenorrhoea were reflective of treatments used in all studies. These herbs may

Table 5.26. Frequently Reported Orally Used Herbs in Meta-Analyses Showing Favourable Effect for Dysmenorrhoea

Herbs	Scientific Name	Frequency of Use
Dang gui 当归	*Angelica sinensis* (Oliv.) Diels	36
E zhu 莪术	*Curcuma* spp.	31
Gan cao 甘草	*Glycyrrhiza* spp.	27
Yan hu suo 延胡索	*Corydalis yanhusuo* W.T. Wang	27
Chi shao 赤芍	*Paeonia* spp.	25
San leng 三棱	*Sparganium stoloniferum* Buch. -Ham.	25
Chuan xiong 川芎	*Ligusticum chuangxiong* Hort.	21
Xiang fu 香附	*Cyperus rotundus* L.	21
Dan shen 丹参	*Salvia miltiorrhiza* Bge.	20
Tao ren 桃仁	*Prunus* spp.	17

For details of meta-analyses, see Tables 5.4, 5.5, and 5.7 and the following sections of Dysmenorrhoea: 'Oral Chinese herbal medicine versus no treatment' and 'Oral Chinese herbal medicine plus pharmacotherapy versus pharmacotherapy'.

Note: The use of some herbs may be restricted in some countries. Readers are advised to comply with relevant regulations.

have contributed to the positive results shown in meta-analyses, and practitioners may consider formulas that include these herbs for women with endometriosis who also report dysmenorrhoea.

Among the 12 meta-analyses and 39 RCTs that showed favourable effects of oral CHM for the prevention of recurrence, studies included in these analyses used 110 different herbs. The most frequently used herbs were *dang gui*当归, *e zhu* 莪术, and *tao ren* 桃仁 (Table 5.27). Many of the frequently used herbs were also seen in studies that contributed to reductions in dysmenorrhoea, albeit with lower frequency in studies that documented recurrence.

Fewer studies were included in meta-analyses of pregnancy outcomes. Four meta-analyses involving 18 RCTs showed benefits with oral CHM in improving the pregnancy rate and reducing the miscarriage rate. The most frequently used herbs in studies included in these meta-analyses were *dang gui* 当归 and *yan hu suo* 延胡索 (Table 5.28). These herbs may contribute to positive pregnancy outcomes, although the frequency of use for all herbs was limited by the number of studies included in the analyses. Practitioners should use their

Table 5.27. Frequently Reported Orally Used Herbs in Meta-Analyses Showing Favourable Effect for Recurrence

Herbs	Scientific Name	Frequency of Use
Dang gui 当归	*Angelica sinensis* (Oliv.) Diels	21
E zhu 莪术	*Curcuma* spp.	20
Tao ren 桃仁	*Prunus* spp.	20
Dan shen 丹参	*Salvia miltiorrhiza* Bge.	19
San leng 三棱	*Sparganium stoloniferum* Buch. -Ham.	17
Gan cao 甘草	*Glycyrrhiza* spp.	16
Chi shao 赤芍	*Paeonia* spp.	15
Xiang fu 香附	*Cyperus rotundus* L.	15
Yan hu suo 延胡索	*Corydalis yanhusuo* W.T. Wang	14
Tu si zi 菟丝子	*Cuscuta* spp.	13

For details of meta-analyses, see Tables 5.8, 5.9, and 5.10.
Note: The use of some herbs may be restricted in some countries. Readers are advised to comply with relevant regulations.

Table 5.28. Frequently Reported Orally Used Herbs in Meta-Analyses Showing Favourable Effect for Pregnancy Outcomes

Herbs	Scientific Name	Frequency of Use
Dang gui 当归	Angelica sinensis (Oliv.) Diels	10
Yan hu suo 延胡索	Corydalis yanhusuo W.T. Wang	9
Bai shao 白芍	Paeonia lactiflora Pall.	8
Dan shen 丹参	Salvia miltiorrhiza Bge.	8
Pu huang 蒲黄	Typha spp.	8
Tu si zi 菟丝子	Cuscuta spp.	8
Wu ling zhi 五灵脂	Trogopterus xanthipes Milne-Edwards	8
Shu di huang 熟地黄	Rehmannia glutinosa Libosch.	7
Xiang fu 香附	Cyperus rotundus L.	7

For details of meta-analyses, see Tables 5.12, 5.13, and 5.14.
Note: The use of some herbs may be restricted in some countries. Readers are advised to comply with relevant regulations.

Table 5.29. Frequently Reported Orally Used Herbs in Meta-Analyses Showing Favourable Effect for Sonographic Measures

Herbs	Scientific Name	Frequency of Use
Dang shen 党参	Codonopsis spp.	5
Dang gui 当归	Angelica sinensis (Oliv.) Diels	4
E zhu 莪术	Curcuma spp.	4
Huang qi 黄芪	Astragalus spp.	4

For details of meta-analyses, see the following sections of Ovarian cyst size: 'Oral Chinese herbal medicine versus placebo' and 'Oral Chinese herbal medicine plus hormone therapy versus hormone therapy'.
Note: The use of some herbs may be restricted in some countries. Readers are advised to comply with relevant regulations.

clinical judgement when prescribing formulas for women who wish to conceive.

Fewer studies documented sonographic measures (two meta-analyses with eight RCTs) and health-related quality of life (five meta-analyses with six RCTs) compared with dysmenorrhoea. *Dang shen* 党参 was the most frequently used herb in studies that showed benefits for reducing ovarian cyst size and uterine volume (Table 5.29),

Table 5.30. Frequently Reported Orally Used Herbs in Meta-Analyses Showing Favourable Effect for Health-related Quality of Life

Herbs	Scientific Name	Frequency of Use
Chi shao 赤芍	Paeonia spp.	5
E zhu 莪术	Curcuma spp.	4
Dan shen 丹参	Salvia miltiorrhiza Bge.	3
Mu dan pi 牡丹皮	Paeonia suffruticosa Andr.	3
Tao ren 桃仁	Prunus spp.	3

For details of meta-analyses, see Tables 5.16 and 5.17 and the following section of Health-related quality of life: 'Oral Chinese herbal medicine versus hormone therapy'.
Note: The use of some herbs may be restricted in some countries. Readers are advised to comply with relevant regulations.

while *chi shao* 赤芍 was the most frequently used herb in studies that showed benefits in improving health-related quality of life (Table 5.30). While it is possible that these herbs may be beneficial in reducing cyst size and uterine volume and improving health-related quality of life, the small number of studies and meta-analyses limits certainty. Practitioners may consider using these herbs when appropriate for each individual's CM syndrome diagnosis.

Safety of oral Chinese herbal medicine in randomised controlled trials

Ninety-six RCTs reported on the safety of oral CHM (H1, H6–H14, H16, H22–H25, H27, H30, H33–H35, H37, H40, H43–H45, H49–H53, H55, H56, H58, H60, H61, H64–H66, H70, H75, H76, H81–H83, H85, H86, H90, H93, H94, H96–H99, H101, H102, H104–H107, H113–H115, H118, H119, H121, H128–H132, H136, H138–H140, H143, H145, H146, H148–H152, H154–H157, H162–H170, H173). Many of these studies compared oral CHM with HT; the AEs in these studies have been described (see the sections on 'Assessment using Grading of Recommendations Assessment, Development and Evaluation' subsections 'Oral Chinese herbal medicine versus placebo', 'Oral Chinese herbal medicine versus hormone therapy', and 'Oral Chinese herbal medicine plus hormone therapy versus hormone therapy').

Two RCTs that compared oral CHM with non-HT treatments reported on safety (H13, H121). No AEs were reported in either group when oral CHM was compared to ibuprofen (H13). In one RCT (H121), AEs with oral CHM included eight cases of irregular vaginal bleeding, eight cases of vasomotor symptoms, six cases of insomnia, six cases of vaginal dryness, and five cases of constipation. In the same study, AEs among women who received unspecified conventional therapy included 25 cases of vasomotor symptoms, 22 cases of irregular vaginal bleeding, 20 cases of vaginal dryness, 18 cases of insomnia, and 16 cases of constipation.

Thirteen RCTs that compared oral CHM with no treatment reported on safety (H7–H9, H11, H12, H14, H16, H22, H24, H25, H45, H168, H152), of which five reported that no AEs occurred in either group (H7, H8, H11, H45, H152). Not surprisingly, more AEs were reported in women who received treatment than in women who did not. Adverse events with oral CHM included 25 cases of irregular vaginal bleeding, 15 cases of gastrointestinal reactions, 10 cases of breast tenderness, eight cases of hot flushes, six cases of weight gain, five cases of abnormal liver function, four cases of amenorrhoea, and one case of rash. In addition, three cases of various AEs were reported, including pruritus, fever, dizziness, and gastrointestinal discomfort. One study documented AEs among women who received no treatment (H14), which included eight cases of irregular vaginal bleeding, five cases of hot flushes, and three cases of amenorrhoea.

Controlled Clinical Trials of Oral Chinese Herbal Medicine for Endometriosis

Oral CHM was evaluated in 27 CCTs involving 2,668 women (H176–H202). All studies were conducted in China, with women recruited from hospital inpatient or outpatient departments; however, many studies did not specify the study setting. Six CCTs included three study arms (H176, H178, H181, H183, H185, H200). Some included two control arms (HT in one and no treatment in the other), while others included two treatment arms (CHM alone in one and CHM plus HT in the other).

All studies that assessed the duration of endometriosis reported a mean duration of fewer than 10 years. Women in 17 studies had undergone surgery prior to enrolling in the study (H176, H177, H179, H181–H185, H187, H188, H190–H192, H197, H199, H201, H202), and laparoscopy was used for diagnosis in 14 of these studies. The rASRM stage was reported in 14 studies; six included women with stage II or III endometriosis (H176, H185, H190, H192, H201, H202), three included women with stage II, III, or IV endometriosis (H184, H186, H199), and five included women of all rASRM stages (H177, H181, H182, H188, H198). Two studies included only women with endometriosis-related infertility (H182, H197).

Five CCTs documented CM syndromes (H181, H189, H194, H195, H197). Two syndromes were described in two CCTs: cold coagulation with Blood stasis and Kidney deficiency with Blood stasis. Other syndromes included internal phlegm-damp, Blood stasis, *qi* stagnation with Blood stasis, Liver stagnation alone or with Blood deficiency, and the combination of phlegm-dampness with Blood stasis.

Treatment was provided for between three and six months, and most studies conducted follow-up assessment for up to three years. Two CCTs reported loss to follow-up (H178, H195). Seven studies tailored oral CHM according to the time of the menstrual cycle (H178, H180–H183, H197, H202), which involved either adding to and/or removing herbs from a base formula or using a new formula for each phase of the menstrual cycle. Three traditional formulas or manufactured products were common to two CCTs: *Fu fang e zhu san* 复方莪术散 (H185, H186), *Gui zhi fu ling jiao nang* 桂枝茯苓胶囊 (H176, H198), and *San jie zhen tong jiao nang* 散结镇痛胶囊 (H188, H199; Table 5.31). The most frequently used herbs in oral CHM formulas are described in Table 5.32. The most frequently used herbs were *bai shao* 白芍, *yan huo suo* 延胡索, *dang gui* 当归, *huang qi* 黄芪, and *chi shao* 赤芍.

Nine studies tested the combination of oral CHM and pharmacotherapy (H177, H179, H180, H185, H190, H193, H197, H198, H200), most of which used HT. Comparators included no treatment (H176, H181–H183, H192), menstrual pain relief (H193), and HT.

Table 5.31. Frequently Reported Oral Formulas in Controlled Clinical Trials

Most Common Formulas	No. of Studies	Ingredients
Fu fang e zhu san 复方莪术散	2	San leng 三棱, e zhu 莪术, yin yang huo 淫羊藿, huang qi 黄芪, yan hu suo 延胡索 (H185, H186)
Gui zhi fu ling jiao nang 桂枝茯苓胶囊	2	Gui zhi 桂枝, fu ling 茯苓, tao ren 桃仁, dan pi 丹皮, chi shao 赤芍 (H176, H198)
San jie zhen tong jiao nang 散结镇痛胶囊	2	Long xue jie 龙血竭, san qi 三七, zhe bei mu 浙贝母, yi yi ren 薏苡仁 (H188, H199)

Note: the use of some herbs may be restricted in some countries. Readers are advised to comply with relevant regulations.

Table 5.32. Frequently Reported Orally Used Herbs in Controlled Clinical Trials

Most Common Herbs	Scientific Name	Frequency of Use
Bai shao 白芍	Paeonia lactiflora Pall.	13
Yan hu suo 延胡索	Corydalis yanhusuo W.T. Wang	12
Dang gui 当归	Angelica sinensis (Oliv.) Diels	11
Huang qi 黄芪	Astragalus membranaceus (Fisch.) Bge.	11
Chi shao 赤芍	Paeonia spp.	10
E zhu 莪术	Curcuma spp.	9
Shu di huang 熟地黄	Rehmannia glutinosa Libosch.	9
Chuan xiong 川芎	Ligusticum chuangxiong Hort.	8
San leng 三棱	Sparganium stoloniferum Buch. -Ham.	8
Tao ren 桃仁	Prunus spp.	8
Dan shen 丹参	Salvia miltiorrhiza Bge.	7
Gan cao 甘草	Glycyrrhiza spp.	6
Gui zhi 桂枝	Cinnamomum cassia Presl	6
Shan zhu yu 山茱萸	Cornus officinalis Sieb. et Zucc.	6
Xiang fu 香附	Cyperus rotundus L.	6
Yin yang huo 淫羊藿	Epimedium spp.	6
Ba ji tian 巴戟天	Morinda officinalis How	5
Wu ling zhi 五灵脂	Trogopterus xanthipes Milne-Edwards	5
Xue jie 血竭	Daemonorops draco Bl.	5

Note: the use of some herbs may be restricted in some countries. Readers are advised to comply with relevant regulations.

Outcomes

Recurrence was the most frequently documented clinical outcome measure, which was reported in 17 CCTs (H176, H177, H179, H181–H188, H190, H192, H199, H200–H202). Thirteen studies documented dysmenorrhoea (H179, H181, H183, H185, H186, H189, H191, H193–H196, H198, H202); however, data for two studies could not be re-analysed (H181, H185). Five studies reported ovarian cyst size (H178, H180, H195, H196, H198); four of these were included in the analyses.

Two CCTs documented dyspareunia (H191, H196) and one study each reported pelvic pain (H191) and uterine volume (H196). Both studies that included women with endometriosis-related infertility reported on pregnancy outcomes (H182, H197). None of the studies reported on changes in menstrual volume, fatigue, or health-related quality of life. Seventeen CCTs reported on the safety of oral CHM.

Dysmenorrhoea

Results for assessments of dysmenorrhoea were analysed for 11 CCTs (H179, H183, H185, H186, H189, H191, H193–H196, H202). Studies assessed dysmenorrhoea using a 10 cm VAS, the 1993 Guideline, or the simplified McGill Pain Questionnaire (MPQ).[37] Meta-analyses were conducted where possible and results are presented according to the comparison.

Oral Chinese herbal medicine versus no treatment

One CCT (H183) that compared cycle-specific oral CHM with no treatment found a lower mean score on the 1993 Guideline at the end of treatment with oral CHM than with no treatment (34 women, MD −3.10 points [−4.21, −1.99]). While dysmenorrhoea scores were lower, the same study found no difference in the number of women with dysmenorrhoea at the end of treatment (34 women, RR 0.44 [0.14, 1.33]).

Oral Chinese herbal medicine versus pharmacotherapy

Meta-analysis was conducted for four studies that assessed dysmenorrhoea using the 1993 Guideline (H189, H194, H195, H202). Oral CHM was not statistically different from HT in reducing dysmenorrhoea scores at the end of treatment (276 women, MD 0.07 points [−0.39, 0.53], I^2 = 27%). Results for other studies could not be pooled in meta-analyses, and results are presented for individual studies.

One CCT, involving 92 women, assessed dysmenorrhoea using a 10 cm VAS (H186). Women who received *Fu fang e zhu san* 复方莪术散 scored lower on the VAS than women who received diphereline (MD −0.43 cm [−0.64, −0.22]). A similar finding was seen when the effects of *Dang gui si ni tang* 当归四逆汤 were measured using the simplified MPQ; women who received *Dang gui si ni tang* 当归四逆汤 scored 2.16 points lower at the end of treatment than women who received gestrinone (74 women, [−2.76, −1.56]; H191). Another oral CHM formula, *Yi wei kang chong ji* 异位康冲剂, did not significantly reduce the number of women with dysmenorrhoea at the end of treatment compared to danazol (100 women, RR 1.33 [0.50, 3.56]; H196).

Oral Chinese herbal medicine plus pharmacotherapy versus pharmacotherapy

Meta-analysis of two studies showed that combining oral CHM with HT was more effective than HT alone in reducing pain scores on a 10 cm VAS (200 women, MD −1.44 cm [−1.61, −1.27], I^2 = 27%; H179, H198). When dysmenorrhoea was assessed using the 1993 Guideline, the mean score at the end of treatment was also lower among women who received oral CHM plus pain relief compared to women who received pain relief alone (150 women, MD −3.02 points [−3.80, −2.24]; H193).

Pelvic pain

Results from one CCT showed no difference in the number of women with pelvic pain at the end of treatment between women who received *Dang gui si ni tang* 当归四逆汤 and those who received gestrinone (74 women, RR 0.25 [0.06, 1.10]; H191).

Dyspareunia

Two CCTs (H191, H196) assessed the number of women with dyspareunia at the end of treatment, and results from both were pooled for meta-analysis. Women who received oral CHM alone were no more or less likely to have dyspareunia at the end of treatment than women who received HT (174 women, RR 0.72 [0.24, 2.17], I^2 = 25%).

Recurrence

Studies that assessed recurrence did so in a variety of ways and at different time points. The decision was made to keep results separate for analyses where different criteria were used to assess recurrence.

Oral Chinese herbal medicine versus no treatment

Meta-analysis was conducted with two CCTs that assessed the recurrence of signs and symptoms at the end of treatment and at two follow-up assessments (H182, H183). The chance of recurrence at the end of treatment was not statistically different between the groups (450 women, RR 0.16 [0.02, 1.39], I^2 = not estimable). This finding primarily represents the study by Zhang (2016; H182), as the second study reported that no recurrence occurred in either group; hence, statistical heterogeneity could not be calculated. When recurrence of signs and symptoms was assessed six months after the end of treatment, women who received oral CHM had a lower chance of recurrence than women who received no treatment (450 women, RR 0.21 [0.11, 0.42]). One study that assessed recurrence of signs and symptoms 12 months after the end of treatment found no difference between the groups (43 women, RR 0.46 [0.10, 2.12]; H192).

Among individual studies, the chance of pain recurrence, assessed six months after the end of treatment, was lower among women who received *Jing tong yu shu fang* 经痛愈舒方 than among those who received no treatment (28 women, RR 0.19 [0.05, 0.75]; H181). In the same study, the chance of cyst recurrence was also lower among women who received oral CHM (28 women, RR 0.11 [0.01, 0.82]). Two studies assessed recurrence of signs and symptoms at different time points. Nine months after the end of treatment, women who received oral CHM treatment tailored to the menstrual cycle were less likely to have recurrence of signs and symptoms (81 women, RR 0.91 [0.31, 2.70]; H184). No such benefit was seen when recurrence was assessed between one and three years after the end of treatment (81 women, RR 0.65 [0.11, 3.69]; H176).

Oral Chinese herbal medicine versus hormone therapy

Analysis of two studies that assessed the recurrence of signs and symptoms at the end of treatment showed no statistical difference between those who received oral CHM and those who received HT (122 women, RR 1.23 [0.35, 4.30]; H185, H199). Results for individual studies showed no benefit of oral CHM over HT when recurrence of signs and symptoms was assessed at:

- Six months (45 women, RR 1.25 [0.27, 5.70]; H202);
- Twelve months (84 women, RR 0.65 [0.22, 1.88]; H187);
- Two years (116 women, RR 0.91 [0.31, 2.70]; H184);
- Between one and three years (83 women, RR 1.28 [0.37, 4.44]; H176);
- At a mean of 25 months after the end of treatment (89 women, RR 0.68 [0.04, 10.51]; H185).

Other studies determined recurrence based on specific criteria. No statistical difference was seen between an unspecified oral CHM formula and goserelin in the chance of recurrence of endometriosis after six months (65 women, RR 1.10 [0.07, 16.80]; H201) or 12 months (65 women, RR 0.91 [0.31, 2.70]; H201). The chance of pain recurrence was not different between women who received *Jing tong yu shu fang* 经痛愈舒方 and those who received leuprolin (28 women, RR 0.63 [0.12, 3.32]; H181).

Similar findings were seen for recurrence of cysts. There was no statistical difference in the chance of cyst recurrence six months after the end of treatment when *Jing tong yu shu fang* 经痛愈舒方 was compared with leuprolin (28 women, RR 0.56 [0.04, 7.96]; H181). Finally, the chance of cyst recurrence between 14 and 25 months was not different between *San jie zhen tong jiao nang* 散结镇痛胶囊 and gestrinone (140 women, RR 0.40 [0.06, 2.74]; H188).

Oral Chinese herbal medicine plus hormone therapy versus hormone therapy

The chance of recurrence of signs and symptoms was not lower among women who received oral CHM plus HT compared with those who received HT alone (122 women, RR 0.17 [0.02, 1.30], I^2 = not estimable; H177, H185). As one of the two studies in this meta-analysis reported no recurrence in either group (H185), this result essentially represents the result of the second study. Results from single studies showed no difference between groups when recurrence of signs and symptoms was assessed one year after the end of treatment (80 women, RR 0.14 [0.02, 1.11]; H179), but a lower chance of recurrence of signs and symptoms three years after surgery among women who received the combination of *Fu zheng xiao yi tang* 扶正消异方 and goserelin, compared with goserelin alone (60 women, RR 0.08 [0.01, 0.60]; H177). One study that assessed recurrence of signs and symptoms at a mean of 25 months after the end of treatment showed no benefit of adding *Fu fang e zhu san* 复方莪术散 to triptorelin (62 women, RR 0.46 [0.02, 10.79]; H185). A final study that tested the combination of *Nuan gong qi wei wan* 暖宫七味丸 and menstrual pain relief found no difference compared to menstrual pain relief alone in reducing the recurrence of cysts one year after the end of treatment (62 women, RR 0.24 [0.05, 1.04]; H190).

Pregnancy outcomes

Pregnancy outcomes were reported in two CCTs (H182, H197). As different comparisons were made across the studies, results were analysed separately.

Oral Chinese herbal medicine versus no treatment

Women who received *Bu shen huo xue fang* 补肾活血方, modified according to the phase of the menstrual cycle, had a higher pregnancy rate than women who received no treatment (416 women, RR 1.73 [1.34, 2.23]; H182). In the same study, the miscarriage rate was not statistically different between the groups (188 women, RR 0.41 [0.16, 1.08]).

Oral Chinese herbal medicine plus hormone therapy versus hormone therapy

The second study that assessed pregnancy outcomes tailored CHM treatment according to the phase of the menstrual cycle (H197). In this study, there was no difference between groups in the pregnancy rate (62 women, RR 1.22 [0.84, 1.78]) or miscarriage rate (62 women, RR 0.17 [0.01, 3.24]). The live birth rate was, however, higher among women who received tailored CHM treatment, letrozole, and triptorelin than in women who received letrozole plus triptorelin alone (62 women, RR 1.43 [1.02, 2.01]).

Ovarian cyst size

Among the four CCTs that assessed ovarian cyst size, two tested the same comparison and used the same method for calculating cyst size; these two studies were pooled for analysis. Results are reported according to comparisons.

Oral Chinese herbal medicine versus hormone therapy

Results from one CCT showed that the cyst area was not statistically different between women who received *Wen shen xiao zheng tang* 温肾消癥汤 and those who received mifepristone (50 women, MD −0.24 cm^2 [−2.45, 1.97]; H195). In a second study, there was no difference in cyst volume between *Yi wei kang chong ji* 异位康冲剂 and danazol (100 women, MD −0.80 cm^3 [−2.18, 0.58]; H196).

Oral Chinese herbal medicine plus hormone therapy versus hormone therapy

Meta-analysis of two CCTs found that the combination of oral CHM plus HT reduced the diameter of ovarian cysts by 0.61 cm (196 women, [−1.09, −0.12], I^2 = 81%; H180, H198). Considerable statistical heterogeneity lowers confidence in the results.

Uterine volume

Uterine volume was measured in one study of 100 women (H196). There was no difference in uterine volume between women who received Yi wei kang chong ji 异位康冲剂 and those who received danazol (MD −0.07 cm^3 [−1.91, 1.77]).

Safety of oral Chinese herbal medicine in controlled clinical trials

The safety of oral CHM was reported in 17 CCTs (H176, H178, H181, H182, H184–H188, H194–H196, H198–H202), three of which reported that no AEs occurred (H181, H198, H201). Among women who received oral CHM alone, AEs included 32 cases of gastrointestinal reactions such as nausea, vomiting, diarrhoea, and constipation, eight cases of weight gain, seven cases of hot flushes, five cases of irregular vaginal bleeding, two cases of rash, two cases of increased hair growth and acne, and one case each of amenorrhoea, abnormal liver function, vaginal dryness, irritability, and fatigue. In addition, an unspecified number of events were reported in two studies, which included loss of taste, unpleasant smell, haemorrhoids, mild gastrointestinal discomfort and diarrhoea, increased menstrual flow, and irregular vaginal bleeding.

Adverse events in two studies (H185, H200) that combined oral CHM with HT included 23 cases of gastrointestinal and menopausal symptoms and 11 cases of mild nausea, loss of appetite, and upper abdominal discomfort. Among women in the control groups who received pharmacotherapy, AEs included 94 cases of menopausal/

low oestrogen symptoms such as hot flushes, 76 cases of amenorrhoea, 41 cases of irregular vaginal bleeding, 37 cases of abnormal liver function, 35 cases of weight gain, 22 cases of increased hair growth and acne, 15 cases of vaginal dryness, hot flushes, and insomnia, seven cases of irritability, five cases of nausea, five cases of vaginal dryness, four cases of insomnia, three cases of vomiting, three cases of fatigue, two cases of acne, two cases of early pregnancy symptoms, two cases of decrease in breast size, two cases of palpitations, and one case each of weight loss and osteoporosis. In addition, there were 26 cases of various combinations of AEs, including vaginal dryness, muscle cramps, oedema, hot flushes, amenorrhoea and others, and an unspecified number of cases of amenorrhoea, hot flushes, night sweats, vaginal dryness, and emotional changes.

Non-controlled Studies of Oral Chinese Herbal Medicine for Endometriosis

Oral CHM was tested in 1,267 women in 53 non-controlled studies (H203–H255). One case report was from Korea (H255), one prospective observational study was conducted in Hong Kong (H254), and remaining studies were either case series or case reports from mainland China. Women in 10 studies had surgery prior to enrolling (H206–H209, H212, H215, H216, H219, H222, H237), six studies focused on women with endometriosis-related infertility (H205, H217, H219, H228, H245, H252), and two studies examined the role of oral CHM in adolescents with endometriosis (H219, H226). Participants had lived with endometriosis for between one month (H246) and 38 years (H253). Diagnosis was confirmed by laparoscopy in three studies (H216, H237, H253); one of these studies reported that women had rASRM stage II or III endometriosis (H216).

Forty-four studies documented CM syndromes, which were either used as an inclusion criterion or to guide treatment (H203, H205–H210, H212–H218, H220–H232, H234–H242, H244–H249, H251, H252). The most frequently reported syndromes included Kidney deficiency and Blood stasis (11 studies), *qi* stagnation and Blood stasis (10 studies), cold coagulation and Blood stasis (seven studies), Kidney *yang* deficiency (four studies), and Blood stasis with phlegm (four studies). Treatment with oral CHM was provided for as little as one month (H236), while others provided treatment for up to one year (H219, H253). Close to half of the studies (24 of 53, 45%) prescribed oral CHM for three months. Follow-up assessments ranged from one week (H207) to four years (H218) after the end of treatment.

Nineteen studies adapted treatments according to the time of the menstrual cycle (H206, H222–H224, H226, H227, H229, H232, H234, H235, H239, H243–H245, H248–H252), and many more used investigator-developed formulas. Among traditional CHM formulas, only six were tested in multiple studies; *Gui zhi fu ling jiao nang/wan* 桂枝茯苓胶囊/丸 was used in three studies (Table 5.33).

For studies that used different oral CHM formulas during different times of the menstrual cycle, herbs used in each formula were counted once. This meant that any given herb may have been counted twice or more from one study in herb frequency analyses.

Table 5.33. Frequently Reported Oral Formulas in Non-controlled Studies

Most Common Formulas	No. of Studies	Ingredients
Gui zhi fu ling jiao nang/ wan 桂枝茯苓胶囊/丸	3	*Gui zhi* 桂枝, *fu ling* 茯苓, *mu dan* 牡丹, *tao ren* 桃仁, *shao yao* 芍药
Dan chi yin 丹赤饮	2	*Chai hu* 柴胡, *chi shao* 赤芍, *e zhu* 莪术, *wu ling zhi* 五灵脂, *can shen* 参审 (H213); *chai hu* 柴胡, *chi shao* 赤芍, *e zhu* 莪术, *dan shen* 丹参, *zao jiao ci* 皂角刺, *zhi xiang fu* 制香附 (H245)
Hua yu xiao zheng fang 化瘀消癥方	2	*Dang shen* 党参, *san leng* 三棱, *dan shen* 丹参, *zhe bei mu* 浙贝母 (H227); *chao lu dang* 炒潞党, *sheng huang qi* 生黄芪, *fu ling* 茯苓, *gui zhi* 桂枝, *chi shao* 赤芍, *dan pi* 丹皮, *tao ren* 桃仁, *zao jiao ci* 皂角刺, *zhi bie jia* 炙鳖甲 (H243)

(*Continued*)

Table 5.33. (*Continued*)

Most Common Formulas	No. of Studies	Ingredients
Hua yu zhi tong fang 化瘀止痛方	2	*Dang gui* 当归, *chuan xiong* 川芎, *yan hu suo* 延胡索, *wu ling zhi* 五灵脂, *xue jie* 血竭 (H227); *chao dang gui* 炒当归, *dan shen* 丹参, *chi shao* 赤芍, *chuan niu xi* 川牛膝, *zhi xiang fu* 制香附, *yan hu suo* 延胡索, *zhi mo yao* 制没药, *sheng pu huang* 生蒲黄, *hua rui shi* 花蕊石 (H243)
Nei yi 2 hao fang 内异2号方	2	*Zhi ke* 枳壳, *wu yao* 乌药, *pu huang* 蒲黄, *wu ling zhi* 五灵脂, *yi mu cao* 益母草, *qian cao gen* 茜草根, *yan hu suo* 延胡索, *bai shao* 白芍, *xiang fu* 香附, *gan cao* 甘草 (H244); *fu ling* 茯苓, *gui zhi* 桂枝, *chi shao* 赤芍, *dan pi* 丹皮, *tao ren* 桃仁, *xia ku cao* 夏枯草, *zao jiao ci* 皂角刺, *zhi jia pian* 炙甲片, *lu lu tong* 路路通, *xiang ling pi* 仙灵脾, *chao du zhong* 炒杜仲, *bai ji rou* 巴戟肉 (H222)
Yi qi huo xue fang 益气活血方	2	*Sheng huang qi* 生黄芪, *dang shen* 党参, *shui zhi* 水蛭, *san leng* 三棱, *e zhu* 莪术 (H241); *dang shen* 党参, *chao bai zhu* 炒白术, *huang qi* 黄芪, *chuan niu xi* 川牛膝, *san leng* 三棱, *e zhu* 莪术, *jiu xiang chong* 九香虫, *zhi mu* 知母, *lian qiao* 连翘, *zhi shi* 枳实, *yu jin* 郁金, *ji nei jin* 鸡内金, *zhi gan cao* 炙甘草, *zhi da huang* 制大黄, *zhi fu zi* 制附子, *jing qian jia* 经前加, *yan hu suo* 延胡索, *chuan xiong* 川芎 (H228)

Ingredients are referenced to the original studies where possible. If herb ingredients varied across studies, the herb ingredients were sourced from *Zhong Yi Fang Ji Da Ci Dian* 中医方剂大辞典.

Note: the use of some herbs may be restricted in some countries. Readers are advised to comply with relevant regulations.

Table 5.34. Frequently Reported Orally Used Herbs in Non-controlled Studies

Most Common Herbs	Scientific Name	Frequency of Use
Dang gui 当归	Angelica sinensis (Oliv.) Diels	37
E zhu 莪术	Curcuma spp.	31
Chi shao 赤芍	Paeonia spp.	28
San leng 三棱	Sparganium stoloniferum Buch. -Ham.	28
Yan hu suo 延胡索	Corydalis yanhusuo W.T. Wang	25
Gan cao 甘草	Glycyrrhiza spp.	22
Bai shao 白芍	Paeonia lactiflora Pall.	21
Dan shen 丹参	Salvia miltiorrhiza Bge.	18
Pu huang 蒲黄	Typha spp.	18
Wu ling zhi 五灵脂	Trogopterus xanthipes Milne-Edwards	18
Xiang fu 香附	Cyperus rotundus L.	18
Chuan xiong 川芎	Ligusticum chuangxiong Hort.	17
Fu ling 茯苓	Poria cocos (Schw.) Wolf	17
Huang qi 黄芪	Astragalus membranaceus (Fisch.) Bge.	17
Niu xi 牛膝	Achyranthes bidentata Bl.	17
Tao ren 桃仁	Prunus spp.	17
Wu yao 乌药	Lindera aggregata (Sims) Kosterm.	17
Gui zhi 桂枝	Cinnamomum cassia Presl	16
Mu dan pi 牡丹皮	Paeonia suffruticosa Andr.	13

Note: The use of some herbs may be restricted in some countries. Readers are advised to comply with relevant regulations.

The most frequently used herbs were *dang gui* 当归, *e zhu* 莪术, *chi shao* 赤芍, *san leng* 三棱, and *yan hu suo* 延胡索 (Table 5.34).

Safety of oral Chinese herbal medicine in non-controlled studies

Of the five non-controlled studies that documented the safety of oral CHM, three reported that no AEs occurred (H240, H254, H255). In the remaining two studies, AEs included eight unspecified events in one study (H216), and 11 cases of mild nausea in the other (H253).

Topical Chinese Herbal Medicine for Endometriosis

Fifteen clinical studies evaluated the potential role of topical CHM for women with endometriosis. Of these, 12 were RCTs (H256–H267), two were CCTs (H268, H269), and one was a non-controlled study (H270).

Randomised Controlled Trials of Topical Chinese Herbal Medicine for Endometriosis

Topical CHM was tested in 12 RCTs that included 975 adult women (H256–H267). All studies were conducted in China. Women in three RCTs had previous surgery for endometriosis (H260, H262, H267). Two studies reported on the rASRM stage: one included women with stage II, III, or IV endometriosis (H262), while the other included women with any of the four rASRM stages (H260). Three studies confirmed endometriosis by laparoscopy (H260, H262, H267). The duration of endometriosis ranged from six months (H257, H265) to 10 years (H257), and the median of the mean duration was 4.1 years. One study included older women (mean age 56.8 years; H256), while other studies reported a mean age in the late 20s to mid 30s.

Two RCTs used CM syndrome differentiation as an inclusion criterion or to guide treatment (H261, H266). The syndrome *qi* stagnation and Blood stasis was reported in both; other syndromes included cold coagulation and Blood stasis, damp-heat stasis, Kidney deficiency and Blood stasis, *qi* deficiency and Blood stasis, and burning heat and Blood stasis. Many studies tested investigator-developed formulas, and no traditional formula was used in two or more studies. The most frequently used herbs were *dan shen* 丹参, *e zhu* 莪术, and *chi shao* 赤芍 (Table 5.35).

Two studies compared topical CHM with the non-steroidal anti-inflammatory drug (NSAID) indomethacin (H258, H266), while all others used HT in the control group. Three RCTs tested topical CHM as integrative medicine with HT (H259, H260, H261). One study provided treatment for three weeks (H259), in contrast with other studies of either three (H257, H258, H263, H265–H267), six (H256,

Table 5.35. Frequently Reported Topically Used Herbs in Randomised Controlled Trials

Most Common Herbs	Scientific Name	Frequency of Use
Dan shen 丹参	Salvia miltiorrhiza Bge.	8
E zhu 莪术	Curcuma spp.	8
Chi shao 赤芍	Paeonia spp.	7
Dang gui 当归	Angelica sinensis (Oliv.) Diels	5
San leng 三棱	Sparganium stoloniferum Buch. -Ham.	5
Tao ren 桃仁	Prunus persica (L.) Batsch	5
Gui zhi 桂枝	Cinnamomum cassia Presl	4
Hong hua 红花	Carthamus tinctorius L.	4
Huang qi 黄芪	Astragalus membranaceus (Fisch.) Bge.	4
Mo yao 没药	Commiphora spp.	4
Ru xiang 乳香	Boswellia spp.	4
Bai jiang 败酱	Patrinia villosa Juss.	3
Bai shao 白芍	Paeonia lactiflora Pall.	3
Mu dan pi 牡丹皮	Paeonia suffruticosa Andr.	3
Hong teng 红藤	Spatholobus suberectus Dunn	3
Tu si zi 菟丝子	Cuscuta spp.	3

Note: The use of some herbs may be restricted in some countries. Readers are advised to comply with relevant regulations.

H260, H262, H264), or nine months duration (H261). Seven studies conducted follow-up assessment (H256, H258, H260, H262–H264, H267) ranging from three months (H258, H263) to three years (H256). Three studies reported loss to follow-up (H262, H264, H267), which was small and generally balanced across groups.

Risk of bias assessment

Lack of blinding and inadequate reporting were potential sources of bias in all 12 studies (Table 5.36). Four RCTs that used a random number generator for sequence generation were judged as having low risk of bias for sequence generation (H256, H258, H259, H267). None of

Table 5.36. Risk of Bias Assessment of Randomised Controlled Trials: Topical CHM

Risk of Bias Domain	Low Risk n (%)	Unclear Risk n (%)	High Risk n (%)
Sequence generation	4 (33.3)	8 (66.7)	0 (0)
Allocation concealment	0 (0)	12 (100)	0 (0)
Blinding of participants	0 (0)	0 (0)	12 (100)
Blinding of personnel	0 (0)	0 (0)	12 (100)
Blinding of outcome assessors	0 (0)	0 (0)	12 (100)
Incomplete outcome data	10 (83.3)	2 (16.7)	0 (0)
Selective outcome reporting	0 (0)	12 (100)	0 (0)

the studies documented the method used to conceal group allocation or blinded participants, personnel, and outcome assessors to group allocation. In two RCTs, reasons for participant loss to follow-up were not described (H264, H267). The studies neither reported trial registration nor published the trial protocol; as such, all were judged as posing unclear risk of bias for selective outcome reporting.

Outcomes

Dysmenorrhoea was the most common clinical outcome, reported in seven RCTs (H256–H258, H261, H263, H265, H266). Despite this, not all studies documented the data in a way that allowed for analysis, and data for two studies were excluded (H257, H266). Ovarian cyst volume was reported in four RCTs (H257, H259, H263, H264), recurrence was reported in three RCTs (H260, H262, H267), and both dyspareunia and pelvic pain were reported in one RCT (H264). Eight RCTs reported on the safety of topical CHM (H256–H258, H260, H262–H265).

Dysmenorrhoea

Five RCTs that tested topical CHM documented dysmenorrhoea using a range of outcome scales (H256, H258, H261, H263, H265).

Results are reported separately for studies that compared topical CHM with pharmacotherapy, as well as those that tested the combination of topical CHM with pharmacotherapy.

Topical Chinese herbal medicine versus pharmacotherapy

Meta-analysis was conducted with two RCTs that measured dysmenorrhoea using the 1993 Guideline (H263, H265). Among the 114 participants, women who received topical CHM enema reported a similar score at the end of treatment compared to women who received pharmacotherapy (MD 0.11 [-6.19, 6.40], I^2 = 94%). Results for individual studies showed no difference between *Nei yi xiao* 内异消 and danazol on the 1993 Guideline at follow-up three months after surgery (34 women, MD 0.39 [-2.05, 2.83]; H263).

One RCT that used a VAS to assess the severity of dysmenorrhoea found a greater score reduction — indicating less pain — in women who received *Hong teng ye* enema 红藤汤灌肠 than in those who received sustained-release ibuprofen (H258). This result was found both at the end of treatment (64 women, MD -1.19 [-1.81, -0.57]) and at follow-up (-2.59 [-3.19, -1.99]). When dysmenorrhoea was assessed using the VRS, women who received *Hong teng tang* enema 红藤汤 scored lower than women who received gestrinone (70 women, MD -0.64 [-0.75, -0.53]; H256).

Topical Chinese herbal medicine plus hormone therapy versus hormone therapy

One RCT compared the combination of *Nei yi tong jing fang* enema 内异痛经方 and gestrinone with gestrinone alone (H261). The addition of topical CHM to gestrinone did not result in greater pain relief (60 women, MD -0.42 [-1.24, 0.40]).

Pelvic pain

The number of women with pelvic pain was assessed in one RCT (H264). Topical application of *Tong yu tie* 痛愈帖 to the umbilicus did not reduce the number of women with pelvic pain more than danazol did (100 women, RR 1.40 [0.61, 3.21]).

Dyspareunia

The study that assessed the number of women with pelvic pain also determined the number of women with dyspareunia (H264). Women who received topical *Tong yu tie* 痛愈帖 were no less likely to have dyspareunia than women who received danazol (100 women, RR 0.70 [0.29, 1.68]).

Recurrence

Three studies that documented recurrence differed in the comparisons made and the timing and criteria for assessment of recurrence. Results were not suitable for meta-analysis, and results of individual studies are described.

Topical Chinese herbal medicine versus no treatment

One three-arm study compared an investigator-developed CHM enema with no treatment (H267). Fewer cases of recurrence of symptoms and lesions were seen one year after surgery in women who received CHM than in those who received no treatment (85 women, RR 0.26 [0.08, 0.84]).

Topical Chinese herbal medicine versus hormone therapy

When an investigator-developed CHM enema was compared with gestrinone one year after surgery, women who received topical CHM were as likely to experience recurrence of symptoms and lesions as women who received gestrinone (82 women, RR 0.71 [0.17, 2.99]; H267). In a second RCT, recurrence of pain and cysts was assessed six months after the end of treatment (H262). There was no statistical difference between topical CHM and gestrinone in this study (65 women, RR 1.09 [0.37, 3.23]).

Topical Chinese herbal medicine plus hormone therapy versus hormone therapy

One study tested the combination of *Fu fang da xue teng guan chang ji* enema 复方大血藤灌肠剂 and leuprolin (H260). Compared with leuprolin alone, the combination of topical CHM and HT resulted in a lower chance of recurrence based on symptoms, signs, ultrasound assessment, and CA125 levels one year after the end of treatment (90 women, RR 0.20 [0.05, 0.86]).

Ovarian cyst size

Ovarian cyst size was reported in different ways, which prevented meta-analysis. Results are reported separately for studies that compared topical CHM with HT and those that compared the combination of topical CHM plus HT with HT alone.

Topical Chinese herbal medicine versus hormone therapy

In one RCT, danazol was more effective at reducing ovarian cyst diameter than *Yi wei er hao fang* enema 异位二号方 (60 women, MD 0.28 cm [0.10, 0.46]; H257). Among women with ovarian cysts, ovarian cyst volume was not statistically different between women who received *Nei yi xiao* enema 内异消 and those who received danazol (H263). This result was found at the end of treatment (25 women, MD −3.64 cm^3 [−21.92, 14.64]) and at follow-up three months after surgery (25 women, MD −5.26 cm^3 [−20.10, 9.58]). Finally, the ovarian cyst area was larger at the end of treatment among women who received topical CHM applied to the umbilicus compared to women who received danazol (100 women, MD 0.84 cm^2 [0.15, 1.53]; H264).

Topical Chinese herbal medicine plus hormone therapy versus hormone therapy

One RCT that used topical CHM as integrative medicine with HT documented ovarian cyst size (H259). At the end of treatment, the mean ovarian cyst diameter was smaller in women who received *Huo xue san yu* enema 活血散瘀灌肠 plus medroxyprogesterone acetate than in women who received medroxyprogesterone acetate alone (86 women, MD −1.00 cm [−1.30, −0.70]).

Safety of topical Chinese herbal medicine in randomised controlled trials

Eight RCTs that tested topical CHM reported on its safety (H256–H258, H260, H262–H265). Five reported that AEs occurred in women who received topical CHM (H258, H260, H262–H264), including seven cases of allergic reaction, six cases of mild gastrointestinal symptoms, and one case of local skin irritation. In women who received topical CHM as integrative medicine, an unknown number of cases of hot flushes, night sweats, irritability, and other perimenopausal symptoms were reported (H260). Adverse events in women who received pharmacotherapy included 30 cases of abnormal liver function such as elevated alanine aminotransferase (AAT), 10 cases of weight gain, eight cases of nausea or vomiting, six cases of haemorrhoids, five cases of acne, five cases of gastrointestinal discomfort, four cases of obesity and haemorrhoids, three cases of vaginal bleeding, three cases of increased hair growth, two cases of rash, two cases of hot flushes, two cases of headache, and two cases of oedema. Five cases of a variety of symptoms — including weight gain, oedema, haemorrhoids, increased hair growth, and facial flushing — were reported in one study (H263), while another documented an unspecified number of cases of hot flushes, night sweats, irritability, and other perimenopausal symptoms (H260).

Controlled Clinical Trials of Topical Chinese Herbal Medicine for Endometriosis

Two CCTs tested topical CHM formulations in 234 women with endometriosis (H268, H269), with one examining effects in women with endometriosis-related infertility (H269). Both studies were conducted in China and recruited adult women. Women in the study by Wang et al. (2015; H269) had surgery prior to enrolling in the trial.

Neither study described CM syndrome diagnosis. One study compared 90 days of treatment with *San jie zhi tong tang* 散结止痛汤 enema to medroxyprogesterone acetate (H268), while the other compared one month of treatment with the combination of *Hong hua jin ye* 红花浸液 and gestrinone to gestrinone alone (H269). A topical preparation of *Hong hua jin ye* 红花浸液 was applied to the abdomen and vagina for 30 minutes per application. One herb was common to both studies: *hong hua* 红花.

Outcomes

Outcomes assessed in the two CCTs related to endometriosis recurrence and pregnancy outcomes. Data from the study that described recurrence reported on recurrence for all women (H268). As it was not clear whether all women achieved resolution of endometriosis, these data were excluded from further analysis.

Pregnancy outcomes

The study by Wang et al. (2015; H269) reported the cumulative pregnancy rate at three, six, nine, and 12 months, and the number of pregnancies at 12 months was analysed. The combination of *Hong hua jin ye* 红花浸液 and gestrinone resulted in a higher pregnancy rate than did gestrinone alone (98 women, RR 1.55 [1.08, 2.22]).

Safety of topical Chinese herbal medicine in controlled clinical trials

Both studies reported on the safety of topical CHM. No AEs were reported in women who received topical CHM alone. Adverse events among women who received topical CHM and gestrinone (H269) included three cases of irregular menstruation, two cases of nausea and vomiting, and one case of wound infection. Adverse events in the control groups included eight cases of lengthened menstrual cycle, four cases of irregular menstruation, three cases of irregular uterine bleeding, three cases of nausea and vomiting, two cases of significant weight gain, and one case of wound infection.

Non-controlled Studies of Topical Chinese Herbal Medicine for Endometriosis

Topical CHM was evaluated in one case series of 46 adult women who had lived with endometriosis for between three and nine years and had not previously undergone surgery as treatment (H270). Treatment with an enema made from *Hong teng tang* 红藤汤 was provided for six months. The authors did not report on the CM syndromes of patients and or any safety data.

Oral plus Topical CHM for Endometriosis

Twenty-two studies tested the combination of oral plus topical CHM for women with endometriosis. Twelve of these were RCTs (H271–H282), two were CCTs (H183, H283), and eight were non-controlled studies (H284–H291).

Randomised Controlled Trials of Oral plus Topical Chinese Herbal Medicine for Endometriosis

All 12 RCTs that evaluated the combination of oral plus topical CHM were conducted in China (H271–H282). In total, 840 adult women with endometriosis participated in these studies. Three RCTs were three-arm studies (H275, H276, H278); each of these included a treatment arm of oral CHM alone and another of oral plus topical CHM. Eight RCTs included women who had received surgery prior to enrolling in the trial (H271, H273–H277, H280, H282). Five RCTs documented the rASRM stage: one RCT included women with stage I or II endometriosis (H277); another included women with stage II, III, or IV endometriosis (H271); and three studies included all rASRM stages of endometriosis (H273, H275, H276). Among studies that reported the setting, women were recruited from both inpatient and outpatient departments.

Seven studies used CM syndrome differentiation as an inclusion criterion. Syndromes included Blood stasis (H274), Kidney deficiency and Blood stasis (H273, H282), *qi* stagnation and Blood stasis (H275), *qi* stagnation and Blood stasis with Kidney deficiency (H276), Kidney deficiency and phlegm stasis (H277), and cold coagulation and Blood stasis (H281). Four studies provided treatment for six months (H275, H277, H279, H280), while other studies provided treatment for three months. Seven RCTs conducted follow-up assessments after the end of treatment (H273, H275, H277, H279–H282), which ranged from six months (H277, H279–H281) to two years (H273).

Most studies tested investigator-developed oral and/or topical formulas or treatment according to the menstrual cycle. One formula, *Nei yi fang/wan* 内异方/内异丸, was used three times in one study (H276); no other traditional formulas were used in multiple RCTs. Most topical CHMs were administered as enemas. Herbs that were used in multiple RCTs included *dan shen* 丹参, *e zhu* 莪术, *chi shao* 赤芍, *dang gui* 当归, and *san leng* 三棱 (Table 5.37). One RCT tested the combination of oral and topical CHM and gestrinone (H275).

Risk of bias assessment

Over half of the RCTs used random number tables to allocate participants to intervention and control groups (7 of 12 RCTs) and were judged as having low risk of bias for sequence generation (Table 5.38). Allocation concealment was poorly reported; one RCT (H273) used methods that were unlikely to conceal group allocation and was judged to carry high risk of bias. One RCT (H276) stated that participants were blind to group allocation, but because the nature of the intervention (oral and topical CHM) and control (danazol) suggested that achieving blinding would be unlikely, this study was

Table 5.37. Frequently Reported Oral plus Topical Herbs in Randomised Controlled Trials

Most Common Herbs	Scientific Name	Frequency of Use
Dan shen 丹参	Salvia miltiorrhiza Bge.	20
E zhu 莪术	Curcuma spp.	16
Chi shao 赤芍	Paeonia spp.	14
Dang gui 当归	Angelica sinensis (Oliv.) Diels	14
San leng 三棱	Sparganium stoloniferum Buch. -Ham.	14
Hong hua 红花	Carthamus tinctorius L.	9
Tao ren 桃仁	Prunus persica (L.) Batsch	9
Yan hu suo 延胡索	Corydalis yanhusuo W.T. Wang	9
Gui zhi 桂枝	Cinnamomum cassia Presl	7
Wu ling zhi 五灵脂	Trogopterus xanthipes Milne-Edwards	7
Hong teng 红藤	Spatholobus suberectus Dunn	6
Zao jiao ci 皂角刺	Gleditsia sinensis Lam.	6
Chai hu 柴胡	Bupleurum spp.	5
Huang qi 黄芪	Astragalus membranaceus (Fisch.) Bge.	5
Pu huang 蒲黄	Typha spp.	5
Shu di huang 熟地黄	Rehmannia glutinosa Libosch.	5
Xiang fu 香附	Cyperus rotundus L.	5

Note: the use of some herbs may be restricted in some countries. Readers are advised to comply with relevant regulations.

Table 5.38. Risk of Bias Assessment of Randomised Controlled Trials: Oral plus Topical CHM

Risk of Bias Domain	Low Risk n (%)	Unclear Risk n (%)	High Risk n (%)
Sequence generation	7 (58.3)	3 (25.0)	2 (16.7)
Allocation concealment	0 (0)	11 (91.6)	1 (8.3)
Blinding of participants	0 (0)	1 (8.3)	11 (91.6)
Blinding of personnel	0 (0)	0 (0)	12 (100)
Blinding of outcome assessors	0 (0)	0 (0)	12 (100)
Incomplete outcome data	11 (91.6)	1 (8.3)	0 (0)
Selective outcome reporting	0 (0)	12 (100)	0 (0)

assessed as having unclear risk of bias for blinding of participants. None of the studies blinded personnel or outcome assessors. In one RCT (H279), seven participants in the control group withdrew due to AEs; the study was considered to have unclear risk of bias. All other studies had complete outcome data. Trial registrations and/or published trial protocols were not identified for any of the studies.

Outcomes

Five RCTs reported outcomes relating to dysmenorrhoea (H271– H274, H276) and two RCTs reported dyspareunia (H273, H274), although data could be used only for one study (H274). Six RCTs assessed recurrence (H273, H275, H279–H282), with data from two studies being excluded due to definitions of recurrence. Several outcomes were reported by only one RCT: pregnancy rate (H277), miscarriage rate (H277), ovarian cyst volume (H278), and health-related quality of life (H281). Eight RCTs reported on the safety of the combination of oral plus topical CHM (H271, H273, H276, H278– H282).

Dysmenorrhoea

Dysmenorrhoea was measured in different ways among the five RCTs (H271–H274, H276), and only one meta-analysis was possible. In the four RCTs that assessed dysmenorrhoea using the 1993 Guideline, the combination of oral plus topical CHM was not statistically different from HT in reducing menstrual pain (218 women, MD −0.82 points [−3.01, 1.38], $I^2 = 91\%$; H272, H273, H274, H276). Planned subgroup analyses to explore statistical heterogeneity, including treatment duration and CHM formulas, could not be conducted as all studies provided treatment duration for three months and none of the formulas were used in multiple studies. Confidence in this result is limited.

Results from individual studies showed that *Hua yu tiao jing fang* 化瘀调经方 plus CHM enema resulted in a greater reduction in VAS pain scores than did gestrinone (64 women, MD −1.30 cm [−1.76,

−0.84]; H271). When measured using the CMSS, one study of 60 women (H273) found that the combination of oral *Nei yi fang* 内异方 and an unnamed topical CHM reduced the total duration (MD −1.49 points [−2.58, −0.40]) and the total severity of dysmenorrhoea (MD −2.00 [−3.05, −0.95]) compared to gestrinone.

Dyspareunia

One RCT reported the number of women with dyspareunia at the end of treatment (H274). Fewer women who received oral *Jing dai ning jiao nang* 经带宁胶囊, enema with *E ling guan chang ye* 莪棱灌肠液, and topical *Shuang bai san* 双柏散 reported on dyspareunia at the end of treatment compared with women who received goserelin sustained-release implant (50 women, RR 0.29 [0.11, 0.75]).

Recurrence

Results were analysed for three studies that documented recurrence (H273, H275, H282). Differences in comparisons and criteria for assessing recurrence meant that meta-analysis was not possible.

Oral plus topical Chinese herbal medicine versus hormone therapy

Both studies that reported on recurrence did so in women who had undergone surgery prior to enrolling in the study (H282, H273). Oral plus topical CHM tailored according to the menstrual cycle did not reduce the chance of recurrence as measured by signs, symptoms, ultrasound, and CA125 more than danazol did (60 women, RR 0.42 [0.17, 1.04]; H282). When recurrence was based on signs and symptoms, masses, and CA125, there was no difference between women who received oral *Nei yi fang* 内异方 and an unnamed topical CHM and those who received gestrinone (60 women, RR 0.67 [0.12, 3.71]; H273).

Oral plus topical Chinese herbal medicine plus hormone therapy versus hormone therapy

One RCT that reported on the recurrence of cysts one year after surgery included two CHM arms; as these two arms were considered sufficiently similar, they were merged for analysis (H275). Analysis showed that the investigator-developed oral and topical CHM combined with gestrinone was no more effective than gestrinone alone (40 women, RR 0.40 [0.09, 1.83]).

Ovarian cyst volume

Investigator-developed CHM treatments did not result in a greater reduction in ovarian cyst volume compared to danazol (62 women, MD 0.52 cm^3 [-0.33, 1.37]; H278).

Pregnancy outcomes

Among 90 women with endometrosis-related infertility, the pregnancy rate, confirmed by the presence of fetal heartbeat on ultrasound, was higher in women who received CHM as both an oral and enema preparation than in women who received no treatment (RR 1.43 [1.03, 2.01]; H277). The same study found no difference in the miscarriage rate between groups (RR 1.39 [0.13, 14.48]).

Health-related quality of life

One study of 120 women assessed health-related quality of life using the EHP-5 (H281). Results were reported for the core five scales and the six supplementary modules. While no benefit of oral CHM plus CHM enema over gestrinone was found for the pain scale (MD −5.18 points [−10.77, 0.41]), benefit was seen for the following: control and powerlessness (MD −8.82 points [−12.56, −5.08]), emotional wellbeing (MD −6.99 points [−10.21, −3.77]), social support (MD −6.66 points [−9.69, −3.63]), and self-image (MD −5.11 points

[−8.15, −2.07]). Benefits of CHM treatment were seen in four of the six supplementary modules: work (MD −6.75 points [−9.59, −3.91]), relationships with children (MD −9.73 points [−13.46, −6.00]), sexual relationship (MD −6.37 points [−9.27, −3.47]), and feelings about the medical profession (MD −7.58 points [−12.77, −2.39]). No differences were seen in the supplementary modules: feelings about treatment (MD −4.21 points [−9.75, 1.33]) and feelings about infertility (MD −1.63 points [−7.24, 3.98]).

Safety of oral plus topical Chinese herbal medicine in randomised controlled trials

Of the eight RCTs that documented the safety of oral plus topical CHM (H271, H273, H276, H278–H282), one reported that no AEs occurred in either group (H280). Among women who received oral plus topical CHM, AEs included four cases of irregular vaginal bleeding or increased menstrual flow, three cases of gastrointestinal discomfort, two cases of mild nausea, two cases of abnormal liver function, and one case of weight gain. Adverse events among women who received HT included 51 cases of weight gain, 32 cases of abnormal liver function including six that were accompanied by gastrointestinal symptoms, 20 cases of irregular vaginal bleeding, 14 cases of acne with or without hirsuitism, 11 cases of hot flushes, eight cases of gastrointestinal discomfort, three cases of headache, two cases of hot flushes and vaginal dryness, and one case of menopause.

Controlled Clinical Trials of Oral plus Topical Chinese Herbal Medicine for Endometriosis

Two non-randomised CCTs used both oral and topical CHM in 110 women with endometriosis (H183, H283). Both studies were conducted in China. One study examined oral plus topical CHM for 50 women with endometriosis-related infertility (H283), and women in both studies had undergone surgery prior to study enrolment. In women in the three-arm CCT, which compared oral CHM alone, oral

CHM plus topical CHM, and no treatment (H183), diagnosis of endometriosis was made by laparoscopy.

Neither study described CM syndrome differentiation, but both selected CHM according to the time of the menstrual cycle. Both studies administered treatment for three months, and follow-up assessments were conducted at either nine months (H183) or one year (H283) after the end of treatment. Several herbs were common to both studies: *dan shen* 丹参, *shan zhu yu* 山茱萸, *ba ji tian* 巴戟天, *shu di* 熟地, and *bai jiang cao* 败酱草.

Outcomes

As the two studies tested the combination of oral and topical CHM in different populations and for different purposes, meta-analyses could not be conducted. Results for each study are reported according to the outcome measured.

Dysmenorrhoea

One CCT assessed dysmenorrhoea in two ways: as a score using the 1993 Guideline and as the number of people with dysmenorrhoea at the end of treatment (H183). Women who received oral and topical CHM according to the time of the menstrual cycle reported lower scores on the 1993 Guideline than women who received no treatment (38 women, MD −5.50 points [−6.36, −4.64]). Further, the number of women with dysmenorrhoea at the end of treatment was lower in women who received oral plus topical CHM (RR 0.18 [0.04, 0.82]).

Recurrence

In one study that documented the recurrence of signs and symptoms (H183), there was no recurrence in either group at the end of treatment. Endometriosis recurred in both groups at follow-up after nine months, but there was no statistical difference in the chance of recurrence (38 women, RR 0.15 [0.02, 1.33]).

Pregnancy outcomes

Pregnancy outcomes were reported in one CCT of 50 women (H283). Neither the pregnancy rate (RR 1.08 [0.65, 1.80]), miscarriage rate (RR 0.93 [0.15, 5.67]), nor live birth rate (RR 1.01 [0.74, 1.39]) were statistically different between women who received oral plus topical CHM and those who received goserelin.

Safety of oral plus topical Chinese herbal medicine in controlled clinical trials

One CCT reported on the safety of oral plus topical CHM in CCTs (H183). Two cases of diarrhoea were reported in women who received the combination of oral plus topical CHM.

Non-controlled Studies of Oral plus Topical Chinese Herbal Medicine for Endometriosis

Eight non-controlled studies tested the combination of oral plus topical CHM in 315 women with endometriosis (H284–H291). Five were case series (H286, H287, H288, H290, H291) and three were case reports (H284, H285, H289). Women in four of the eight studies had undergone surgery prior to study enrolment (H284, H285, H288, H290). One study included both adults and adolescents (H286), while the remaining studies included only adults. The duration of endometriosis ranged from one month (H286) to 20 years (H286).

Half of the studies used CM syndrome as an inclusion criterion (H284, H285, H289, H290). Syndromes included Kidney deficiency and Blood stasis (H285), Kidney deficiency and phlegm stasis (H290), cold coagulation and Blood stasis (H284), and *qi* stagnation and Blood stasis (H289). Treatment was provided for between three months (H285, H286, H291) and one year (H284). All studies tested CHM alone.

Each study used a different oral CHM formula (or formulas, in studies that used treatment according to the menstrual cycle) and a different topical formula. Most topical formulas were used as enemas.

Table 5.39. Frequently Reported Orally plus Topically Used Herbs in Non-controlled Studies

Most Common Herbs	Scientific Name	Frequency of Use
Huang qi 黄芪	Astragalus spp.	8
Chi shao 赤芍	Paeonia spp.	7
E zhu 莪术	Curcuma spp.	7
Dang gui 当归	Angelica sinensis (Oliv.) Diels	6
Mo yao 没药	Commiphora spp.	6
Ru xiang 乳香	Boswellia spp.	6
San leng 三棱	Sparganium stoloniferum Buch. -Ham.	6
Gan cao 甘草	Glycyrrhiza spp.	5
Pu huang 蒲黄	Typha spp.	5
Ai ye 艾叶	Artemisia argyi Lévl. et Vant.	4
Dan shen 丹参	Salvia miltiorrhiza Bge.	4
Dang shen 党参	Codonopsis spp.	4
Ji xue teng 鸡血藤	Spatholobus suberectus Dunn	4
Shan yao 山药	Dioscorea opposita Thunb.	4
Shui zhi 水蛭	Whitmania pigra Whitman; Hirudo nipponica Whitman; Whitmania acranulata Whitman	4
Tu si zi 菟丝子	Cuscuta spp.	4
Wu jia pi 五加皮	Acanthopanax gracilistylus W. W. Smith	4
Wu ling zhi 五灵脂	Trogopterus xanthipes Milne-Edwards	4
Xue jie 血竭	Daemonorops draco Bl.	4

Note: The use of some herbs may be restricted in some countries. Readers are advised to comply with relevant regulations.

The most frequently used herbs were *huang qi* 黄芪, *chi shao* 赤芍, and *e zhu* 莪术 (Table 5.39). None of the studies reported on safety of the combination of oral and topical CHM.

Part 2. Adenomyosis

Ninety-six studies evaluated the efficacy of CHM for women with adenomyosis. The majority of studies evaluated oral CHM as a treatment for women with adenomyosis (88 of the 96 studies). Five studies tested topical CHM and three studies investigated the combination of oral plus topical CHM (H380–H384). Results are presented according to the route of administration and by study design.

Oral Chinese Herbal Medicine for Adenomyosis

Fifty-five were RCTs (H292–H346), six were CCTs (H347–H352), and 27 were non-controlled studies (H353–H379).

Randomised Controlled Trials of Oral Chinese Herbal Medicine for Adenomyosis

All RCTs were conducted in China and 5,034 adult women participated. The mean age of participants was in the 30s in most studies, and the mean duration of endometriosis ranged from 11 months (H294) to almost nine years (8.9 years; H305). None of the studies reported using laparoscopy for diagnosis, nor did they report the rASRM stage of participants. Twenty-six studies recruited women from hospital outpatient departments (H292, H294–H296, H299–H301, H304, H306, H307, H309, H310, H311, H314, H315, H318, H322, H324–H326, H331, H335, H339, H342, H344, H346), two recruited women from inpatient departments (H320, H336), and the remaining studies did not report this information. Two studies reported that women had undergone surgery prior to the trial (H300, H336).

Twenty-two RCTs used CM syndrome differentiation as an inclusion criterion (H292, H294, H296, H304, H307, H309, H310, H314, H315, H318, H321, H322, H327, H329, H331, H333, H335, H337, H340, H342, H344, H346). Syndromes documented in two or more studies were *qi* stagnation and Blood stasis (H294, H309, H318, H327, H342, H344), cold coagulation and Blood stasis (H292, H314, H333, H337, H346), Kidney deficiency and Blood stasis (H307, H321, H331, H335), and blinding of (Blood) stasis and heat (H296, H304, H315).

Most studies (35 of the 55 RCTs) provided treatment for 12 weeks/three months (H292–H297, H299, H303, H304, H306, H308, H309, H311, H313, H314, H316, H318, H321, H324–H326, H329, H331–H337, H341–H346); other studies provided treatment for 28 days (H322), between three and six months (H339, H340), four months (H307), or six months (H298, H300–H302, H305, H310, H312, H315, H317, H319, H320, H323, H327, H328, H330, H338). Nineteen studies conducted follow-up assessment after the end of treatment. Additional assessments were conducted from between two months (H307) and two years (H304). A total of 31 participants were lost to follow-up in four studies (H322, H331, H335, H342).

Oral CHM was used alone as the intervention in 24 RCTs (H296, H297, H300, H304, H306–H308, H310, H314, H315, H321, H322, H324–H326, H329, H331, H335, H336, H339, H342, H344–H346) and as integrative medicine with conventional medical treatments in 32 RCTs (H292–H295, H298, H299, H301–H303, H305, H309, H311–H313, H316–H320, H323, H327, H328, H330, H332–H334, H337, H338, H340–H343). One three-arm study included two treatments arms (H342): one arm received oral CHM alone and another received oral CHM as integrative medicine. Five oral CHM formulas were used in multiple studies (Table 5.40); *Gui zhi fu ling* capsules (*jiao nang*) or pills (*wan*) 桂枝茯苓胶囊/丸 were tested in 10 RCTs. The most frequently used herb was *dang gui* 当归, followed by *yan hu suo* 延胡索, *chi shao* 赤芍, and *dan shen* 丹参 (Table 5.41).

Risk of bias assessment

None of the studies were free from bias (Table 5.42). Twenty-one studies used appropriate methods for sequence generation (low risk of bias), while 10 used methods such as alternate allocation (high risk). Two studies were considered to have high risk of bias for allocation concealment, as participants were allocated to groups according to the visit order (H295, H318). One RCT blinded study participants and personnel through the use of a placebo in the control group, but

Table 5.40. Frequently Reported Oral Formulas in Randomised Controlled Trials for Adenomyosis

Most Common Formulas	No. of Studies	Ingredients
Gui zhi fu ling jiao nang/wan 桂枝茯苓胶囊/丸	10	Gui zhi 桂枝, fu ling 茯苓, mu dan 牡丹, tao ren 桃仁, shao yao 芍药
San jie zhen tong jiao nang 散结镇痛胶囊	6	Xue jie 血竭, san qi 三七, zhe bei mu 浙贝母, yi yi ren 薏苡仁 (H316, H319, H332, H336, H340, H345)
Shao fu zhu yu tang/jiao nang 少腹逐瘀汤/胶囊	2	Xiao hui xiang 小茴香, gan jiang 干姜, yuan hu 元胡, mo yao 没药, dang gui 当归, chuan xiong 川芎, guan gui 官桂, chi shao 赤芍, pu huang 蒲黄, ling zhi 灵脂
Xiao yi fang/tang 消异方/汤	2	E zhu 莪术, dan shen 丹参, dang gui 当归, yin yang huo 淫羊藿, xiang fu 香附, zhi gan cao 炙甘草 (H341); fu ling 茯苓, tu si zi 菟丝子, chao wang bu liu xing 炒王不留行, hong teng 红藤, cu xiang fu 醋香附, san qi 三七, bai jiang cao 败酱草 (H346)
Ge gen er xian tang 葛根二仙汤	2	Ge gen 葛根, tu si zi 菟丝子, gou teng 钩藤, shi jue ming 石决明, ba ji tian 巴戟天, xian mao 仙茅, yin yang huo 淫羊藿, bu gu zhi 补骨脂, huang bai 黄柏, zhi zi 栀子, huang qin 黄芩, zhi mu 知母, gu sui bu 骨碎补, tian ma 天麻, rou cong rong 肉苁蓉, gan cao 甘草 (H311, H343)

Ingredients are referenced to the original studies where possible. If herb ingredients varied across studies, the herb ingredients were sourced from *Zhong Yi Fang Ji Da Ci Dian* 中医方剂大辞典.

Note: The use of some herbs may be restricted in some countries. Readers are advised to comply with relevant regulations.

insufficient detail was provided as to whether outcome assessors were blinded to group allocation (H335). All other RCTs were considered to have high risk of bias for blinding of participants, personnel, and outcome assessors. There was unclear risk of bias for four RCTs that described loss to follow-up but did not describe the

Table 5.41. Frequently Reported Herbs in Randomised Controlled Trials for Adenomyosis

Most Common Herbs	Scientific Name	Frequency of Use
Dang gui 当归	Angelica sinensis (Oliv.) Diels	36
Yan hu suo 延胡索	Corydalis yanhusuo W.T. Wang	22
Chi shao 赤芍	Paeonia spp.	17
Dan shen 丹参	Salvia miltiorrhiza Bge.	17
Bai shao 白芍	Paeonia lactiflora Pall.	15
E zhu 莪术	Curcuma spp.	15
Fu ling 茯苓	Poria cocos (Schw.) Wolf	15
Gan cao 甘草	Glycyrrhiza spp.	15
Pu huang 蒲黄	Typha spp.	15
San leng 三棱	Sparganium stoloniferum Buch. -Ham.	14
Wu ling zhi 五灵脂	Trogopterus xanthipes Milne-Edwards	13
Xiang fu 香附	Cyperus rotundus L.	13
Chuan xiong 川芎	Ligusticum chuangxiong Hort.	12
Gui zhi 桂枝	Cinnamomum cassia Presl	12
Tu si zi 菟丝子	Cuscuta spp.	12
Mu dan pi 牡丹皮	Paeonia suffruticosa Andr.	11
Shu di huang 熟地黄	Rehmannia glutinosa Libosch.	11
San qi 三七	Panax notoginseng (Burk.) F.H. Chen	10
Tao ren 桃仁	Prunus persica (L.) Batsch	10

Note: The use of some herbs may be restricted in some countries. Readers are advised to comply with relevant regulations.

Table 5.42. Risk of Bias Assessment of Randomised Controlled Trials for Adenomyosis: Oral CHM

Risk of Bias Domain	Low Risk n (%)	Unclear Risk n (%)	High Risk n (%)
Sequence generation	21 (38.2)	24 (43.6)	10 (18.2)
Allocation concealment	1 (1.8)	52 (94.5)	2 (3.6)
Blinding of participants	1 (1.8)	0 (0)	54 (98.2)
Blinding of personnel	1 (1.8)	0 (0)	54 (98.2)
Blinding of outcome assessors	0 (0)	1 (1.8)	54 (98.2)
Incomplete outcome data	51 (92.7)	4 (7.3)	0 (0)
Selective outcome reporting	0 (0)	55 (100)	0 (0)

reasons for missing data (H322, H331, H335, H342), and published trial protocols or trial registrations were also not identified for the RCTs.

Outcomes

The most frequently documented outcome was dysmenorrhoea, which was measured in 43 of the 55 RCTs (H292–H295, H297, H298, H300–H308, H310–H314, H316, H318, H320, H321, H323, H324, H326–H335, H337, H338, H342–H346). Thirty-nine RCTs assessed uterine volume (H292, H295–H297, H299–H301, H303, H305–H307, H309–H312, H315–H320, H325, H327–H334, H336–H343, H345), 18 RCTs assessed menstrual volume (H292, H295, H300, H301, H308, H310–H312, H317, H320, H323, H330, H331, H332, H334, H336, H340, H343), three RCTs reported health-related quality of life (H318, H319, H337), two reported on dyspareunia (H299, H306), and two reported on recurrence (H303, H315). Fatigue (H299) and pregnancy rate (H322) were reported in one study each. None of the studies reported pelvic pain, ovarian cyst, bone density, or other pregnancy outcomes. Not all studies reported data in a way that allowed for re-analysis and some studies described incorrect methods for calculating uterine volume; such data were excluded from analyses.

Dysmenorrhoea

Studies used a variety of methods to assess dysmenorrhoea, including VAS, the 1993 Guideline, the CPGQ, the CMSS, VRS, and numerical rating scale (NRS). The VAS was used most frequently.

Oral Chinese herbal medicine versus no treatment

Two RCTs compared oral CHM with no treatment (H300, H346). The dysmenorrhoea score was 1.13 cm lower on the VAS among women who received *Xiao yi fang* 消异方 (60 women, [−1.33, −0.93];

H346). Benefit was also seen with the formula *Hua yu xiao jie fang* 化瘀消结方 when dysmenorrhoea pain intensity was measured using the CPGQ in 40 women who had undergone surgery (MD −22.90 [−31.47, −14.33]; H300).

Oral Chinese herbal medicine versus placebo

One RCT, involving 61 women, that compared oral CHM with placebo measured dysmenorrhoea using both the VAS and the CMSS (H335). Women who received *Yi kun yi tong ping ke li* 益坤抑痛平颗粒 scored 3.77 cm lower on the VAS at the end of treatment than women who received placebo [−4.77, −2.77]). The same study also reported results for items on the CMSS. Benefits were seen for the total duration of pain (MD −17.36 [−19.57, −15.15]) and total severity of pain (MD −30.00 points [−33.22, −26.78]). Women who received *Yi kun yi tong ping ke li* 益坤抑痛平颗粒 scored lower for the following items: abdominal pain (MD −2.67 points [−3.09, −2.25]), nausea (MD −1.73 points [−2.19, −1.27]), vomiting (MD −1.40 points [−1.98, −0.82]), loss of appetite (MD −2.17 points [−2.79, −1.55]), headache (MD −1.04 points [−1.63, −0.45]), back pain (MD −1.94 points [−2.50, −1.38]), leg pain (MD −0.90 points [−1.43, −0.37]), weakness (MD −1.90 points [−2.40, −1.40]), dizziness (MD −2.16 points [−2.70, −1.62]), diarrhoea (MD −1.67 points [−2.27, −1.07]), facial change (MD −1.14 points [−1.70, −0.58]), stomach pain (MD −0.87 points [−1.34, −0.40]), red face (MD −0.70 points [−1.27, −0.13]), insomnia (MD −0.96 points [−1.57, −0.35]), body pain (MD −1.07 points [−1.32, −0.82]), depression (MD −1.07 points [−1.74, −0.40]), irritability (MD −0.80 points [−1.26, −0.34]), and neuroticism (MD −1.10 points [−1.66, −0.54].

Oral CHM versus pharmacotherapy

Dysmenorrhoea was measured using a VAS in six RCTs (H297, H308, H314, H326, H329, H344) and the 1993 Guideline in seven studies (H304, H307, H310, H321, H324, H331, H342). All studies

Table 5.43. Oral Chinese Herbal Medicine versus Pharmacotherapy for Adenomyosis: Dysmenorrhoea

Outcome Measure	No. of Studies (Participants)	Effect Size MD [95% CI], I^2	Included Studies
VAS	6 (501)	−1.32 [−1.86, −0.79]*, 82%	H297, H308, H314, H326, H329, H344
1993 Guideline	7 (499)	−0.29 [−1.34, 0.76]	H304, H307, H310, H321, H324, H331, H342

*Statistically significant, see Statistical Analysis in Chapter 4.
Abbreviations: CI, confidence intervals; MD, mean difference; VAS, visual analogue scale.

that used the VAS provided treatment for three months and, at the end of treatment, VAS score was 1.32 cm lower in women who received oral CHM than in those who received pharmacotherapy (501 women, [−1.86, −0.79], I^2 = 82%; Table 5.43). A substantial amount of statistical heterogeneity was detected in subgroup analyses for studies judged as having low risk of bias for sequence generation (246 women, MD −0.94 cm [−1.78, −0.11], I^2 = 90%; H308, H314, H344) and studies that compared oral CHM with either HT (315 women, MD −1.00 cm [−1.71, −0.29], I^2 = 83%; H297, H308, H314, H329) or NSAIDs (186 women, MD −1.98 cm [−2.90, −1.05], I^2 = 72%; H326, H344).

Follow-up assessment was conducted in one study of 65 women (H314). Women who received *Jue jin jian* plus *Shi xiao san jia wei* 决津煎合失笑散加味 reported VAS scores that were 2.26 cm lower compared to women who received gestrinone, measured three months after the end of treatment ([−3.22, −1.30]).

Among seven RCTs that assessed dysmenorrhoea using the 1993 Guideline (Table 5.43), no statistical difference was found in dysmenorrhoea scores at the end of treatment in women who received oral CHM and those who received HT (499 women, MD −0.29 cm [−1.34, 0.76], I^2 = 91%). Statistical heterogeneity was not reduced in studies judged to pose low risk of bias for sequence generation (190 women, MD −0.32 cm [−2.86, 2.21]; H307, H310, H342). As such, confidence in these results is limited.

One study that assessed dysmenorrhoea using a VRS found that women who received *San jie zhen tong jiao nang* 散结镇痛胶囊 scored 0.54 points lower than women who received gestrinone (82 women, [−0.80, −0.28]; H345).

Oral Chinese herbal medicine plus hormone therapy versus hormone therapy

Among studies that tested the combination of oral CHM and HT, outcome measures used to assess dysmenorrhoea included the VAS, 1993 Guideline, and the CPGQ. Meta-analysis showed the combination to be superior to HT alone in reducing VAS pain scores at the end of treatment (821 women, MD −0.88 cm [−1.54, −0.22], I^2 = 96%; Table 5.44). Considerable statistical heterogeneity remained in sensitivity analysis of studies judged as having low risk of bias for sequence generation (398 women, MD −1.26 cm [−2.33, −0.18], I^2 = 97%); H293, H323, H334). Benefit was no longer evident at follow-up (Table 5.44).

The combination of oral CHM and HT also reduced dysmenorrhoea scores by 1.94 points on the 1993 Guideline (870 women, [−2.42, −1.46], I^2 = 77%; Table 5.44). Again, statistical heterogeneity remained substantial in studies assessed as having low risk of bias for sequence generation (446 women, −2.07 [−2.81, −1.32], I^2 = 75%; H327, H333, H342). Unexplained statistical heterogeneity lowers confidence in these results.

Several studies assessed dysmenorrhoea using the CPGQ. The pain intensity score was reduced by 15.06 points (414 women, [−25.40, −4.72], I^2 = 99%) and the disability points score was reduced by 0.67 points (248 women, [−1.03, −0.31], I^2 = 0%; Table 5.44) in women who received oral CHM plus HT. Findings for the disability points score was influenced by one study (H330) that reported scores of zero, indicating no disability, in both groups at the end of treatment. As such, the statistical analysis was effectively an analysis of two studies, both of which were judged as having low risk of bias for sequence generation. There was no statistical difference

Table 5.44. Oral Chinese Herbal Medicine plus Pharmacotherapy versus Pharmacotherapy for Adenomyosis: Dysmenorrhoea

Outcome Measure	No. of Studies (Participants)	Effect Size MD [95% CI], I^2	Included Studies
VAS – EoT	8 (821)	−0.88 [−1.54, −0.22]*, 96%	H292, H293, H302, H311, H316, H323, H334, H343
VAS – Follow-up	3 (191)	−1.74 [−3.53, 0.05]	H292, H311, H343
1993 Guideline	8 (870)	−1.94 [−2.42, −1.46]*, 77%	H294, H313, H318, H327, H333, H337, H338, H342
CPGQ pain intensity	4 (414)	−15.06 [−25.40, −4.72]*, 99%	H295, H301, H305, H330
CPGQ disability score	4 (414)	−13.93 [−29.14, 1.29], 99%	H295, H301, H305, H330
CPGQ disability points score	3 (248)	−0.67 [−1.03, −0.31]*, 0%	H295, H305, H330

*Statistically significant, see Statistical Analysis in Chapter 4.
Abbreviations: CI, confidence intervals; CPGQ, Chronic Pain Grading Questionnaire; EoT, end of treatment; MD, mean difference; RoB, risk of bias; VAS, visual analogue scale.

between groups in the disability score at the end of treatment. Sensitivity analyses including studies with low risk of bias for sequence generation did not reduce statistical heterogeneity (pain intensity: 291 women, −19.21 points [−27.78, −10.64], I^2 = 93%, H295, H301, H305; disability score: 291 women, −17.50 points [−29.91, −5.09], I^2 = 94%, H295, H301, H305).

When dysmenorrhoea was assessed using the NRS, women who received *Gong liu xiao jiao nang* 宫瘤消胶囊 plus mifepristone scored 0.26 points lower than women who received mifepristone alone (210 women, [−0.49, −0.03]; H303). Finally, women who received *San jie zhen tong jiao nang* 散结镇痛胶囊 in combination with Mirena® scored lower on the VRS — indicating less pain — than women who received Mirena® alone. This finding was seen at the end of treatment (61 women, MD −0.68 points [−0.91, −0.45];

H332) and at three-month follow-up (61 women, MD −0.47 points [−0.58, −0.36]; H332).

Dyspareunia

Two RCTs of women with adenomyosis evaluated the effects of oral CHM on dyspareunia (H299, H306). Meta-analysis was not possible as one RCT tested oral CHM alone while the other combined oral CHM with HT.

Oral Chinese herbal medicine versus hormone therapy

Among 62 women, treatment with *Gui zhi fu ling wan* 桂枝茯苓丸 resulted in a VAS score that was 0.63 cm lower than that of gestrinone ([−1.04, −0.22]; H306). This difference is unlikely to be clinically significant.

Oral Chinese herbal medicine plus hormone therapy versus hormone therapy

In 29 perimenopausal women who reported dyspareunia at baseline, there was no statistical difference in the number of women who continued to report dyspareunia at the end of treatment (RR 0.60 [0.25, 1.44]; H299).

Uterine volume

Twenty-eight RCTs documented uterine volume in women with adenomyosis (H292, H296, H299, H301, H303, H309, H311, H312, H316–H320, H325, H329–H334, H336, H337, H339–H343, H345). Meta-analysis was conducted separately for studies that tested oral CHM alone and those that tested the combination of oral CHM and pharmacotherapy.

Oral Chinese herbal medicine versus no treatment

One RCT that included 38 women who had previously undergone surgery compared the effect of *San jie zhen tong jiao nang* 散结镇痛胶囊

and no treatment on uterine volume (H336). The mean uterine volume at the end of treatment was 21.50 cm^3 lower among women who received San jie zhen tong jiao nang 散结镇痛胶囊 ([−42.13, −0.87]).

Oral Chinese herbal medicine versus hormone therapy

Among the 447 women who participated in seven RCTs (H296, H325, H329, H331, H339, H342, H345), the mean uterine volume at the end of treatment was not statistically different between women who received oral CHM and those who received HT (MD −5.09 cm^3 [−11.95, 1.77], I^2 = 62%). Moderate levels of statistical heterogeneity were detected. As all studies provided oral CHM for three months or more and compared CHM with HT, planned subgroup and sensitivity analyses could not be performed to examine potential causes of heterogeneity.

Oral Chinese herbal medicine plus hormone therapy versus hormone therapy

Twenty-one RCTs, involving 2,159 women, tested the effect of oral CHM plus HT on uterine volume (H292, H299, H301, H303, H309, H311, H312, H316–H320, H330, H332–H334, H337, H340–H343). At the end of treatment, women who received oral CHM plus HT had a smaller uterine volume than women who received HT alone (2,159 women, MD −17.30 cm^3 [−22.44, −12.17], I^2 = 83%; Table 5.45). Meta-analysis of studies judged to pose low risk of bias for sequence generation showed considerable heterogeneity, suggesting that the variation in results is likely to be due to other factors.

Five RCTs that measured uterine volume at the end of treatment performed another assessment after the end of treatment (H292, H311, H332, H340, H343). The combination of oral CHM plus HT resulted in uterine volume that was comparable to that of HT alone (375 women, MD −30.68 cm^3 [−64.33, 2.98], I^2 = 98%; Table 5.46). One RCT that used appropriate methods for sequence generation found a smaller uterine volume at follow-up in women who received

Table 5.45. Oral Chinese Herbal Medicine plus Hormone Therapy versus Hormone Therapy for Adenomyosis: Uterine Volume at the End of Treatment

Time of Assessment	No. of Studies (Participants)	Effect Size MD [95% CI], I^2	Included Studies
EoT	21 (2,159)	−17.30 [−22.44, −12.17]*, 83%	H292, H299, H301, H303, H309, H311, H312, H316–H320, H330, H332–H334, H337, H340–H343
Subgroup: low RoB SG	7 (983)	−24.38 [−37.96, −10.79]*, 91%	H301, H303, H320, H332–H334, H342

*Statistically significant, see Statistical Analysis in Chapter 4.
Abbreviations: CI, confidence intervals; EoT, end of treatment; MD, mean difference; RoB, risk of bias; SG, sequence generation.

Table 5.46. Oral Chinese Herbal Medicine plus Hormone Therapy versus Hormone Therapy for Adenomyosis: Uterine Volume at Follow-up

Time of Assessment	No. of Studies (Participants)	Effect Size MD [95% CI], I^2	Included Studies
EoT	5 (375)	−30.68 [−64.33, 2.98], 98%	H292, H311, H332, H340, H343
Subgroup: low RoB SG	1 (61)	−53.80 [−64.30, −43.30]*, NA	H332

*Statistically significant, see Statistical Analysis in Chapter 4.
Abbreviations: CI, confidence intervals; EoT, end of treatment; NA, not applicable; MD, mean difference; RoB, risk of bias; SG, sequence generation.

oral CHM plus HT (Table 5.46), but statistical heterogeneity remained considerable in subgroup analyses for specific formulas.

Menstrual volume

Seventeen RCTs reported on menstrual volumes (H292, H295, H300, H301, H308, H310–H312, H317, H320, H323, H330–H332, H336, H340, H343). A variety of different methods were used to determine menstrual volume, including the pictorial blood loss assessment chart (PBAC), weight or volume of the sanitary napkin, percentage of napkin filled, and menstrual volume as a percentage of the pre-surgery volume. Meta-analyses were conducted wherever possible.

Oral Chinese herbal medicine versus no treatment

Two studies compared oral CHM with no treatment in women who had undergone surgery before the trial (H300, H336). When *Hua yu xiao jie fang* 化瘀消结方 was compared with no treatment, women who received oral CHM had a combined sanitary napkin weight that was 43.5 mg lighter than that of women who received no treatment (40 women, [-46.41, -40.59]; H300). Another RCT that calculated menstrual volume as a percentage of the pre-surgery volume found that women who received *San jie zhen tong jiao nang* 散结镇痛胶囊 had 13.8% less menstrual volume than women who received no treatment (38 women, [-21.76, -5.90]; H336).

Oral Chinese herbal medicine versus hormone therapy

Meta-analysis of two RCTs showed no difference between women who received oral CHM and those who received HT in menstrual volume as assessed with the PBAC (130 women, MD 14.21 [-35.04, 63.45], $I^2 = 99\%$; H308, H310). A similar finding was seen in a single study that assessed the weight of menstrual volume (55 women, MD 0.33 [-8.19, 8.85]; H331).

Oral Chinese herbal medicine plus hormone therapy versus hormone therapy

Thirteen studies that compared the combination of oral CHM plus HT with HT alone assessed menstrual volume using different techniques (H292, H295, H301, H311, H312, H317, H320, H323, H330, H332, H334, H340, H343). Meta-analysis was possible for six

Table 5.47. Oral Chinese Herbal Medicine plus Hormone Therapy versus Hormone Therapy for Adenomyosis: Pictorial Blood Loss Assessment Chart

Time of Assessment	No. of Studies (Participants)	Effect Size MD [95% CI], I^2	Included Studies
EoT	6 (547)	−30.98 [−60.71, −1.25]*, 99%	H312, H317, H320, H323, H332, H340
Subgroup: low RoB SG	3 (143)	−9.30 [−17.81, −0.78]*, 77%	H320, H323, H332

*Statistically significant, see Statistical Analysis in Chapter 4.
Abbreviations: CI, confidence intervals; EoT, end of treatment; MD, mean difference; RoB, risk of bias; SG, sequence generation.

RCTs that measured menstrual volume using the PBAC (H312, H317, H320, H323, H332, H340). At the end of treatment, women who received oral CHM plus HT had smaller menstrual volume than women who received HT alone (547 women, MD −30.98 [−60.71, −1.25], I^2 = 99%). The large range of the confidence intervals produced considerable statistical heterogeneity. Sensitivity and subgroup analyses were conducted to examine potential causes of heterogeneity (Table 5.47), although this did not reduce statistical heterogeneity. The presence of statistical heterogeneity in all analyses lowers confidence in the result.

One RCT conducted follow-up assessment (H332) and found that the PBAC was lower in women who received *San jie zhen tong jiao nang* 散结镇痛胶囊 plus HT than in those who received HT alone (61 women, MD −16.20 [−22.44, −9.96]).

When menstrual volume at the end of treatment was assessed as a percentage of the baseline menstrual volume, meta-analysis of three RCTs showed no difference between women who received oral CHM as integrative medicine and those who received HT alone (349 women, MD −0.29% [−23.58, 23.00], I^2 = 99%; H292, H301, H330). Subgroup analysis excluding one study that included self-reported change in menstrual volume favoured oral CHM as integrative medicine over HT alone (183 women, MD −11.05 [−17.60, −4.49], I^2 = 0%; H292, H330). Follow-up assessment in one

RCT showed no difference between *Tong jing tang* 痛经汤 plus Mirena® and Mirena® alone (60 women, MD −4.87 [−14.32, 4.58]; H292).

Two RCTs used other methods to determine menstrual volume (H295, H343). In one RCT with 60 women, women who received *Dan leng fu kang jian gao* 丹莪妇康煎膏 plus medroxyprogesterone acetate and methyltestosterone used a similar number of sanitary napkins as women who received medroxyprogesterone acetate and methyltestosterone alone (MD 1.00 napkins [−7.11, 9.11]; H295). The volume of menstrual blood was 8.90 mL lower in women who received *Ge gen er xian tang* 葛根二仙汤 as integrative medicine than in women who received triptorelin and Mirena® (52 women, [−12.15, −5.65]; H343).

Pregnancy outcomes

Results from one RCT with 99 women showed that the pregnancy rate was higher among women who received *Zi shen shu gan tang* 滋肾疏肝汤 than among women who received no treatment (RR 1.59 [1.02, 2.47]; H322).

Fatigue

One RCT assessed the number of women with fatigue (H299). There was no difference between women who received *Hua yu xiao zheng fang* 化瘀消癥方 plus mifepristone and those who received mifepristone alone in the number of women with fatigue at the end of treatment (60 women, RR 0.60 [0.25, 1.44]).

Health-related quality of life

Three RCTs assessed health-related quality of life for women with adenomyosis (H318, H319, H337), all of whom used oral CHM as integrative medicine with HT. When health-related quality of life was assessed in 68 women using the SF-36, the combination of *Xi huang jiao nang* 西黄胶囊 and Mirena® resulted in higher scores — indicating better quality of life — than Mirena® alone for the domains of general health (MD 7.65 points [1.53, 13.77]) and vitality (MD 6.18 points [0.99, 11.37]). No difference was seen between groups for the domains of physical role function (MD 1.47 points [−6.19, 9.13]), bodily pain (MD 2.22 points [−5.28, 9.72]), social function (MD 4.05 points [−1.52, 9.62]), emotional role function (MD 9.81 points [−2.00, 21.62]), mental health (MD 4.00 points [−2.44, 10.44]), and physical function (MD 1.47 points [−4.02, 6.96]).

The Psychological General Well-Being Index (PGWB) was used to measure health-related quality of life in one RCT (H319). The scale includes 22 items scored from 0–5. Item scores are summed to provide a total score, for which higher scores indicate better quality of life. Women who received *San jie zhen tong jiao nang* 散结镇痛胶囊 and Mirena® scored higher on the PGWB than women who received Mirena® alone (70 women, MD 12.30 points [7.54, 17.06]).

One RCT reported the effect of *Shao fu zhu yu tang* 少腹逐瘀汤 plus gestrinone on health-related quality of life using the Nottingham Health Profile (NHP). Among the 96 participants, women who received *Shao fu zhu yu tang* 少腹逐瘀汤 plus gestrinone scored lower on the NHP — indicating better outcomes — for all six domains: pain (MD −1.50 points [−1.85, −1.15]), emotional reaction (MD −0.58 points [−0.77, −0.39]), sleep (MD −2.50 points [−3.04, −1.96]), physical abilities (MD −0.60 points [−0.79, −0.41]), energy levels (MD −2.12 points [−2.62, −1.62]), and social isolation (MD −0.48 points [−0.73, −0.23]).

Randomised controlled trial evidence for individual oral formulas

Several RCTs that tested the same formula reported on the same outcomes, and meta-analyses were possible. Evidence revealed that the combination of *Gui zhi fu ling jiao nang* 桂枝茯苓胶囊 and pharmacotherapy resulted in a dysmenorrhoea VAS score that was 2.08 cm lower than that of pharmacotherapy alone (Table 5.48). The pill

Table 5.48. Oral Chinese Herbal Medicine plus Pharmacotherapy versus Pharmacotherapy for Adenomyosis: Dysmenorrhoea

Formula	No. of Studies (Participants)	Effect Size MD [95% CI], I^2	Included Studies
VAS – EoT			
Gui zhi fu ling jiao nang 桂枝茯苓胶囊	2 (252)	−2.08 [−2.61, −1.56]*, 58%	H302, H323
Ge gen er xian tang 葛根二仙汤	2 (132)	−0.27 [−0.69, 0.16], 0%	H311, H343
VAS – follow-up			
Ge gen er xian tang 葛根二仙汤	3 (191)	−1.74 [−3.53, 0.05], 96%	H292, H311, H343
1993 Guideline			
Gui zhi fu ling wan 桂枝茯苓丸	2 (138)	−1.40 [−2.13, −0.68]*, 11%	H294, H313
Shao fu zhu yu tang/jiao nang 少腹逐瘀汤/胶囊	2 (396)	−1.97 [−3.05, −0.89]*, 89%	H333, H337

*Statistically significant, see Statistical Analysis in Chapter 4.
Abbreviations: CI, confidence intervals; EoT, end of treatment; MD, mean difference; VAS, visual analogue scale.

formulation, *Gui zhi fu ling wan* 桂枝茯苓丸, combined with pharmacotherapy also reduced dysmenorrhoea; the dysmenorrhoea score was 1.4 points lower among those who received *Gui zhi fu ling wan* 桂枝茯苓丸 plus pharmacotherapy when measured using the 1993 Guideline (Table 5.48). Two studies that combined *Shao fu zhu yu tang/jiao nang* 少腹逐瘀汤/胶囊 with pharmacotherapy also showed reduction of dysmenorrhoea by 1.97 points when measured with the 1993 Guideline. *Ge gen er xian tang* 葛根二仙汤 plus pharmacotherapy did not result in a statistically different VAS score when compared to pharmacotherapy alone both at the end of treatment and at follow-up.

Meta-analyses of results for menstrual volume change measured with the PBAC were also conducted for two CHM formulas that were combined with HT: *Gui zhi fu ling jiao nang/wan* 桂枝茯苓胶囊/丸 and *San jie zhen tong jiao nang* 散结镇痛胶囊 (Table 5.49). Neither

Table 5.49. Oral Chinese Herbal Medicine plus Hormone Therapy versus Hormone Therapy for Adenomyosis: Pictorial Blood Loss Assessment Chart

Formula	No. of Studies (Participants)	Effect Size MD [95% CI], I^2	Included Studies
Gui zhi fu ling jiao nang/wan 桂枝茯苓胶囊/丸	4 (426)	−13.76 [−29.41, 1.89], 95%	H312, H317, H320, H323
San jie zhen tong jiao nang 散结镇痛胶囊	2 (121)	−65.49 [−156.24, 25.25], 100%	H332, H340

*Statistically significant, see Statistical Analysis in Chapter 4.
Abbreviations: CI, confidence intervals; MD, mean difference.

Table 5.50. Oral Chinese Herbal Medicine plus Hormone Therapy versus Hormone Therapy for Adenomyosis: Uterine Volume at End of Treatment

Formula	No. of Studies (Participants)	Effect Size MD [95% CI], I^2	Included Studies
Gui zhi fu ling jiao nang/wan 桂枝茯苓胶囊/丸	4 (374)	−14.96 [−21.31, −8.60]*, 67%	H309, H312, H317, H320
Shao fu zhu yu jiao nang/Shao fu zhu yu tang 少腹逐瘀胶囊/少腹逐瘀汤	2 (396)	−9.35 [−12.74, −5.96]*, 0%	H333, H337
San jie zhen tong jiao nang 散结镇痛胶囊	4 (344)	−26.43 [−46.38, −6.49]*, 91%	H316, H319, H332, H340
Ge gen er xian tang 葛根二仙汤	2 (132)	−4.23 [−11.33, 2.88], 0%	H311, H343

*Statistically significant, see Statistical Analysis in Chapter 4.
Abbreviations: CI, confidence intervals; MD, mean difference.

formula resulted in a statistically significant change in the PBAC when combined with HT compared with HT alone.

When combined with HT, three formulas reduced uterine volume at the end of treatment more than HT alone did (Table 5.50). Uterine volume was reduced by 15 cm³ for *Gui zhi fu ling jiao nang/wan* 桂枝茯苓胶囊/丸 plus HT, 9.4 cm³ for *Shao fu zhu yu jiao nang/Shao fu zhu yu tang* 少腹逐瘀胶囊/少腹逐瘀汤, and 26.4 cm³ for *San jie zhen tong jiao nang* 散结镇痛胶囊. *Ge gen er xian tang* 葛根二仙汤 used with HT provided no greater benefit than HT alone.

Table 5.51. Oral Chinese Herbal Medicine plus Hormone Therapy versus Hormone Therapy for Adenomyosis: Uterine Volume at Follow-up

Formula	No. of Studies (Participants)	Effect Size MD [95% CI], I^2	Included Studies
San jie zhen tong jiao nang 散结镇痛胶囊	2 (183)	−16.88 [−37.16, 3.41], 91%	H332, H340
Ge gen er xian tang 葛根二仙汤	2 (132)	−55.32 [−138.52, 27.88], 99%	H311, H343

*Statistically significant, see Statistical Analysis in Chapter 4.
Abbreviations: CI, confidence intervals; MD, mean difference.

Meta-analyses of individual formulas were also possible for uterine volume at follow-up. The benefits seen with *San jie zhen tong jiao nang* 散结镇痛胶囊 plus HT at the end of treatment were no longer evident at follow-up assessment (Table 5.51). Uterine volume at follow-up assessment was not different between *Ge gen er xian tang* 葛根二仙汤 plus HT and HT alone. This was not surprising as no benefit of the combination was seen at the end of treatment.

Frequently reported herbs in meta-analyses showing favourable effect

Several meta-analyses indicated that the combination of oral CHM and pharmacotherapy was superior to pharmacotherapy alone in reducing dysmenorrhoea for women with adenomyosis. Among the five meta-analyses and 26 RCTs, the most frequently used herbs were *dang gui* 当归 and *yan hu suo* 延胡索 (Table 5.52). These herbs have actions that activate Blood, dispel stasis, and alleviate pain. Such actions may explain their high frequency of use in studies that were included in positive meta-analyses.

One meta-analysis with 21 RCTs showed that the combination of oral CHM plus HT was superior to HT alone in reducing the uterine volume for women with adenomyosis. The most frequently used herbs among the 21 RCTs were *dang gui* 当归, *wu ling zhi* 五灵脂, and *chi shao* 赤芍 (Table 5.53). These herbs may contribute to the positive effects seen.

Table 5.52. Frequently Reported Orally Used Herbs in Meta-Analyses Showing Favourable Effect for Dysmenorrhoea

Herbs	Scientific Name	Frequency of Use
Dang gui 当归	*Angelica sinensis* (Oliv.) Diels	19
Yan hu suo 延胡索	*Corydalis yanhusuo* W.T. Wang	13
Wu ling zhi 五灵脂	*Trogopterus xanthipes* Milne-Edwards	10
Bai shao 白芍	*Paeonia* spp.	10
Chi shao 赤芍	*Paeonia* spp.	10
Dan shen 丹参	*Salvia miltiorrhiza* Bge.	9
Chuan xiong 川芎	*Ligusticum chuangxiong* Hort.	8
Gan cao 甘草	*Glycyrrhiza* spp.	8
E zhu 莪术	*Curcuma* spp.	8
Pu huang 蒲黄	*Typha* spp.	8

For details of meta-analyses, see Tables 5.43 and 5.44.
Note: The use of some herbs may be restricted in some countries. Readers are advised to comply with relevant regulations.

Table 5.53. Frequently Reported Orally Used Herbs in Meta-Analyses Showing Favourable Effect for Sonographic Measures

Herbs	Scientific Name	Frequency of Use
Dang gui 当归	*Angelica sinensis* (Oliv.) Diels	9
Wu ling zhi 五灵脂	*Trogopterus xanthipes* Milne-Edwards	8
Chi shao 赤芍	*Paeonia* spp.	7
Gan cao 甘草	*Glycyrrhiza* spp.	5
Tu si zi 菟丝子	*Cuscuta* spp.	5
Yan hu suo 延胡索	*Corydalis yanhusuo* W.T. Wang	5
Yin yang huo 淫羊藿	*Epimedium* spp.	5
Chuan xiong 川芎	*Ligusticum chuangxiong* Hort.	4
Pu huang 蒲黄	*Typha* spp.	4

For details of meta-analyses, see Table 5.45.
Note: The use of some herbs may be restricted in some countries. Readers are advised to comply with relevant regulations.

One meta-analysis including six RCTs showed that the combination of oral CHM plus HT was beneficial over HT alone in reducing menstrual blood loss (Table 5.47). Among these six RCTs, only one listed the herbal ingredients of the treatments used. As such, it was not possible to determine which herbs may have contributed to the positive effects seen in the meta-analysis.

Safety of oral Chinese herbal medicine for adenomyosis in randomised controlled trials

Thirty-four RCTs reported on the safety of oral CHM (H292–H294, H297, H299, H301, H302, H304–H307, H309–H312, H316–H319, H322–H324, H326, H328, H330–H332, H334, H335, H337, H338, H340, H342, H343), with nine RCTs stating that no AEs occurred during the conduct of the trial (H292, H297, H299, H301, H309, H322, H328, H335, H337).

In the 11 RCTs that tested oral CHM alone, two RCTs reported 22 AEs (H307, H342). Adverse events in women who received oral CHM included three cases of loss of appetite, two cases of vaginal bleeding, two cases of weight gain, and one case of ovarian cyst. In studies that used oral CHM as integrative medicine, 149 AEs were reported. Adverse events with oral CHM as integrative medicine included 40 cases of irregular vaginal bleeding, 22 cases with symptoms of low oestrogen such as hot flushes and sweating, 15 cases of weight gain, 13 cases of nausea, 11 cases of amenorrhoea, seven cases of breast pain, six cases of headache, five cases of acne, five cases of menstrual disorders, five cases of unnamed AEs, four cases of headache, insomnia, mood swings, and vaginal dryness, three cases of ovarian cyst, three cases of nausea, vomiting, headache, fatigue, and hot flushes, three cases of nausea, vomiting, and loss of appetite, two cases of lower limb oedema, two cases of abnormal liver function, two cases of abdominal or gastrointestinal discomfort, and one case of dizziness, nausea, breast pain, and irregular vaginal bleeding.

Among women who received HT, 526 AEs were reported. These included 108 cases of irregular vaginal bleeding, 98 cases of low oestrogen symptoms such as hot flushes and sweating, 63 cases of abnormal liver function, 20 cases of weight gain, 20 cases of weight gain with increased sebum production and prolonged acne, 17 cases of amenorrhoea, 17 cases of nausea, 17 cases of gastrointestinal discomfort, 15 cases of acne, 14 cases of breast pain, 14 cases of nausea and loss of appetite, 12 cases of dizziness, nausea, vomiting, general malaise, and lethargy, 12 cases of amenorrhoea, weight gain, acne, and increase in sebum, 12 cases of haemorrhoids, nine cases of headache, insomnia, mood swings, and vaginal dryness, eight cases of nausea, vomiting, headache, fatigue, and hot flushes, seven cases of ovarian cysts, six cases of headache, six cases of lower limb oedema, five cases of menstrual disorders, five cases of haemorrhoids and oily skin, five cases of loss of appetite, five cases of nausea and vomiting, five cases of nausea, vomiting, and loss of appetite, four cases of dizziness, nausea, breast pain, and irregular vaginal bleeding, four cases of loss of libido, three cases of change in breast size, three cases of headache and painful phlegm, two cases of weight gain and breast pain, two cases of dizziness, and one case each of vomiting, fatigue, and mild constipation. Five other unspecified events were reported, as was an unknown number of cases of prolonged menstrual period and irregular vaginal bleeding.

Controlled Clinical Trials of Oral Chinese Herbal Medicine for Adenomyosis

Oral CHM for women with adenomyosis was evaluated in six CCTs (H347–H352). One study included two treatment arms: one treatment arm tested oral CHM alone while the other tested oral CHM used in combination with oral contraceptives (H349). All studies were conducted in China and included 978 adult women. None of the women had undergone surgery prior to treatment. The mean age of women ranged from the low to high 30s for four of the five studies that documented participant age, while the fifth study reported a mean age of 42.

Two studies included women with Kidney deficiency and Blood stasis (H348, H352). Three studies tested the combination of oral CHM and oral contraceptives (H349–H351) and four studies compared oral CHM with either NSAIDs or HT (H347–H349, H352). The commercially manufactured product *San jie zhen tong jiao nang* 散结镇痛胶囊 was used in two CCTs (H347, H351), and there was no overlap in other oral CHM formulas used. Forty-five different herbs were used in the six studies, with the most frequently used herbs being *e zhu* 莪术, *san leng* 三棱, *shan yao* 山药, and *xiang fu* 香附 (three uses each).

Treatment was provided for between three and six months, and three CCTs conducted follow-up assessments, which ocurred from three to 21 months. One large study of 587 women reported high numbers of dropouts (H349), although the number of dropouts was not reported by group allocation.

Dysmenorrhoea

Three studies assessed dysmenorrhoea using either the 1993 Guideline (H348, H352) or the CPGQ (H350). Meta-analysis was possible for the two studies that used the 1993 Guideline.

Oral Chinese herbal medicine versus hormone therapy

Two studies involving 154 women found no difference between oral CHM and HT in reducing dysmenorrhoea measured with the 1993 Guideline (MD 0.08 points, [–2.19, 2.34], I^2 = 95%; H348, H352).

Oral Chinese herbal medicine plus hormone therapy versus hormone therapy

Results from a single study (H350) found that the combination of *Gui zhi fu ling jiao nang* 桂枝茯苓胶囊 and Mirena® did not reduce pain intensity, measured using the CPGQ, more than Mirena® alone did at the end of treatment (MD –0.10 points [–0.55, 0.35]). At follow-up, women who received *Gui zhi fu ling jiao nang* 桂枝茯苓胶囊 and Mirena® had lower pain intensity than women who received Mirena® (MD –0.40 points [–0.59, –0.21]). The difference between groups was small, and the clinical significance of this result remains unclear.

Uterine volume

Three studies measured uterine volume (H347, H349, H351). Meta-analysis could be conducted when oral CHM was used alone and as integrative medicine.

Oral Chinese herbal medicine versus pharmacotherapy

Meta-analysis of two CCTs showed no benefit of oral CHM over pharmacotherapy at the end of treatment, with considerable statistical heterogeneity (318 women, MD −77.52 cm^3 [−214.32, 59.28], I^2 = 99%; H347, H349). Due to the small number of studies, statistical heterogeneity could not be examined and confidence in the results is limited. One study that conducted follow-up assessment three months after the end of treatment found the uterine volume to be 13.2 cm^3 lower in women who received *Qu yu xiao yi tang* 祛瘀消异汤 compared with those who received oral contraceptives (244 women, [−17.43, −8.97]; H349).

Oral Chinese herbal medicine plus hormone therapy versus hormone therapy

Two studies that evaluated oral CHM plus HT (H349, H351) found no benefit of the combination over HT alone for uterine volume. This result was seen at the end of treatment (291 women, MD −1.97 cm^3 [−12.86, 8.92], I^2 = 58%) and at follow-up (291 women, MD −7.26 cm^3 [−18.44, 3.92], I^2 = 62%).

Menstrual volume

One CCT assessed menstrual volume using the PBAC in 68 women with adenomyosis (H351). While menstrual volume was lower at the end of treatment in women who received the combination of *San jie zhen tong jiao nang* 散结镇痛胶囊 plus Mirena® (MD −2.70 points [−5.31, −0.09]), the effect was no longer statistically significant at six-month follow-up (MD −1.30 points [−3.61, 1.01]).

Safety of oral Chinese herbal medicine in controlled clinical trials for women with adenomyosis

Four CCTs reported on the safety of oral CHM (H347, H348, H350, H351), with one reporting that no AEs occurred (H348). Adverse events in women who received oral CHM were 11 cases of irregular bleeding, nine cases of breast pain, two cases of gastrointestinal discomfort, and two cases where the Mirena® had dislodged. Adverse events in women who received pharmacotherapy were 28 cases of irregular vaginal bleeding, 14 cases of breast pain, and two cases where the Mirena® had dislodged.

Non-controlled Studies of Oral Chinese Herbal Medicine for Adenomyosis

Twenty-seven non-controlled studies used oral CHM for 511 women with adenomyosis (H353–H379). All studies were conducted in China and included adult women with no prior surgery. Thirteen were case series (H354, H356, H358–H362, H366–H368, H374, H375, H379) and 14 were case reports (H353, H355, H357, H363–H365, H369, H370–H373, H376–H378). Three studies did not specify how women were recruited (H356, H362, H379) and the remaining studies recruited women through hospital outpatient departments. Duration of adenomyosis ranged from one (H377) to 10 years (H355, H363, H373).

Nineteen studies used CM syndrome differentiation to select participants (H353, H354, H357, H359–H365, H369, H370–H373, H376–H379). Four syndromes were described in multiple studies: *qi* stagnation and Blood stasis (seven studies), cold coagulation and Blood stasis (three studies), Kidney deficiency and Blood stasis (two studies), and phlegm and Blood stasis (two studies). Ten studies tailored

Table 5.54. Frequently Reported Orally Used Herbs in Non-controlled Studies for Adenomyosis

Most Common Herbs	Scientific Name	Frequency of Use
E zhu 莪术	Curcuma spp.	17
Chi shao 赤芍	Paeonia spp.	15
Fu ling 茯苓	Poria cocos (Schw.) Wolf	15
Yan hu suo 延胡索	Corydalis yanhusuo W.T. Wang	15
Bai shao 白芍	Paeonia lactiflora Pall.	13
Tao ren 桃仁	Prunus spp.	12
Dan shen 丹参	Salvia miltiorrhiza Bge.	11
Dang gui 当归	Angelica sinensis (Oliv.) Diels	11
San leng 三棱	Sparganium stoloniferum Buch. -Ham.	11
Wu ling zhi 五灵脂	Trogopterus xanthipes Milne-Edwards	11
Gan cao 甘草	Glycyrrhiza spp.	10
Huang qi 黄芪	Astragalus spp.	10
Mu dan pi 牡丹皮	Paeonia suffruticosa Andr.	10
Shan yao 山药	Dioscorea opposita Thunb.	10
Xia ku cao 夏枯草	Prunella vulgaris L.	10
Xu duan 续断	Dipsacus asper Wall. ex Henry	10

Note: The use of some herbs may be restricted in some countries. Readers are advised to comply with relevant regulations.

treatment according to the time of the menstrual cycle (H355, H357, H359, H365, H368, H369, H371–H373, H376) and many oral CHM formulas were investigator-developed treatments. One formula was used in two studies: *Hu po san* 琥珀散. There was considerable diversity in formula ingredients, with 147 different herbs described in the 27 studies. The most frequently used herbs were *e zhu* 莪术, *chi shao* 赤芍, *fu ling* 茯苓, and *yan hu suo* 延胡索 (Table 5.54).

Treatment with oral CHM was provided for between one (H355) and 24 months (H372); the median duration of treatment was three months. Six studies conducted follow-up assessment (H361, H363, H370–H372, H378) up to one year. None of the studies reported on the safety of oral CHM for women with adenomyosis.

Topical Chinese Herbal Medicine for Adenomyosis

Five studies that tested topical CHM in women with adenomyosis were included in this section. Three were RCTs (H380–H382) and two were non-controlled studies (H383, H384). None of the CCTs met the inclusion criteria.

Randomised Controlled Trials of Topical Chinese Herbal Medicine for Adenomyosis

Three RCTs used topical CHM for 198 adult women with adenomyosis (H380–H382). All studies were conducted in China; one study recruited women from the hospital outpatient department, while the remaining studies did not specify the setting. The median of the mean age of participants was 35.3 years. All women completed the study.

Chinese medicine syndrome differentiation was used to select study participants in two studies (H380, H382). Syndromes included hot Blood stasis (H380) and cold coagulation and Blood stasis (H382). Topical CHM was administered as an enema for three months in all studies, none of which conducted follow-up assessments beyond the end of treatment. Each study used a different CHM enema, although six herbs were common to two studies: *san leng* 三棱, *dan shen* 丹参, *chuan xiong* 川芎, *dang gui* 当归, *e zhu* 莪术, and *chi shao* 赤芍.

One RCT compared CHM enema with oral contraceptives (H380). The remaining studies tested the combination of topical CHM and conventional medical management; topical CHM was combined with mifepristone in one study (H382), while the other study combined topical CHM with ultrasound treatment (H381).

Risk of bias assessment

Potential sources of bias were identified in all three studies. One study used a random number table to allocate participants to groups and was judged as having low risk of bias (H380). No details were reported about the method of sequence generation in the remaining two studies, and none of the studies described how group allocation was concealed (unclear risk of bias). None of the studies reported blinding of participants, personnel, or outcome assessors, and all three were judged as having high risk for these domains. The studies posed low risk of bias for incomplete outcome assessment as there was no missing data. No trial protocols or trial registrations were reported or located, and all studies were considered to have an unclear risk of bias in terms of selective outcome reporting.

Dysmenorrhoea

All three studies reported the effect of CHM enema on dysmenorrhoea. One study reported results based on the CPGQ (H382); however, results were not consistent with the standard scoring for this outcome tool. Thus, results for this outcome were excluded from analysis. The remaining two studies assessed dysmenorrhoea using a 10 cm VAS. Due to differences in comparisons, results could not be pooled for meta-analysis.

Topical Chinese herbal medicine versus hormone therapy

One study with 62 women found *Hua yu san jie guan chang ye* 化瘀散结灌肠液 to be superior to desogestrel ethinylestradiol in reducing VAS pain scores at the end of treatment (MD −0.50 cm [−0.95, −0.05]; H380).

Topical Chinese herbal medicine plus ultrasound therapy versus ultrasound therapy

An investigator-developed CHM enema used in combination with ultrasound therapy resulted in a VAS score that was 2.30 cm lower at the end of treatment than that of ultrasound therapy alone (60 women, [−3.29, −1.31]; H381).

Uterine volume

At the end of treatment, the uterine volume of women who received Hua yu san jie guan chang ye 化瘀散结灌肠液 was 14 cm³ lower than in women who received desogestrel ethinylestradiol (62 women, [−24.13, −3.87]; H380).

Ovarian cyst volume

The combination of CHM enema with ultrasound therapy reduced ovarian cyst volume by 18.4 cm³ at the end of treatment compared with ultrasound therapy alone (60 women, [−36.56, −0.24]; H381).

Menstrual volume

At the final assessment, there was no statistical difference in menstrual volume, assessed using the PBAC, between women who received Hua yu san jie guan chang ye 化瘀散结灌肠液 and those who received desogestrel ethinylestradiol (62 women, MD −7.30 [−18.11, 3.51]; H380).

Safety of topical Chinese herbal medicine in randomised controlled trials for women with adenomyosis

One RCT reported on the safety of topical CHM for women with adenomyosis (H381). Two cases of a small amount of vaginal bleeding were reported among the 30 women who received topical CHM as integrative medicine, while one case of vaginal bleeding was reported among the 30 women who received ultrasound treatment.

Non-controlled Studies of Topical Chinese Herbal Medicine for Adenomyosis

Sixty-three adult women with no previous surgery for adenomyosis participated in the two case series included in this section (H383, H384). Studies were conducted in Chinese hospital outpatient departments. One study documented the duration of adenomyosis, which ranged from eight months to 12 years (H383). Women with the CM syndrome of Kidney deficiency with Blood stasis were selected in the study by Liu (H383), while the other study did not report CM syndromes.

Topical CHM treatment was provided for three months in both studies, and women were followed up for an additional three months in one study (H383). The topical CHM formulas used in the two studies were different: *Zhe chong yin* 折冲饮 (H383) and *Yi qi san jie ji* 益气散结剂 (H384). *E zhu* 莪术 and *chuan xiong* 川芎 were used in both formulas. One study reported that seven cases of mild bloating and diarrhoea occurred (H384), while the other study did not state whether AEs occurred.

Oral plus Topical Chinese Herbal Medicine for Adenomyosis

Three studies were included that tested the combination of oral plus topical CHM for adenomyosis. One study was an RCT (H385) and two studies were case series (H386, H387). No CCTs were identified that met the eligibility criteria for inclusion.

Randomised Controlled Trials of Oral plus Topical Chinese Herbal Medicine for Adenomyosis

The combination of oral plus topical CHM for adenomyosis was tested in one RCT with 60 women who had not undergone surgery prior to enrolling in the study (H385). The women were recruited from hospital outpatient departments in China and received treatment for three months, with an additional follow-up assessment conducted three months after the end of treatment. The mean duration of adenomyosis was 3.5 years and the mean age of participants was 37.7 years.

Women with the CM syndrome of *qi* stagnation and Blood stasis were included, and women in the CHM group received oral *Hu po san* 琥珀散, consisting of ingredients *san leng* 三棱, *e zhu* 莪术, *dan pi* 丹皮, *chi shao* 赤芍, *rou gui* 肉桂, *dang gui* 当归, *xiang fu* 香附,

shu di 熟地, *yan hu suo* 延胡索, *wu yao* 乌药, *liu ji nu* 刘寄奴, and *hu po* 琥珀; *san qi fen* 三七粉 was added during menstruation. An unnamed herbal formula was applied topically to the umbilicus; herb ingredients included *shui zhi* 水蛭, *tu chong* 土虫, *di long* 地龙, *wu gong* 蜈蚣, and *xue jie* 血竭. Oral plus topical CHM was compared with mifepristone.

The study was described as a randomised controlled trial, but the methods used to allocate participants to groups and to conceal group allocation were not described (unclear risk of bias). As neither participants, personnel, nor outcome assessors were blind to group allocation, the study was judged to pose high risk of bias for these domains. Outcome data were available for all participants (low risk of bias). No trial protocol or trial registration was identified, so the study was considered to have unclear bias for selective outcome reporting.

The study reported on two clinical outcomes: dysmenorrhoea and uterine volume. Dysmenorrhoea was assessed using the 1993 Guideline. A reduction of 2.10 points, suggesting an improvement in dysmenorrhoea, was found in women who received oral *Hu po san* 琥珀散 plus topical CHM compared with those who received mifepristone ([−3.71, −0.49]). Uterine volume was 11.8 cm^3 greater among women who received oral plus topical CHM ([1.24, 22.28]), indicating worse outcomes than mifepristone.

The study also reported on the safety of oral plus topical CHM for women with adenomyosis. No AEs occurred in the treatment group, while an unspecified number of cases of nausea and vomiting occurred in the control group.

Non-controlled Studies of Oral plus Topical Chinese Herbal Medicine for Adenomyosis

Both case series were conducted in China and included 180 women who were recruited from hospital outpatient departments (H386, H387). The average duration of adenomyosis was 69 months. Studies included women with the CM syndrome damp-heat stasis (H386) or damp-heat toxin (H387). Women received treatment with CHM for three months, which was tailored according to the time of the menstrual cycle. In both case series, women received *Si ni jin ling shi xiao san* 四逆金铃失笑散 and *Du yi wei jiao nang* 独一味胶囊 during menstruation. One formula used at other times of the menstrual cycle was common to both studies: *Nei yi kang fu pian* 内异康复片. Other formulas included *Pu qiao xiao luo shi xiao san* 蒲翘消瘰失笑散 (H386) and *Fu an ning* 妇安宁 (H387). Two herbs, *pu huang* 蒲黄 and *wu ling zhi* 五灵脂, were used in three formulas, while 10 herbs were used in two formulas: *bai shao* 白芍, *chai hu* 柴胡, *chuan lian zi* 川楝子, *lian qiao* 连翘, *sheng mu li* 生牡蛎, *xuan shen* 玄参, *yan hu suo* 延胡索, *zhe bei* 浙贝, *zhi gan cao* 炙甘草, and *zhi qiao* 枳壳. Neither study reported on the safety of the combination of oral plus topical CHM for women with adenomyosis.

Part 3. Endometriosis and Adenomyosis

Thirty studies included women with endometriosis and those with adenomyosis (H388–H415). Of these, 28 investigated the benefits of oral CHM and two tested the combination of oral plus topical CHM. Results are presented according to the route of administration and study design.

Oral Chinese Herbal Medicine for Endometriosis and Adenomyosis

Among the 28 studies of oral CHM, seven were RCTs (H388–H394), four were CCTs (H395–H398), and 17 were non-controlled studies (H399–H415).

Randomised Controlled Trials of Oral Chinese Herbal Medicine for Endometriosis and Adenomyosis

Oral CHM was tested in seven RCTs with 624 women (H388–H394). Two RCTs were three-arm studies that included two CHM arms (H390, H391); the CHM interventions were considered sufficiently similar that results for the two groups were merged for statistical analysis. Remaining studies were two-arm, parallel RCTs.

Most women were in their 30s (the median of the mean age was 34.5 years). The mean age in one RCT was 48.4 years (H393), and the mean ages of women in two studies were in the 20s (25.3 years, H392; 27.4 years, H394). Women were recruited from hospital inpatient and outpatient departments in China and had lived with endometriosis or adenomyosis for an average of 2.1 years (H393) to 10.3 years (H392). None of the participants received surgery prior to enrolling in the trials. Women in one RCT had laparoscopic diagnosis of endometriosis/adenomyosis (H393).

Three RCTs used CM syndromes to select participants (H388, H390, H394). Syndromes included *yang* deficiency cold, Blood stasis obstructing the *Chong* 冲 and *Ren* 任 vessels and uterus (H388), *qi* stagnation and Blood stasis (H390), and Blood stasis (H394). Two RCTs varied the oral CHM according to the time of the menstrual cycle (H390, H392), while two studies tested oral CHM as integrative medicine with HT (H392, H393). One manufactured product, *San jie zhen tong jiao nang* 散结镇痛胶囊, was evaluated in three studies (H389, H393, H394); there was no overlap in formulas used in the other studies. The most frequently used herbs were *chuan xiong* 川芎 and *san qi* 三七 (four uses each), followed by *chai hu* 柴胡, *dang gui* 当归, *xue jie* 血竭, *yi yi ren* 薏苡仁, and *zhe bei mu* 浙贝母 (three uses each).

Six of the seven RCTs provided oral CHM treatment for three months (H388–H392, H394), and the remaining study provided treatment for six months (H393). Three studies conducted follow-up assessment at either one month (H391) or three months (H390, H392) after the end of treatment. One RCT reported loss to follow-up, with four dropouts in both the treatment and control groups (H394).

Risk of bias assessment

Several potential sources of bias were identified in the seven RCTs. Two studies used a random number table to allocate participants (H390, H391); these were judged as having low risk of bias for sequence generation. One RCT used a method that could not ensure random allocation (H394) and was judged as having high risk of bias. Two studies failed to adequately conceal group allocation (high risk of bias; H391, H394), and there was insufficient information available for the method of allocation concealment in remaining studies.

The lack of blinding meant that all studies were assessed as having high risk of bias for blinding of participants, personnel, and outcome assessors. The effect of missing data on results from one RCT could not be determined (unclear risk; H394); there were no missing data in the remaining studies. All studies were assessed as having unclear risk of bias for selective outcome reporting, as no trial protocols or trial registrations were identified.

Dysmenorrhoea

All studies measured dysmenorrhoea using either the VAS or the 1993 Guideline. Studies that tested oral CHM alone were analysed separately from those that tested oral CHM as integrative medicine with pharmacotherapy.

Oral Chinese herbal medicine versus pharmacotherapy

Five studies compared oral CHM with either analgesics or HT (H388–H391, H394). Meta-analysis of studies showed no statistical difference between oral CHM and pharmacotherapy in reducing pain scores on the VAS (266 women, MD −0.63 cm [−4.56, 3.30], $I^2 = 99\%$; H389, H390) and the 1993 Guideline (132 women, MD −0.42 points [−1.69, 0.84], $I^2 = 20\%$; H391, H394). Results from a single study showed that VAS pain scores were 1.62 cm lower at three-month follow-up among women who received the oral formula *Tong jing ning* 痛经宁 compared with women who received paracetamol ([−2.21, −1.03]; H390).

Oral Chinese herbal medicine plus hormone therapy versus hormone therapy

Two studies that tested oral CHM plus HT assessed dysmenorrhoea at the end of treatment; however, due to differences in outcome scales, results could not be pooled for meta-analysis. Findings from one RCT showed no difference between *San jie zhen tong jiao nang* 散结镇痛胶囊 and goserelin when dysmenorrhoea was assessed using a VAS (80 women, MD −0.23 cm [−0.70, 0.24]; H393). When the 1993 Guideline was used to assess dysmenorrhoea, women who received the formula *Hua yu zhi tong tang* 化瘀止痛汤 reported lower pain scores than women who received mifepristone (92 women, MD −2.84 points [−3.61, −2.07]; H392).

Safety of oral Chinese herbal medicine in randomised controlled trials for endometriosis and adenomyosis

Safety of oral CHM was documented in five RCTs (H388, H390–H393), four of which reported that no AEs occurred during the trial (H388, H390–H392). In the final study of 80 women (H393), the four AEs in women who received CHM as integrative medicine were two cases of rash and itch and one case each of thirst and diarrhoea. Eleven AEs in the control group were three cases of rash and itch, two cases of dizziness and headache, two cases of diarrhoea, two cases of constipation, one case of abnormal liver function, and one case of weight gain.

Controlled Clinical Trials of Oral Chinese Herbal Medicine for Endometriosis and Adenomyosis

Four CCTs tested oral CHM in 424 women with endometriosis or adenomyosis (H395, H396, H397, H398). One study compared oral CHM alone or in combination with GnRHa (H395), while other studies compared a treatment arm with a HT control arm. Studies were conducted in either outpatient (H396, H397, H398) or both inpatient and outpatient (H395) hospital departments in China.

One study included women with laparoscopically confirmed endometriosis (H395), while others used other methods for diagnosis. The mean duration of endometriosis ranged from 4.2 years (H395) to 8.5 years (H398), and the mean age of participants was

32.6 years. One study reported on stages based on the rASRM (H395), and women with all four stages were included. Treatment duration ranged from three months (H397, H398) to 6.3 months (H395), and 10 participants were lost to follow-up in one study (H398). One study conducted follow-up assessments at six and 12 months (H396).

Three studies reported selecting women with a diagnosis of Kidney deficiency and Blood stasis (H395), *qi* stagnation and Blood stasis (H397), or *qi* deficiency and Blood stasis (H398). Two studies used different treatments according to the time of the menstrual cycle (H395, H398), and there was no overlap in formulas used. Herbs used in multiple studies are shown in Table 5.55.

Table 5.55. Frequently Reported Herbs in Controlled Clinical Trials for Endometriosis and Adenomyosis

Most Common Herbs	Scientific Name	Frequency of Use
Dan shen 丹参	*Salvia miltiorrhiza* Bge.	5
Yan hu suo 延胡索	*Corydalis yanhusuo* W.T. Wang	5
Chi shao 赤芍	*Paeonia* spp.	4
Dang gui 当归	*Angelica sinensis* (Oliv.) Diels	4
Gui jian yu 鬼箭羽	*Euonymus alatus* (Thunb.) Sieb.	4
Ba ji tian 巴戟天	*Morinda officinalis* How	2
Bai shao 白芍	*Paeonia lactiflora* Pall.	2
Chuan xiong 川芎	*Ligusticum chuanxiong* Hort.	2
E zhu 莪术	*Curcuma* spp.	2
Nv zhen zi 女贞子	*Ligustrum lucidum* Ait.	2
San leng 三棱	*Sparganium stoloniferum* Buch. -Ham.	2
Shan yao 山药	*Dioscorea opposita* Thunb.	2
Sheng di huang 生地黄	*Rehmannia glutinosa* Libosch.	2
Tu si zi 菟丝子	*Cuscuta* spp.	2
Yi mu cao 益母草	*Leonurus japonicus* Houtt.	2
Zi shi ying 紫石英	Calcium fluoride	2

Note: The use of some herbs may be restricted in some countries. Readers are advised to comply with relevant regulations.

Outcomes

Dysmenorrhoea was the main outcome assessed in CCTs of oral CHM for endometriosis or adenomyosis, assessed in all four studies. One study also assessed recurrence of signs and symptoms (H395).

Dysmenorrhoea

All four studies reported on dysmenorrhoea. Analyses were conducted according to comparisons: oral CHM versus HT and oral CHM plus HT versus HT alone.

Oral Chinese herbal medicine versus hormone therapy

Meta-analysis was possible for four studies that assessed dysmenorrhoea using the 1993 Guideline (H395–H398). Results of analysis showed that oral CHM alone was superior to HT in reducing dysmenorrhoea scores (674 women, MD −2.25 points [−3.56, −0.94], I^2 = 96%). Statistical heterogeneity was detected that was lower in subgroup analysis with women who had not undergone surgery for endometriosis previously (3 studies, 594 women, MD −0.96 points [−1.31, −0.60], I^2 = 53%; H396, H397, H398). One study that assessed dysmenorrhoea using a 10 cm VAS found no difference between oral CHM, tailored according to the menstrual cycle, and Marvelon® (50 women, MD −0.11 cm [−0.71, 0.49]; H398).

Oral Chinese herbal medicine plus hormone therapy versus hormone therapy

One study that tested oral CHM plus HT found a greater reduction in dysmenorrhoea scores on the 1993 Guideline in women who received cycle-related treatment than in those who received GnRHa (40 women, MD −6.33 points [−7.92, −4.74]; H395).

Recurrence

Eighty women were assessed for recurrence of signs and symptoms at the end of treatment in one study (H395). There was no difference between the two groups in the chance of recurrence (RR 0.88 [0.37, 2.07]).

Safety of oral Chinese herbal medicine in controlled clinical trials for endometriosis and adenomyosis

Safety of oral CHM was documented in three of the four studies (H395–H398). One study reported that no AEs occurred during the trial (H396). Adverse events among women who received oral CHM included three cases of stomach discomfort, three cases of menopausal symptoms due to low oestrogen levels, two cases of vaginal bleeding, and one case each of constipation and irregular vaginal bleeding. Adverse events in the control group included six cases of menopausal symptoms, five cases of irregular vaginal bleeding, and two cases of breast pain.

Non-controlled Studies of Oral Chinese Herbal Medicine for Endometriosis and Adenomyosis

Seventeen non-controlled studies tested oral CHM for 617 women with endometriosis or adenomyosis (H399–H415). Four were case reports (H403, H404, H408, H413) and the remaining studies were case series. One study was conducted in Japan (H415) and the rest were conducted in China. The duration of disease ranged from one month (H409) to 25 years (H409). Two studies confirmed diagnosis by laparoscopy (H403, H415), and women in two studies had previously undergone surgery (H403, H404).

Twelve studies used CM syndrome differentiation as an inclusion criterion (H399–H401, H403–H411). The most frequently reported syndromes were Blood stasis (four studies; H400, H404, H401, H408), *qi* stagnation and Blood stasis (three studies; H405, H407, H409), *qi* deficiency and Blood stasis (two studies; H399, H409), and *yang* deficiency cold coagulation with Blood stasis (two studies; H406, H411).

There was diversity in the duration of treatment; the shortest (two months) and longest durations (20 months) were both reported in one study that described the range (H415). Four studies tested investigator-developed formulas (H402, H403, H408, H412, H413); these were excluded from frequency analysis. Only one traditional formula was tested in multiple studies: *Dan chi yin* 丹赤饮 (two studies). *Dan shen* 丹参 was the most frequently used herb (15 uses), followed by *e zhu* 莪术 (11 uses), *bai shao* 白芍, and *chi shao* 赤芍 (10 uses) (Table 5.56). Safety of oral CHM was reported in one study (H415), with no AEs occurring.

Table 5.56. Frequently Reported Orally Used Herbs in Randomised Controlled Trials for Endometriosis and Adenomyosis

Most Common Herbs	Scientific Name	Frequency of Use
Dan shen 丹参	*Salvia miltiorrhiza* Bge.	15
E zhu 莪术	*Curcuma* spp.	11
Bai shao 白芍	*Paeonia* spp.	10
Chi shao 赤芍	*Paeonia* spp.	10
Dang gui 当归	*Angelica sinensis* (Oliv.) Diels	9
Chai hu 柴胡	*Bupleurum* spp.	8
Fu ling 茯苓	*Poria cocos* (Schw.) Wolf	8
San leng 三棱	*Sparganium stoloniferum* Buch. -Ham.	8
Gui zhi 桂枝	*Cinnamomum cassia* Presl	6
Yan hu suo 延胡索	*Corydalis yanhusuo* W.T. Wang	6
Bai zhu 白术	*Atractylodes macrocephala* Koidz.	5
Gan cao 甘草	*Glycyrrhiza* spp.	5
Pu huang 蒲黄	*Typha* spp.	5
Wu yao 乌药	*Lindera aggregata* (Sims) Kosterm.	5
Xiang fu 香附	*Cyperus rotundus* L.	5
Zhe bei mu 浙贝母	*Fritillaria thunbergii* Miq.	5

Note: The use of some herbs may be restricted in some countries. Readers are advised to comply with relevant regulations.

Oral plus Topical Chinese Herbal Medicine for Endometriosis and Adenomyosis

Two studies evaluated oral plus topical CHM in women with endometriosis or adenomyosis. One was an RCT (H416) and the other was a non-controlled study (H417).

Randomised Controlled Trials of Oral plus Topical Chinese Herbal Medicine for Endometriosis and Adenomyosis

One RCT tested the combination of oral plus topical CHM against guideline-recommended treatments for laparoscopically confirmed endometriosis/adenomyosis (H416). The study was conducted in China and included 80 women between 23 and 50 years of age who had lived with symptoms for between one and 20 years. All women had undergone surgery prior to enrolling in the trial.

Treatment was provided for three months and the women were followed up for six months. Chinese medicine syndrome diagnosis was not used to select participants or guide treatment. *Qu yu zhen tong he ji* 祛瘀镇痛合剂 was administered between cycle day 20 and the next menstrual period and was compared with mifepristone.

The study was not free from bias. There was insufficient detail about the method of randomisation and allocation concealment (both judged to pose unclear risk of bias), neither participants, personnel, nor outcome assessors were blind to group allocation (high risk), and no trial protocol or trial registration was available to assess whether there was selective outcome reporting (unclear risk). As the study reported no missing data, it was judged to pose low risk of bias for incomplete outcome data.

The study measured dysmenorrhoea using the 1993 Guideline. *Qu yu zhen tong he ji* 祛瘀镇痛合剂 resulted in a score of 2.28 points lower than that of mifepristone ([−2.69, −1.87]). An unspecified number of AEs in the CHM group included mild gastrointestinal reactions, nausea, and loss of appetite. Adverse events with mifepristone included seven cases of abnormal liver function.

Non-controlled Studies of Oral plus Topical Chinese Herbal Medicine for Endometriosis and Adenomyosis

One case series involving 36 Chinese women with endometriosis or adenomyosis tested oral *Xiao yi zhi tong tang* 消异止痛汤 during the menstrual period and *Xiao yi zhi tong guan chang fang* 消异止痛灌肠方 (enema) at other times of the menstrual cycle (H417). The women had lived with symptoms for between two and 20 years and did not undergo surgery prior to enrolling in the study. Treatment was provided for three months, and whether any AEs occurred was not specified.

Part 4. Side Effects of Gonadotropin-releasing Hormone Agonists

Seventeen studies examined the potential role of CHM in the treatment of menopausal side effects following treatment with GnRHa. Thirteen RCTs (H418–H430) and four CCTs are described in this part (H431–H434).

Randomised Controlled Trials of Oral Chinese Herbal Medicine for Side Effects of Gonadotropin-releasing Hormone Agonists

All 13 RCTs, involving 910 women with endometriosis, were conducted in China (H418–H430). Three studies included three arms (H425, H427, H430): one included two CHM treatment arms (H427), and two included one group that received no treatment and one group that received GnRHa (H425, H430). All remaining studies used a two-arm, parallel group design.

All but one study (H424) included women who had undergone surgery for endometriosis before study enrolment. Twelve of the 13 RCTs reported laparoscopic diagnosis of endometriosis (H418, H419, H421–H430). The rASRM stage was reported in 11 RCTs (H418–H420, H422–H426, H428–H430), with all but one (H428) including women with stage III or IV endometriosis. One study did not specify whether age was an inclusion criterion (H430). All of the remaining studies included adult women, and the median of the mean age was 32.3 years.

The duration of endometriosis was reported in one RCT (H420), which was 24 months in the treatment group and 25 months in the comparator group. Women were recruited from hospital outpatient (H418, H422, H430) or inpatient departments (H419–H421, H423, H425–H428). Two studies did not specify the setting (H424, H429).

Ten RCTs used CM syndrome differentiation as an inclusion criterion (H418–H422, H424, H425, H427–H429). While the names of syndromes varied, most described similar concepts. The syndrome of Kidney *yin* deficiency was used as an inclusion criterion in four studies (H418, H419, H424, H427), Kidney deficiency was described in two RCTs (H422, H429), Kidney deficiency with Blood stasis used in two RCTs (H420, H421), and one study each used an inclusion criterion of Liver and Kidney *yin* deficiency (H425) and Liver stagnation with Kidney deficiency (H428).

One RCT tested oral CHM alone (H425) while the remaining studies tested oral CHM as integrative medicine with pharmacotherapy. Both traditional formulas and manufactured products were tested in included RCTs. Only two treatments were tested in multiple studies; *Kun tai jiao nang* 坤泰胶囊 (capsules) was tested in three RCTs (H423, H427; H430), as was *Zuo gui wan* 左归丸 (H418, H424, H429). Not all studies documented the herb ingredients. Among those that did, *shu di huang* 熟地黄 was the most frequently used herb, followed by *shan yao* 山药 and *shan zhu yu* 山茱萸 (Table 5.57).

Treatment duration ranged from one month (H422) to three months/12 weeks (H420, H421, H423–H428, H430). Four studies conducted follow-up assessment, which was conducted at one month (H422), three months (H428, H429) or six months (H420). Eight studies reported loss to follow-up (H418, H421–H423, H427–H430), with similar numbers of dropouts in both treatment and comparator groups.

Table 5.57. Frequently Reported Herbs in Randomised Controlled Trials for Side Effects of Gonadotropin-releasing Hormone Agonists

Most Common Herbs	Scientific Name	Frequency of Use
Shu di huang 熟地黄	Rehmannia glutinosa Libosch.	9
Shan yao 山药	Dioscorea opposita Thunb.	7
Shan zhu yu 山茱萸	Cornus officinalis Sieb. et Zucc.	5
Huang bai 黄柏	Phellodendron chinense Schneid.	4
Lu jiao jiao 鹿角胶	Cervus spp.	4
Tu si zi 菟丝子	Cuscuta spp.	4
Zhi mu 知母	Anemarrhena asphodeloides Bge.	4
Dang gui 当归	Angelica sinensis (Oliv.) Diels	3
Fu ling 茯苓	Poria cocos (Schw.) Wolf	3
Fu xiao mai 浮小麦	Triticum aestivum L.	3
Gou qi zi 枸杞子	Lycium barbarum L.	3
Mu dan pi 牡丹皮	Paeonia suffruticosa Andr.	3
Niu xi 牛膝	Achyranthes bidentata Bl.	3

Note: The use of some herbs may be restricted in some countries. Readers are advised to comply with relevant regulations.

Risk of Bias Assessment

None of the studies were free from bias (Table 5.58). Eight RCTs posed low risk of bias for the risk of bias domain sequence generation, due to the use of random number tables (H418, H421–H423, H425, H427–H429). Remaining studies did not report the details for how the allocation sequence was generated. Two RCTs used central allocation to conceal group allocation (H421, H422) and were judged as having low risk of bias, while one RCT that used an open randomisation schedule was judged as having high risk of bias (H428). One RCT that was described as double-blinded did not specify who was blinded and was judged to pose unclear risk of bias for blinding of participants, personnel and outcome assessors (H430). Participants, personnel and outcome assessors in remaining studies were not blind to group allocation, and these studies were judged high risk of bias for these domains. Nine RCT had either no missing

Table 5.58. Risk of Bias Assessment of Randomised Controlled Trials for Side Effects of Gonadotropin-releasing Hormone Agonists

Risk of Bias Domain	Low Risk n (%)	Unclear Risk n (%)	High Risk n (%)
Sequence generation	8 (61.5)	5 (38.5)	0 (0)
Allocation concealment	2 (15.4)	10 (76.9)	1 (7.7)
Blinding of participants	0 (0)	1 (7.7)	12 (92.3)
Blinding of personnel	0 (0)	1 (7.7)	12 (92.3)
Blinding of outcome assessors	0 (0)	1 (7.7)	12 (92.3)
Incomplete outcome data	9 (69.2)	3 (23.1)	1 (7.7)
Selective outcome reporting	0 (0)	13 (100)	0 (0)

data, or a small amount of missing data that was considered unlikely to influence the outcomes, and were judged as having low risk of bias (H418–H422, H424–H426, H429). Three RCTs described either participant withdrawal due to side effects of either CHM or GnRHa, or a small number of dropouts that may or may not have influenced outcomes. These studies were judged as having unclear risk of bias for incomplete outcome data. One study that withdrew participants who discontinued treatment before 12 weeks was considered to pose high risk of bias for the same domain. Published trial protocols or trial registrations were not available for any of the RCTs included in this section, and all studies were judged as having unclear risk for selective outcome reporting.

Outcomes

Global assessment of symptom severity using the KI was the most common outcome measure and was reported in 11 RCTs (H419–H423, H425–H430). Three studies each documented recurrence (H420, H425, H428) and bone density (H418, H423, H424), two studies reported dysmenorrhoea (H419, H420), and one reported health-related quality of life (H429). Safety of CHM was reported in 10 of the 13 RCTs (H418, H420–H425, H427, H428, H430).

Dysmenorrhoea

Two studies examined dysmenorrhoea using the VAS (H419, H420). When dysmenorrhoea was assessed at the end of treatment, women who received *Qing xin xiao yin tang* 清心消瘾汤 plus tibolone reported VAS scores that were not statistically different compared to those for women who received tibolone alone (40 women, MD −0.05 cm [−0.45, 0.35]; H419). The second study reported dysmenorrhoea at follow-up (H420). Women who received *Bu shen qu yu fang* 补肾祛瘀方 plus HT scored 1.42 cm lower on the VAS than women who received triptorelin (60 women, [−1.81, −1.03]).

Recurrence

Three RCTs reported on recurrence (H420, H425, H428). Differences in timing and criteria for assessment meant that meta-analysis was not possible, and results are reported for single studies. Recurrence of pelvic pain six months after treatment was not statistically different between women who received *Bu shen qu yu fang* 补肾祛瘀方 plus triptorelin and those who received triptorelin alone (60 women, RR 0.25 [0.06, 1.08]; H420). When recurrence was assessed based on presence of any two of four factors (signs, symptoms, ultrasound assessment, or elevation in CA125), *Zi shen shu gan huo xie tang* 滋肾疏肝活血汤 plus leuprolide was not statistically different from leuprolide alone (60 women, RR 0.50 [0.05, 5.22]; H428). One study that compared *Yi shen ning kun fang* 益肾宁坤方 with no treatment and with tibolone reported no cases of recurrence of cysts or elevation in CA125 in any of the three groups (H425).

Endometriosis Health Profile-5

One RCT with 60 women documented the effect of oral CHM on health-related quality of life (H429). Assessment was made at the end of treatment and at three-month follow-up. *Zuo gui wan* 左归丸 plus leuprolide, oestradiol valerate, and medroxyprogesterone acetate was more effective than leuprolide, oestradiol valerate, and medroxyprogesterone acetate alone in improving scores on the control and powerlessness scale (MD −9.00 points [−16.75, −1.25]) and the self-image scale (MD −10.87 points [−21.43, −0.31]) at the end of treatment. Women who received *Zuo gui wan* 左归丸 as integrative medicine also scored lower — indicating better quality of life — on the sexual relationships supplementary module at the end of treatment (MD −11.32 points [−19.78, −2.86]). No differences were seen between the two groups for the remaining three core scales and supplementary modules at the end of treatment (Table 5.59). Benefits of CHM at the end of treatment were not sustained at three-month follow-up, with no statistically significant differences between groups on any of the core scales or supplementary modules.

Menopausal Symptoms

Global assessment of menopausal symptom severity using the KI was undertaken in 11 RCTs (H419–H423, H425–H430). One study did not report data in a way that could be re-analysed (H430), and data were excluded. As the Chinese version of the KI is modified to add or remove some of the original items, data were analysed using SMD. Results are presented according to the comparison.

Oral Chinese herbal medicine versus no treatment

One three-arm RCT of 60 women compared oral CHM with no treatment (H425) and six items from the KI were reported. The formula *Yi shen ning kun fang* 益肾宁坤方 produced lower scores compared to no treatment — indicating better quality of life — for all six items: hot flushes (MD −3.07 points [−4.32, −1.82]), insomnia (MD −1.20 points [−1.80, −0.60]), nervousness (MD −1.13 points [−1.85, −0.41]), weakness (MD −0.80 points [−1.19, −0.41]), dyspareunia (MD −1.07 points [−1.73, −0.41]), and arthralgia (MD −0.53 points [−0.87, −0.19]).

Table 5.59. Oral Chinese Herbal Medicine versus Gonadotropin-releasing Hormone Agonists: Endometriosis Health Profile-5

Item	Time of Assessment	No. of Studies (Participants)	Effect Size MD [95% CI]	Included Studies
Pain	EoT	1 (60)	−1.83 [−11.56, 7.90]	H429
	Follow-up	1 (60)	0.43 [−9.36, 10.22]	H429
Control and powerlessness	EoT	1 (60)	−9.00 [−16.75, −1.25]*	H429
	Follow-up	1 (60)	−0.07 [−9.01, 8.87]	H429
Emotional wellbeing	EoT	1 (60)	−2.03 [−11.62, 7.56]	H429
	Follow-up	1 (60)	−1.73 [−11.01, 7.55]	H429
Social support	EoT	1 (60)	2.37 [−7.98, 12.72]	H429
	Follow-up	1 (60)	0.60 [−9.94, 11.14]	H429
Self-image	EoT	1 (60)	−10.87 [−21.43, −0.31]*	H429
	Follow-up	1 (60)	−0.07 [−9.87, 9.73]	H429
Work	EoT	1 (60)	−1.47 [−10.03, 7.09]	H429
	Follow-up	1 (60)	−2.13 [−9.27, 5.01]	H429
Feelings about the medical profession	EoT	1 (60)	0.70 [−8.55, 9.95]	H429
	Follow-up	1 (60)	−1.06 [−9.11, 6.99]	H429
Feelings about treatment	EoT	1 (60)	−6.67 [−15.38, 2.04]	H429
	Follow-up	1 (60)	−3.04 [−10.98, 4.90]	H429
Relationship with children	EoT	1 (60)	−2.60 [−10.62, 5.42]	H429
	Follow-up	1 (60)	−1.17 [−7.89, 5.55]	H429
Sexual relationship	EoT	1 (60)	−11.32 [−19.78, −2.86]*	H429
	Follow-up	1 (60)	−0.12 [−7.98, 7.74]	H429
Feelings about infertility	EoT	1 (60)	−0.23 [−7.98, 7.52]	H429
	Follow-up	1 (60)	−1.05 [−8.00, 5.90]	H429

*Statistically significant, see Statistical Analysis in Chapter 4.
Abbreviations: CI, confidence intervals; EoT, end of treatment; MD, mean difference.

Oral Chinese herbal medicine versus pharmacotherapy

The RCT that compared *Yi shen ning kun fang* 益肾宁坤方 with no treatment also compared CHM to tibolone. Among the 60 participants, women who received *Yi shen ning kun fang* 益肾宁坤方 reported scores at the end of treatment that were not statistically different from tibolone in terms of hot flushes (MD 0.13 points [−1.12, 1.38]), insomnia (MD 0.20 points [−0.34, 0.74]), nervousness (MD 0.13 points [−0.48, 0.74]), weakness (MD 0.03 points [−0.29, 0.35]), dyspareunia (MD 0.06 points [−0.46, 0.58]), and arthralgia (MD 0.10 points [−0.17, 0.37]).

Oral Chinese herbal medicine plus pharmacotherapy versus pharmacotherapy

Nine RCTs that compared oral CHM as integrative medicine with pharmacotherapy alone assessed menopause symptoms using the KI (H419–H423, H426–H429). The addition of CHM to pharmacotherapy produced a lower score on the KI — indicating better quality of life — than did pharmacotherapy alone (547 women, SMD −1.81 [−2.80, −0.82], I^2 = 96%). Subgroup analyses according to the version of KI used did not reduce statistical heterogeneity, nor did subgroup analysis according to duration of treatment (Table 5.60). Confidence in these results is limited.

One RCT documented modified KI (MKI) scores at follow-up (H429). Women who received *Zuo gui wan* 左归丸 plus leuprolide, oestradiol, and medroxyprogesterone had similar scores at three-month follow-up to women who received leuprolide, oestradiol, and medroxyprogesterone (60 women, MD −0.13 points [−2.03, 1.77]). The study also reported scores for individual items of the MKI. Women who received *Zuo gui wan* 左归丸 as integrative medicine scored lower on the MKI than women who received leuprolide, oestradiol, and medroxyprogesterone for items relating to vertigo (MD −0.27 points [−0.51, −0.03]), weakness (MD −0.40 points [−0.78, −0.02]), palpitation (MD −0.40 points [−0.77, −0.03]), and vaginal dryness (MD −0.93 points [−1.70, −0.16]). No difference was

Table 5.60. Oral Chinese Herbal Medicine plus Pharmacotherapy versus Pharmacotherapy Alone: Kupperman Index

Category	No. of Studies (Participants)	Effect Size MD/ SMD [95% CI], I^2	Included Studies
KI/MKI – EoT	9 (547)	SMD −1.81 [−2.80, −0.82]*, 96%	H419–H423, H426–H429
Subgroup: KI	2 (150)	MD −6.31 [−17.71, 5.09], 99%	H420, H427
Subgroup: MKI	7 (397)	SMD −1.75 [−2.86, −0.63]*, 95%	H419, H421–H423, H426, H428, H429
Subgroup: treatment duration 3 m	6 (409)	SMD −2.64 [−3.96, −1.32]*, 96%	H420, H421, H423, H426–H427, H428
Subgroup: treatment duration < 3 m	3 (138)	SMD −0.22 [−1.10, 0.66], 84%	H419, H422, H429

Abbreviations: CI, confidence intervals; EoT, end of treatment; KI, Kupperman Index; m, months; MD, mean difference; MKI, modified Kupperman Index; SMD, standardised mean difference.

seen between groups for vasomotor symptoms (MD −0.13 points [−1.13, 0.87]), insomnia (MD −0.06 points [−0.55, 0.43]), nervousness (MD 0.10 points [−0.35, 0.55]), melancholia (MD −0.03 points [−0.30, 0.24]), arthralgia (MD 0.03 points [−0.11, 0.17]), headache (MD 0.07 points [−0.11, 0.25]), and formication (MD 0.07 points [−0.12, 0.26]).

In addition to reporting end of treatment results, four RCTs also reported KI/MKI scores during treatment (H419, H421, H426, H427). Meta-analysis of two studies that reported KI/MKI scores after four weeks of treatment showed that CHM as integrative medicine resulted in lower KI/MKI scores than did pharmacotherapy alone (134 women, SMD −0.83 [−1.53, −0.14], I^2 = 69%; H421, H427). Results from one RCT favoured CHM as integrative medicine when MKI was assessed after two months of treatment (60 women, MD −17.08 points [−18.27, −15.89]; H426) and after four months of treatment (40 women, MD −6.00 points [−7.52, −4.48]; H419).

Bone Density

Three RCTs documented assessments of bone density (H418, H423, H424). Meta-analysis of data from these three RCTs showed no difference between oral CHM plus pharmacotherapy and pharmacotherapy alone in lumbar vertebral bone density (240 women, MD 0.29 standard deviations [SD] [−0.29, 0.86], $I^2 = 79\%$). Results from one RCT with 96 women showed no difference in hip joint bone density between women who received *Zuo gui wan* 左归丸 as integrative medicine and those who received oestradiol valerate plus dydrogesterone alone (MD 0.03 SD [−0.00, 0.06], p = 0.05). Another study (H424) found that women who received *Zuo gui wan* 左归丸 plus leuprolide had better bone density scores at the end of treatment compared with leuprolide alone. This was found for bone density of the femoral neck (49 women, MD 0.95 SD [0.25, 1.65]) and the trochanter major (49 women, MD 0.96 SD [0.29, 1.63]).

Safety of Oral Chinese Herbal Medicine for Side Effects of Gonadotropin-releasing Hormone Agonists in Randomised Controlled Trials

Ten RCTs reported on the safety of oral CHM in women who experienced side effects from GnRHa (H418, H420–H425, H427, H428, H430). One study reported that no AEs occurred in women who received either CHM or tibolone (H425). In women who received both oral CHM and pharmacotherapy, 112 AEs were reported. Adverse events included 24 cases of mood changes, 20 cases of sleep disturbance, 18 cases of hot flushes with or without sweating, 16 cases of joint, bone, or muscle pain, 11 cases of fatigue, five cases of paraesthesia, five cases of vaginal dryness, three cases of nausea, vomiting, or abdominal discomfort, three cases of vaginal bleeding or spotting, two cases of nose bleeds, two cases of distending breast pain, and three cases of unspecified events.

No AEs were reported in women who received no treatment (H430). Two-hundred and fifty AEs were reported in women who received pharmacotherapy, which included 62 cases of hot flushes with or without night sweats, 45 cases of mood changes, 37 cases of sleep disturbance, 29 cases of joint, bone, or muscle pain, 21 cases of vaginal dryness, 15 cases of weakness or fatigue, 13 cases of paraesthesia, 12 cases of vaginal bleeding or spotting, eight cases of distending breast pain, one case each of dyspareunia, palpitations, and headache, and five cases of unspecified events.

Of note, AEs in both groups were predominantly symptoms seen during menopause. It is not clear whether these AEs were due to treatment or were the side effects of GnRHa for which CHM was being tested. While these data suggest that CHM resulted in fewer side effects, there is a need for further research that assesses not only the safety of CHM in terms of GnRHa-related side effects, but also the causality of AEs.

Controlled Clinical Trials of Oral Chinese Herbal Medicine for Side Effects of Gonadotropin-releasing Hormone Agonists

Four CCTs, involving 276 women with endometriosis, assessed the effect of oral CHM on menopausal symptoms from GnRHa (H431–H434). One study included three arms that compared oral CHM as integrative medicine with a placebo (vitamin E) and with conjugated equine oestrogens (CEE) plus medroxyprogesterone (H433), while the remaining studies compared oral CHM with HT. All studies were conducted in inpatient departments in China.

The mean age of participants was 32.8 years. One study documented the mean duration of endometriosis (3.7 years; H432), while three studies diagnosed endometriosis by laparoscopy (H431, H433, H434). Two studies reported on the rASRM stage, with one study including women with stage III or IV endometriosis (H431) and the other including women with stage I–IV endometriosis (H434). Treatment duration ranged from three months/12 weeks (H433, H434) to six months (H432), but was not specified in the fourth study (H431). One study conducted follow-up assessment after six months (H434). None of the studies reported participant withdrawals.

Two studies reported CM syndrome differentiation, with Kidney *yin* deficiency included in one study (H431) and Liver stagnation and Kidney deficiency in the other (H434). There was no overlap in formulas used, and only one herb ingredient was used in two or more studies: *wu ling zhi* 五灵脂.

Outcomes

Three studies assessed menopausal symptoms using the original or modified KI (H431–H433), two assessed dysmenorrhoea (H432, H431), and one study each measured recurrence (H434) and bone density (H433). Results for KI were combined for one meta-analysis, while analysis of other outcomes included single studies.

Dysmenorrhoea

The two studies that measured dysmenorrhoea using a VAS differed in the time at which dysmenorrhoea was assessed (H431, H432), meaning that meta-analysis could not be conducted. One study of 82 women that compared *Xiao jin wan* 小金丸 plus goserelin with goserelin alone found that VAS pain scores were 2.50 cm lower at the end of treatment among the CHM group ([−2.62, −2.38]); H432). In the second study, which assessed dysmenorrhoea when menstruation resumed, no such difference was seen in VAS scores when *Qing xin xiao jia tang* 清心消瘕汤 plus tibolone was compared with tibolone alone (40 women, MD −0.05 cm [−0.45, 0.35]; H431).

Recurrence

One study assessed recurrence six months after the end of treatment (H434). Among the 34 women, treatment with an investigator-developed oral CHM and GnRHa did not reduce the chance of recurrence more than GnRHa alone did (RR 0.72 [0.26, 2.02]).

Menopausal Symptoms

Three studies assessed menopausal symptoms using the KI (H431, H432, H433). Meta-analysis of results was possible for two studies that tested oral CHM plus HT (H431, H432).

Oral Chinese herbal medicine versus placebo

Xian ling gu bao jiao nang 仙灵骨葆胶囊 resulted in a greater reduction in KI scores — indicating symptom improvement — than did vitamin E placebo (82 women, MD −7.60 points [−8.25, −6.95]; H433).

Oral Chinese herbal medicine versus hormone therapy

When Xian ling gu bao jiao nang 仙灵骨葆胶囊 was compared with CEE plus medroxyprogesterone, results showed that HT was more effective at improving menopausal symptoms (82 women, 1.30 points [0.76, 1.84]; H433).

Oral Chinese herbal medicine plus hormone therapy versus hormone therapy

Results for two studies that compared oral CHM plus HT with HT alone were analysed using SMD due to differences in the version of KI used to assess menopausal symptoms. Meta-analysis showed no difference between groups at the end of treatment (122 women, SMD −1.25 [−4.77, 2.27], I^2 = 98%; H431, H432). Considerable statistical heterogeneity was detected but could not be explored due to the small number of included studies, which lowers confidence in the results.

One study also assessed menopausal symptoms using the KI after the second and fourth GnRHa injection (H431). The combination of Qing xin xiao jia tang 清心消瘕汤 and tibolone was not statistically different from tibolone alone after the second injection (40 women, MD −0.09 points [−0.71, 0.53]), but was inferior to tibolone after the fourth injection (40 women, MD 2.40 points [1.57, 3.23]).

Bone Density

Bone density of the fourth and fifth lumbar vertebra was assessed in one study with 82 women (H433). At the end of treatment, bone density results for women who received *Xian ling gu bao jiao nang* 仙灵骨葆胶囊 were not statistically different compared to those of women who received either vitamin E placebo (MD 0.10 SD [−0.17, 0.38]) or CEE plus medroxyprogesterone (MD −0.00 SD [−0.31, 0.30]).

Safety of Oral Chinese Herbal Medicine for Side Effects of Gonadotropin-releasing Hormone Agonists

Three CCTs reported on safety (H432–H434), with one reporting that no AEs occurred during the trial (H432). In the remaining two studies, AEs among people who received oral CHM plus HT were one case each of irritability as well as muscle and joint pain. Adverse events in women who received HT were 12 cases of hot flushes, six cases of irritability, six cases of muscle pain, five cases of irregular vaginal bleeding, four cases of dyspareunia, four cases of fatigue, three cases of palpitations, two cases of insomnia, one case of headache, and one case of depression and paranoia.

Part 5. Endometriosis Outside the Pelvic Cavity

Three non-controlled studies from China documented the effects of CHM on endometriosis outside the pelvic cavity (H250–H252). Two were case reports (H251, H252) and the third was a case series of five women (H250). All three studies described cases of thoracic endometriosis of relatively short duration, ranging from four months to one year.

Oral CHM treatment was provided for between three and eight months in two reports (H250, H251); the duration of treatment was not reported in the third study. Chinese medicine syndromes included *qi* stagnation and Blood stasis (H252) and Lung and Kidney *yin* deficiency (H251). Treatments were tailored towards the time of the menstrual cycle, with participants receiving two or more formulas. Several of the formulas were developed by the study authors. Traditional formulas included *Xue fu zhu yu tang* 血府逐瘀汤 (H250), which was used after the menstrual period, and *Ge xia zhu yu tang*

膈下逐瘀汤 (H252), which was used before menstruation. The most frequently used herbs were *dang gui* 当归 and *gan cao* 甘草 (seven uses each), followed by *chuan niu xi* 川牛膝, *tao ren* 桃仁, and *zhi qiao* 枳壳 (four uses each). None of the studies reported on the safety of oral CHM for thoracic endometriosis.

Clinical Evidence for Commonly Used Chinese Herbal Medicine Treatments

Contemporary clinical textbooks and guidelines recommend both traditional CHM formulas and commercially manufactured products according to CM syndrome differentiation. Traditional formulas described in Chapter 2 are:

- *Ge xia zhu yu tang* 膈下逐瘀汤;
- *Xue fu zhu yu tang* 血府逐瘀汤;
- *Shao fu zhu yu tang* 少腹逐瘀汤;
- *Li chong tang* 理冲汤;
- *Qing re tiao xue tang* 清热调血汤;
- *Cang fu dao tan wan* 苍附导痰丸 used with *Tao hong si wu tang* 桃红四物汤;
- *Gui shen wan* 归肾丸 used with *Tao hong si wu tang* 桃红四物汤;
- *Ju yuan jian* 举元煎 used with either *Tao hong si wu tang* 桃红四物汤 or *Shi xiao san* 失笑散.

Commercially manufactured formulas described in Chapter 2 are:

- *San jie zhen tong jiao nang* 散结镇痛胶囊;
- *Dan e kang fu jian gao* 丹莪妇康煎膏;
- *Gui zhi fu ling jiao nang* 桂枝茯苓胶囊;
- *Ai fu nuan gong wan* 艾附暖宫丸.

Several of these formulas have been tested in clinical studies that met the inclusion criteria, and the findings for these formulas are described. There was no evidence from included clinical studies for the following combinations of formulas: *Cang fu dao tan wan* 苍附导痰丸, *Gui shen wan* 归肾丸 or *Ju yuan jian* 举元煎 used with *Tao hong si wu tang* 桃红四物汤, and *Ju yuan jian* 举元煎 used with *Shi xiao san* 失笑散. As such, the clinical effects of these combinations have not been determined in this review. Further, none of the included studies evaluated *Dan e kang fu jian gao* 丹莪妇康煎膏 or *Ai fu nuan gong wan* 艾附暖宫丸, and the effects of these formulas are unclear.

Ge xia zhu yu tang 膈下逐瘀汤

The formula *Ge xia zhu yu tang* 膈下逐瘀汤 was tested in three studies of women with endometriosis: one RCT (H38), one CCT (H200), and one non-controlled study (H252). The RCT compared *Ge xia zhu yu tang* 膈下逐瘀汤 with no treatment and assessed pregnancy rate and recurrence. There was no difference in the pregnancy rate between groups at the end of treatment (40 women, RR 3.00 [0.13, 69.52]) or follow-up assessment (40 women, RR 2.50 [0.94, 6.66]). Similarly, no difference was seen between groups in recurrence when assessed between six and 30 months after treatment (40 women, RR 0.50 [0.05, 5.08]). The authors reported neither the criteria for the assessment of recurrence nor safety.

In the CCT, a modified version of *Ge xia zhu yu tang* 膈下逐瘀汤 was combined with mifepristone and compared to mifepristone alone. Data relating to recurrence were excluded from analyses as recurrence was assessed in women who reported improvements rather than resolution of symptoms. The number of AEs — mild nausea, loss of appetite, and abdominal discomfort — were similar between the two groups: 11 cases with *Ge xia zhu yu tang* 膈下逐瘀汤 and eight cases with mifepristone.

The non-controlled study included women with thoracic endometriosis resulting in infertility. In this study, *Ge xia zhu yu tang* 膈下逐瘀汤 was used before menstruation, and different formulas were used at other times of the menstrual cycle. The study reported pregnancy outcomes but not the safety of *Ge xia zhu yu tang* 膈下逐瘀汤.

Xue fu zhu yu tang 血府逐瘀汤

Seven clinical studies tested *Xue fu zhu yu tang* 血府逐瘀汤: four were RCTs (H43, H137, H160, H390) and three were non-controlled studies (H219, H250, H254). One RCT (H390) used *Xue fu zhu yu tang* 血府逐瘀汤 from the third day of the menstrual cycle until seven days before the menstrual period and *Tong jing ning* 痛经宁 at other times of the menstrual cycle in women with either endometriosis or adenomyosis. As the clinical effects of each formula when both were used could not be distinguished, analyses of results are not presented here.

The three other RCTs tested *Xue fu zhu yu tang* 血府逐瘀汤 combined with HT. Meta-analysis of two RCTs showed that the combination of *Xue fu zhu yu tang* 血府逐瘀汤 and HT did not result in a statistically different mean VAS score at the end of treatment compared with HT alone (158 women, MD −0.86 cm [−2.41, 0.69], I^2 = 100%; H43; H137). Confidence in this result was limited due to statistical heterogeneity.

Results from individual studies showed that *Xue fu zhu yu tang* 血府逐瘀汤 plus HT resulted in a lower VAS score for pelvic pain (68 women, MD −0.14 cm [−0.16, −0.12]; H43) and dyspareunia (68 women, MD −0.05 cm [−0.05, −0.05]; H43) at the end of treatment compared to HT alone. The combination also increased the pregnancy rate (60 women, RR 1.89 [1.01, 3.55]; H160) and decreased menopausal symptoms measured using the KI (68 women, MD −3.10 points [−3.39, −2.81]; H43), but did not reduce the chance of recurrence of cysts at an unspecified time point (60 women, RR 0.67 [0.21, 2.13]; H160).

All three non-controlled studies used *Xue fu zhu yu tang* 血府逐瘀汤 as one of several formulas during different phases of the menstrual cycle for women with endometriosis, with one study focusing on women with lung endometriosis (H250). One study used both *Xue fu zhu yu tang* 血府逐瘀汤 and *Zhi bai di huang wan* 知柏地黄丸 (H219), the second used *Xue fu zhu yu tang* 血府逐瘀汤 outside of the menstrual period (H250), and the third listed

Xue fu zhu yu tang 血府逐瘀汤 as one of many formulas that were used (H254).

Three studies reported on the safety of *Xue fu zhu yu tang* 血府逐瘀汤, with two reporting that no AEs occurred (H254, H390). The third study (H43) documented two cases of low oestrogen symptoms in each group.

Shao fu zhu yu tang 少腹逐瘀汤

Six studies evaluated the effects of *Shao fu zhu yu tang* 少腹逐瘀汤. Four were RCTs (H162, H172, H337, H382) and two were non-controlled studies (H235; H254). Results from RCTs were analysed according to diagnosis. Outcome data on the recurrence rate (H162) and CPGQ (H382) could not be analysed.

All RCTs tested the combination of *Shao fu zhu yu tang* 少腹逐瘀汤 and HT. In women with endometriosis, results from individual studies showed that the ovarian cyst diameter was lower among women who received *Shao fu zhu yu tang* 少腹逐瘀汤 and HT than in women who received HT alone (70 women, MD −0.84 cm [−0.98, −0.70]; H172).

One study of 96 women with adenomyosis assessed dysmenorrhoea, uterine volume, and health-related quality of life (H337). Dysmenorrhoea scores measured with the 1993 Guideline were lower at the end of treatment in the treatment group than in the HT group (96 women, MD −1.39 points [−2.00, −0.78]). Uterine volume was also lower among women who received *Shao fu zhu yu tang* 少腹逐瘀汤 and HT than in women who received HT alone (96 women, MD −7.77 cm^3 [−12.64, −2.90]; H337). Benefits were seen with *Shao fu zhu yu tang* 少腹逐瘀汤 and HT in reducing end of treatment scores on the pain (MD −1.50 points [−1.85, −1.15]), emotional relation (MD −0.58 points [−0.77, −0.39]), sleep (MD −2.50 points [−3.04, −1.96]), physical abilities (MD −0.60 points [−0.79, −0.41]), and energy level domains (MD −2.12 points [−2.62, −1.62]). Scores for the social isolation domain could not be analysed as women in both groups reported no social isolation.

Both non-controlled studies examined the effects of *Shao fu zhu yu tang* 少腹逐瘀汤 for women with endometriosis. In one case series (H254), *Shao fu zhu yu tang* 少腹逐瘀汤 was one of many formulas described.

Three studies reported on the safety of *Shao fu zhu yu tang* 少腹逐瘀汤 (H162, H254, H337). Two studies reported that no AEs occurred during the conduct of the trial (H254, H337). In the third study (H162), the number of AEs was comparable between groups (nine AEs versus eight AEs). Adverse events in women who received *Shao fu zhu yu tang* 少腹逐瘀汤 plus HT were two cases of itchy skin, two cases of hot flushes, two cases of night sweats, and one case each of irregular vaginal bleeding, vaginal dryness, and amenorrhoea. Adverse events in women who received gestrinone were two cases of night sweats, two cases of hot flushes, two cases of irregular vaginal bleeding, and one case each of vaginal dryness and mild gastrointestinal reactions.

Li chong tang 理冲汤

One case report of a woman with endometriosis used *Li chong tang* 理冲汤 as one of several formulas tailored according to the menstrual cycle phase (H222). In this report, the patient received *Li chong tang* 理冲汤 prior to menstruation, *Nei yi 2 hao fang* 内异2号方 after menstruation, and *Yun 1 fang* 孕1方 during ovulation. The study did not report on the safety of *Li chong tang* 理冲汤.

Qing re tiao xue tang 清热调血汤

Qing re tiao xue tang 清热调血汤 was one of several formulas investigated in one RCT that included women with endometriosis (H98). In this study, *Qing re tiao xue tang* 清热调血汤 was used for the CM syndrome phlegm-heat resistance. As results for recurrence of signs and symptoms were reported for all women, regardless of syndrome and treatment, it was not possible to determine the effects of *Qing re tiao xue tang* 清热调血汤 for women with endometriosis.

San jie zhen tong jiao nang 散结镇痛胶囊

The commercially manufactured product *San jie zhen tong jiao nang* 散结镇痛胶囊 was evaluated in 21 clinical studies. Sixteen of these were RCTs (H10, H12, H16, H104–H107, H316, H319, H332, H336, H340, H345, H389, H393, H394), four were CCTs (H188, H199, H347, H351) and one was a case report (H365). Characteristics of these studies are presented according to the diagnosis of study participants.

Endometriosis

Seven RCTs (H10, H12, H16, H104–H107) and two CCTs (H188, H199) tested *San jie zhen tong jiao nang* 散结镇痛胶囊 in women with endometriosis. One RCT used *San jie zhen tong jiao nang* 散结镇痛胶囊 in combination with *Gui zhi fu ling jiao nang* 桂枝茯苓胶囊 (H104), and data were excluded in these analyses.

Evidence from RCTs showed mixed results for the effects of *San jie zhen tong jiao nang* 散结镇痛胶囊 on reducing recurrence of signs and symptoms. At 24-month follow-up, recurrence of signs and symptoms was lower among women who received *San jie zhen tong jiao nang* 散结镇痛胶囊 than among those who received gestrinone (139 women, RR 0.35 [0.18, 0.66], I^2 = 0%; H12, H16). However, *San jie zhen tong jiao nang* 散结镇痛胶囊 was not superior to gestrinone in reducing recurrence of signs and symptoms when measured:

- Six months or less after the end of treatment (97 women, RR 0.55 [0.30, 1.00]; H107);
- Twelve months after surgery (94 women, RR 1.00 [0.38, 2.63]; H106);
- Two years after the end of treatment (144 women, RR 1.03 [0.44, 2.37], I^2 = 0%; H12, H16);
- At an unspecified time (66 women, RR 1.13 [0.12, 10.13]; H105).

When *San jie zhen tong jiao nang* 散结镇痛胶囊 was combined with mifepristone, the rate of recurrence of signs and symptoms was not statistically different from that of mifepristone alone (48 women, RR 0.54 [0.13, 2.13]; H10). While *San jie zhen tong jiao nang* 散结镇痛胶囊 was superior to no treatment in improving the chance of pregnancy at follow-up (37 women, RR 4.95 [1.30, 18.90]; H12), it was not superior to gestrinone (70 women, RR 1.34 [0.83, 2.14], $I^2 = 0\%$; H12, H105).

Findings from CCTs showed that *San jie zhen tong jiao nang* 散结镇痛胶囊 did not reduce the rate of recurrence more than HT did. Recurrence of cysts 14–25 months after treatment was similar between *San jie zhen tong jiao nang* 散结镇痛胶囊 and gestrinone (140 women, RR 0.40 [0.06, 2.74]; H188), and recurrence of signs and symptoms at the end of treatment was similar between *San jie zhen tong jiao nang* 散结镇痛胶囊 and goserelin (33 women, RR 1.23 [0.35, 4.30]; H199).

All nine studies reported on the safety of *San jie zhen tong jiao nang* 散结镇痛胶囊 for women with endometriosis. Some studies described a range of AEs but not the number that occurred; these AEs are not included in the analyses below. Among women who received *San jie zhen tong jiao nang* 散结镇痛胶囊, 34 AEs were reported: 19 cases of stomach discomfort, five cases of rash, three cases of nausea and vomiting, three cases of constipation, one case of abnormal liver function, and three cases of various AEs including pruritus, fever, thirst, constipation, dizzinesss, nausea, diarrhoea, and excessive sweating.

No AEs were reported in women who received no treatment. More AEs were documented in women who received HT than in women who received *San jie zhen tong jiao nang* 散结镇痛胶囊 (267 AEs with HT versus 34 AEs with CHM). Adverse events in women who received HT were 92 cases of abnormal menstruation or irregular vaginal bleeding, 82 cases of amenorrhoea, 47 cases of abnormal liver function, 34 cases of low oestrogen symptoms such as hot flushes, night sweats, and vaginal dryness, five cases of nausea and vomiting, four cases of acne, and three cases of early pregnancy symptoms, such as nausea and lethargy.

Adenomyosis

Nine studies tested *San jie zhen tong jiao nang* 散结镇痛胶囊 in women with adenomyosis. Six were RCTs (H316, H319, H332, H336, H340, H345), two were CCTs (H347, H351), and one was a case report (H365). In RCTs that tested *San jie zhen tong jiao nang* 散结镇痛胶囊 alone, uterine volume was lower with CHM than with no treatment (38 women, MD −21.50 cm^3 [−42.13, −0.87]; H336) or with gestrinone (82 women, MD −12.00 cm^3 [−20.26, −3.74]; H345). Menstrual volume, measured as a percentage of pre-surgery napkin weight, was also less in women who received *San jie zhen tong jiao nang* 散结镇痛胶囊 than in women who received no treatment (38 women, MD −13.83% [−21.76, −5.90]; H336). Verbal rating scale scores for dysmenorrhoea were also lower in women who received *San jie zhen tong jiao nang* 散结镇痛胶囊 than with gestrinone (82 women, MD −0.54 points [−0.80, −0.28]; H345).

The combination of *San jie zhen tong jiao nang* 散结镇痛胶囊 and HT was more effective than HT alone in reducing dysmenorrhoea as measured on several scales: VAS scores were 0.20 cm lower (91 women, [−0.38, −0.02]; H316), while VRS scores were 0.68 points lower at the end of treatment (61 women, [−0.91, −0.45]; H332) and 0.47 points lower at follow-up (61 women, [−0.58, −0.36]; H332).

Menstrual volume assessed by the PBAC was not different at the end of treatment between women who received *San jie zhen tong jiao nang* 散结镇痛胶囊 plus HT and those who received HT alone (121 women, MD −65.49 [−156.24, 25.25], I^2 = 100%; H332, H340). However, results from one study showed that the PBAC was lower at follow-up among women who received both *San jie zhen tong jiao nang* 散结镇痛胶囊 and HT (61 women, MD −16.20 [−22.44, −9.96]; H332).

Conversely, uterine volume was lower at the end of treatment (344 women, MD −26.43 cm^3 [−46.38, −6.49], I^2 = 91%; H316, H319, H332, H340) but not different at follow-up (183 women, MD −16.88 cm^3 [−37.16, 3.41], I^2 = 91%; H332, H340) between *San jie zhen tong jiao nang* 散结镇痛胶囊 plus HT and HT alone. Finally, health-related quality of life was improved in women who received *San jie zhen tong jiao nang* 散结镇痛胶囊 plus HT, with PGWB scores being 12.3 points higher than that of women who received HT alone (70 women, [7.54, 17.06]; H319).

Analysis of results from one CCT showed that treatment with *San jie zhen tong jiao nang* 散结镇痛胶囊 resulted in a smaller uterine volume than for indomethacin (74 women, MD −148.00 cm^3 [−175.29, −120.71]; H347). Findings from the second CCT (H351) showed no difference in uterine volume between the combination of *San jie zhen tong jiao nang* 散结镇痛胶囊 plus HT and HT alone when measured at the end of treatment (68 women, MD 5.00 cm^3 [−7.65, 17.65]) and at follow-up (68 women, MD 0.60 cm^3 [−13.17, 14.37]). The study also showed results favouring *San jie zhen tong jiao nang* 散结镇痛胶囊 plus HT for the PBAC at the end of treatment (68 women, MD −2.70 [−5.31, −0.09]), but not at follow-up (68 women, MD −1.30 [−3.61, 1.01]).

The safety of *San jie zhen tong jiao nang* 散结镇痛胶囊 was reported in four RCTs (H316, H319, H332, H340) and both CCTs. Adverse events among women who received *San jie zhen tong jiao nang* 散结镇痛胶囊 alone were two cases of gastrointestinal upset. Adverse events among women who received *San jie zhen tong jiao nang* 散结镇痛胶囊 plus HT were eight cases of irregular vaginal bleeding, three cases of gastrointestinal symptoms, two cases of breast pain, two cases of dislodged Mirena®, and one case of dizziness, nausea, breast pain, and irregular vaginal bleeding.

The number of AEs was higher with HT alone ($n = 45$). Adverse events included 17 cases of irregular vaginal bleeding, 12 cases of dizziness, nausea, vomiting, malaise, or lethargy, five cases of gastrointestinal symptoms, four cases of dizziness, nausea, breast pain, or irregular vaginal bleeding, three cases of breast pain, two cases of weight gain and breast pain, and two cases of dislodged Mirena®.

Endometriosis and Adenomyosis

Three RCTs tested *San jie zhen tong jiao nang* 散结镇痛胶囊 in women with endometriosis or adenomyosis (H389, H393, H394).

Women who received *San jie zhen tong jiao nang* 散结镇痛胶囊 reported lower levels of dysmenorrhoea on the VAS (176 women, MD −2.64 cm [−3.23, −2.05]; H389), but similar levels of dysmenorrhoea on the 1993 Guideline (62 women, MD −1.60 points [−4.06, 0.86]; H394). When *San jie zhen tong jiao nang* 散结镇痛胶囊 was used in combination with goserelin, there was no difference between the treatment and control groups in dysmenorrhoea as measured using the VAS (80 women, MD −0.23 cm [−0.70, 0.24]; H393).

Gui zhi fu ling jiao nang 桂枝茯苓胶囊

Gui zhi fu ling jiao nang 桂枝茯苓胶囊 was tested in 13 clinical studies: nine RCTs (H14, H92, H104, H108, H298, H302, H317, H320, H323), three CCTs (H176, H198, H350), and one case report (H205). Study results are presented according to diagnosis.

Endometriosis

Four RCTs (H14, H92, H104, H108) and two CCTs (H176, H198) investigated the benefits of *Gui zhi fu ling jiao nang* 桂枝茯苓胶囊 in women with endometriosis. One RCT combined *Gui zhi fu ling jiao nang* 桂枝茯苓胶囊 with *San jie zhen tong jiao nang* 散结镇痛胶囊 (H104); as the individual effects of each formula could not be distinguished, data for this study were not analysed.

The rate of recurrence of signs and symptoms six months after surgery was not statistically different between women who received *Gui zhi fu ling jiao nang* 桂枝茯苓胶囊 and those who received no treatment (60 women, RR 0.33 [0.01, 7.87]; H14), nor were they different from that of women who received triptorelin in the same RCT (60 women, RR 3.00 [0.13, 70.83]; H14). Recurrence of cysts one year after surgery was not lower in women who received *Gui zhi fu ling jiao nang* 桂枝茯苓胶囊 plus GnRHa than in women who received GnRHa alone (84 women, RR 0.50 [0.16, 1.53]; H92). The combination of *Gui zhi fu ling jiao nang* 桂枝茯苓胶囊 and triptorelin reduced the chance of recurrence two years after the end of treatment compared to triptorelin alone (66 women, RR 0.28 [0.08,

0.93]; H108). *Gui zhi fu ling jiao nang* 桂枝茯苓胶囊 plus GnRHa did not improve the pregnancy rate for women with endometriosis (84 women, RR 1.39 [0.90, 2.13]; H92).

Analysis of CCTs showed that *Gui zhi fu ling jiao nang* 桂枝茯苓胶囊 plus gestrinone reduced dysmenorrhoea when measured with the VAS (120 women, MD −1.53 cm [−1.74, −1.32]; H198) and reduced ovarian cyst diameter (120 women, MD −0.40 cm [−0.49, −0.31]; H198) compared with gestrinone alone. One study that measured recurrence of signs and symptoms between one and three years after the end of treatment found no difference between *Gui zhi fu ling jiao nang* 桂枝茯苓胶囊 and no treatment (81 women, RR 0.65 [0.11, 3.69]; H176) or mifepristone (81 women, RR 0.65 [0.11, 3.69]; H176).

One RCT (H14) and two CCTs (H176, H198) reported on safety, with one CCT stating that no AEs occurred during the trial (H198). Adverse events with *Gui zhi fu ling jiao nang* 桂枝茯苓胶囊 were eight cases of hot flushes, seven cases of irregular vaginal bleeding, six cases of gastrointestinal symptoms, and four cases each of amenorrhoea and abnormal liver function. Adverse events in women who received no treatment were eight cases of irregular vaginal bleeding, five cases of hot flushes, and three cases of amenorrhoea. Adverse events with HT were 16 cases of irregular vaginal bleeding, 15 cases of hot flushes, 11 cases of amenorrhoea, 10 cases of abnormal liver function, and nine cases of nausea, dizziness, fatigue, vomiting, hot flushes, and irregular vaginal bleeding.

Adenomyosis

Five RCTs (H298, H302, H317, H320, H323) and one CCT (H350) investigated the effects of *Gui zhi fu ling jiao nang* 桂枝茯苓胶囊 in women with adenomyosis. All studies used *Gui zhi fu ling jiao nang* 桂枝茯苓胶囊 in combination with HT.

Evidence from RCTs showed a lower VAS score for dysmenorrhoea at the end of treatment in women who received *Gui zhi fu ling jiao nang* 桂枝茯苓胶囊 plus HT than with HT alone (252 women,

MD −2.08 cm [−2.61, −1.56], I² = 58%; H302, H323). Uterine volume was also lower in women who received *Gui zhi fu ling jiao nang* 桂枝茯苓胶囊 plus HT (206 women, MD −19.06 cm³ [−24.83, −13.30], I² = 0%; H317, H320), while there was no difference in menstrual volume, measured with the PBAC, between groups (318 women, MD −16.38 [−37.92, 5.16], I² = 97%; H317, H320, H323).

Evidence from one CCT (H350) showed no difference between *Gui zhi fu ling jiao nang* 桂枝茯苓胶囊 plus Mirena® and Mirena® alone when dysmenorrhoea was measured with the pain intensity domain of the CPGQ (100 women, MD −0.10 points [−0.55, 0.35]); however, a lower score — indicating less pain — was seen at follow-up (100 women, MD −0.40 points [−0.59, −0.21]).

The safety of *Gui zhi fu ling jiao nang* 桂枝茯苓胶囊 was reported in four studies (H302, H317, H323, H350). The 46 AEs in women who received *Gui zhi fu ling jiao nang* 桂枝茯苓胶囊 were nine cases of breast pain, nine cases of irregular vaginal bleeding, six cases of headache, six cases of gastrointestinal symptoms, five cases of menstrual disorders, two cases of acne, two cases of weight gain, two cases of abnormal liver function, and five other unspecified AEs.

More AEs were seen with HT than with the combination of *Gui zhi fu ling jiao nang* 桂枝茯苓胶囊 and HT. The 71 AEs were 22 cases of irregular vaginal bleeding, 14 cases of breast pain, 11 cases of gastrointestinal symptoms, six cases of headache, four cases of menstrual disorders, three cases of acne, three cases of weight gain, three cases of abnormal liver function, and five other unspecified AEs.

Summary of Chinese Herbal Medicine Clinical Evidence

Endometriosis and adenomyosis have significant effects on women's health, and many women seek treatment with complementary and alternative medicines to alleviate symptoms. Results from published SRs have shown benefits with CHM in alleviating symptoms and reducing the chance of recurrence; similar findings have been identified in studies presented in this review.

The majority of clinical studies tested oral CHM for women with endometriosis and assessed dysmenorrhoea and recurrence as key outcomes. This was not surprising as more than three-quarters of women with endometriosis report cyclical pain[38] and many women experience recurrence of pain within 12 months of surgery.[39] Topical CHM was used less frequently, and was often used as an enema. Most studies provided treatment for between three and six months, and follow-up assessment was often conducted up to three years after the end of treatment, highlighting the chronic nature of endometriosis and the likelihood of recurrence.

Many studies tested CHM in a way that reflects clinical practice, tailoring the treatment according to the time of the menstrual cycle. Some studies tested a core formula, to which herbs were added or removed according to the cycle phase, while others used different formulas for each phase of the menstrual cycle. While the latter provides insight into the effectiveness of CHM as a whole, it is more difficult to ascertain the relative contribution of each formula to any clinical changes seen.

Studies tested traditional formulas, commercially manufactured herbal medicine products, and investigator-developed formulas. The evidence for traditional formulas and manufactured products that are recommended in the clinical textbooks and guidelines included in Chapter 2 has been presented. Some formulas were not tested in any of the clinical studies that met the inclusion criteria for this review; however, this should not be interpreted to mean that there was no evidence for these formulas. Instead, it suggests that there is a need for high-quality evidence that reports on clinically important outcomes using established scientific methods.

Investigator-developed formulas were challenging to evaluate. Such formulas were either unnamed, named after the doctor who developed the formula, or named according to the action of the formula, such as *Huo xue hua yu tang* 活血化瘀汤 (Blood circulating formula). It is possible that some of these formulas included the same set of herb ingredients as traditional formulas or commercially manufactured products; however, this could not be established purely based on the formula name. Analysis of herb ingredients was not undertaken due to the complexities in determining formula similarity. As such, the frequency of use of some formulas could be higher than reported.

Based on the analysis of formula names, the most frequently tested CHM across all studies — regardless of medical diagnosis — was San jie zhen tong jiao nang 散结镇痛胶囊, which was tested in 21 studies. This manufactured product is recommended in clinical textbooks and guidelines for two syndromes: qi stagnation and Blood stasis, and phlegm and stasis binding. Gui zhi fu ling 桂枝茯苓 formulas (in capsule or pill formulations) were also used frequently (13 studies), and the manufactured product Gui zhi fu ling jiao nang 桂枝茯苓胶囊 is recommended in textbooks and guidelines for the syndrome of cold congealing and Blood stasis. All three syndromes were among the most common in included studies.

Many of the key herbs were consistent across studies of endometriosis, adenomyosis, and studies that included both endometriosis and adenomyosis, which is likely due to similarity in their clinical presentation. In particular, symptoms of dysmenorrhoea, chronic pelvic pain, dyspareunia, and infertility are common to both conditions. The most frequently used herbs across all studies were *dang gui* 当归 (used in 253 studies), *e zhu* 莪术 (217 studies), *dan shen* 丹参 (194 studies), *yan hu suo* 延胡索 (188 studies), and *chi shao* 赤芍 (186 studies). These five herbs were also the most frequently used in RCTs of oral CHM, which — as the biggest group of studies — was likely to influence the overall herb frequency.

Studies that tested the role of CHM for alleviating side effects used different formulas and herbs compared to studies that focused on treating the symptoms of endometriosis and adenomyosis. Formulas used in multiple studies, such as *Kun tai jiao nang* 坤泰胶囊 and *Zuo gui wan* 左归丸, are typically prescribed to alleviate symptoms of menopause. Some of the key herbs used in these studies were *shu di huang* 熟地黄, *shan yao* 山药, and *shan zhu yu* 山茱萸, which have actions to nourish the Kidneys, Liver, Spleen, *yin*, and *jing* 精.

Most studies compared CHM treatments to pharmacotherapy, with HT as the main comparator. Few studies compared CHM with placebo, probably because CM is a well-established medical system in China and efficacy research is not regarded as necessary. Instead, the focus in Chinese clinical studies is on testing the effectiveness of CHM against conventional medical treatments.

The reported outcomes differed according to the diagnosis of endometriosis or adenomyosis. Dysmenorrhoea was a key outcome common to studies involving women with endometriosis and/or adenomyosis. Recurrence was reported more frequently in studies of women with endometriosis, while uterine and menstrual volume were more frequently reported in women with adenomyosis. Naturally, studies that evaluated the role of CHM in reducing the side effects of GnRHa focused on outcome measures related to low oestrogen levels, such as the KI and bone density.

Meta-analyses were conducted where possible. Evidence from RCTs may provide results with a lower risk of bias than other study types. Results from meta-analyses of RCTs are summarised below.

Key Findings for Endometriosis

The benefits of CHM for endometriosis were seen for many comparisons. Meta-analyses showed that oral CHM was superior to placebo in reducing ovarian cyst diameter and better than no treatment in reducing dysmenorrhoea VAS scores at the end of treatment. This result exceeded the minimal clinically important difference (MCID) for endometriosis of 10 mm.[40] Oral CHM was also more effective than no treatment in:

- reducing the chance of recurrence of signs and symptoms at six, 12, and 24 months after surgery;
- increasing the pregnancy rate at the end of treatment and follow-up;
- improving scores on the emotional role function and social function domains of the SF-36.

Benefits were seen when oral CHM was compared with pharmacotherapy. Specifically, oral CHM was more effective than pharmacotherapy in:

- reducing dysmenorrhoea VAS scores at the end of treatment and at six and 12 month follow-up;
- reducing dysmenorrhoea scores on the 1993 Guideline;
- increasing the pregnancy rate at follow-up.

Oral CHM was more effective than HT, specifically, in:

- reducing the chance of recurrence of signs and symptoms after two years;
- reducing the chance of recurrence of pain one year after surgery;
- increasing scores on the general health and physical domains of the WHOQOL-BREF.

Finally, meta-analysis showed that the formula *Qing re hua yu fang* 清热化瘀方 was more effective than HT at improving quality of life as measured using the EHP-30.

When oral CHM was used as integrative medicine with pharmacotherapy, the combination was superior to pharmacotherapy alone in:

- reducing dysmenorrhoea VAS scores at the end of treatment and at follow-up after one year (with both results exceeding the MCID);
- increasing the pregnancy rate in women with endometriosis-related infertility at the end of treatment and at follow-up;
- reducing the miscarriage rate at follow-up.

More specifically, oral CHM was superior to HT in:

- reducing dysmenorrhoea as measured using the 1993 Guideline at the end of treatment;

- reducing the chance of recurrence of signs and symptoms at the end of treatment, as well as at follow-up within six months and at one, two, and three years;
- reducing the chance of recurrence of cysts within six months and at one year;
- reducing cyst diameter at the end of treatment.

Results for individual formulas showed that *San jie zhen tong jiao nang* 散结镇痛胶囊 was better than both no treatment and HT in reducing the chance of recurrence of signs and symptoms at 24-month follow-up, while *Dan leng fu kang jian gao* 丹棱妇康煎膏 plus pharmacotherapy was better than pharmacotherapy alone at reducing dysmenorrhoea scores as measured with the 1993 Guideline.

Results for clinically important comparisons (i.e., those included in GRADE assessments) showed moderate certainty evidence that oral CHM reduced dysmenorrhoea VAS scores compared with placebo and low certainty evidence that oral CHM reduced dysmenorrhoea VAS scores and the EHP-30 total score compared with HT. Very low certainty evidence found the combination of oral CHM and HT to be superior to HT alone in reducing dysmenorrhoea VAS scores. Low certainty evidence showed *Xue fu zhu yu tang* 血府逐瘀汤 plus HT to be more effective than HT alone in reducing pelvic pain VAS scores and the chance of recurrence of signs and symptoms at the end of treatment, and low certainty evidence showed that *Gui zhi fu ling jiao nang* 桂枝茯苓胶囊 plus HT was more effective than HT alone in reducing the recurrence of signs and symptoms two years after treatment.

Key Findings for Adenomyosis

Studies that included women with adenomyosis demonstrated positive effects of CHM, especially when oral CHM was combined with pharmacotherapy. Oral CHM alone resulted in a clinically important reduction in dysmenorrhoea VAS scores, and while oral CHM plus

HT also reduced dysmenorrhoea VAS scores more than HT alone did, the result was unlikely to be clinically important. The combination of oral CHM and HT produced statistically significant results compared to HT alone in:

- reducing dysmenorrhoea based on the 1993 Guideline;
- reducing dysmenorrhoea pain intensity and disability points scores as measured with the CPGQ;
- reducing uterine volume;
- reducing menstrual volume as measured with the PBAC.

Meta-analyses of individual formulas showed greater reductions in dysmenorrhoea VAS scores at the end of treatment with *Gui zhi fu ling jiao nang* 桂枝茯苓胶囊 plus pharmacotherapy compared to pharmacotherapy alone, and lower dysmenorrhoea scores as measured with the 1993 Guideline in women who received *Gui zhi fu ling wan* 桂枝茯苓丸 plus pharmacotherapy compared to pharmacotherapy alone. Meta-analysis showed that *Gui zhi fu ling jiao nang* 桂枝茯苓胶囊 plus HT also resulted in a greater reduction in uterine volume at the end of treatment than did HT alone.

Shao fu zhu yu tang/jiao nang 少腹逐瘀汤/胶囊 resulted in a lower dysmenorrhoea score on the 1993 Guideline when combined with pharmacotherapy, and a smaller uterine volume at the end of treatment compared to pharmacotherapy alone. Finally, *San jie zhen tong jiao nang* 散结镇痛胶囊 plus HT resulted in a smaller uterine volume than HT alone at the end of treatment.

Key Findings for Endometriosis and Adenomyosis

Fewer studies investigated the role of CHM in women with a diagnosis of either endometriosis or adenomyosis, and these studies focused on the effects of CHM on dysmenorrhoea. While several meta-analyses were conducted, none showed that CHM was superior to pharmacotherapy.

Key Findings for Side Effects of Gonadotropin-releasing Hormone Agonists

Among the studies that tested the benefits of oral CHM in alleviating GnRHa side effects, only one meta-analysis showed results that were favourable to the combination of CHM plus pharmacotherapy. Oral CHM used in combination with pharmacotherapy resulted in less severe menopausal symptoms compared to pharmacotherapy alone based on the KI.

Limitations of the Evidence

While there is a large volume of evidence that appears to show that oral CHM was beneficial in reducing dysmenorrhoea for women with endometriosis and those with adenomyosis, there is little evidence for the role of topical CHM or the combination of oral plus topical CHM. Several of the studies that tested topical CHM prescribed it as an enema, but the evidence for this treatment is lacking. Chinese medicine practitioners may consider the suitability of this treatment option for women based on each case.

While we sought to examine the role of CHM in some of the less common types of endometriosis, including endometriosis outside the uterine cavity, very few studies met the eligibility criteria for this review. Three non-controlled studies reported on the use of CHM for thoracic endometriosis; however, as clinical results were not analysed, the efficacy of CHM for thoracic endometriosis remains uncertain.

Although laparoscopy is the 'gold standard' for diagnosis of endometriosis,[41,42] it was not routinely conducted or reported in included studies. In fact, only half of the RCTs that tested oral CHM for endometriosis confirmed diagnosis using laparoscopy, none of the RCTs of oral CHM for adenomyosis reported the use of laparoscopy, and only one of the seven RCTs of oral CHM for both endometriosis and adenomyosis confirmed diagnosis by laparoscopy. The cost of laparoscopy can be prohibitive and cause diagnosis in some countries to be made according to signs and symptoms and physical examination instead. Subgroup analyses were planned for studies that confirmed diagnosis using laparoscopy but, in many cases, could not be conducted. Definitive confirmation of diagnosis is particularly important in clinical trials in order to be more certain about the effects of different treatments and should be considered in future CM clinical trials.

None of the studies were free from bias and many of the meta-analyses showed considerable to substantial levels of statistical heterogeneity, thus lowering confidence in the results. Interestingly, meta-analyses of oral CHM for endometriosis showed statistical heterogeneity for outcomes relating to pain, but homogeneity in meta-analyses of pregnancy outcomes. The reasons for this are not clear but may relate to objectivity in outcome reporting. Patient-reported outcomes, such as pain, frequently had considerable levels of statistical heterogeneity, while objective outcomes, such as recurrence and pregnancy outcomes, generally had little or no statistical heterogeneity. Adequate blinding of outcome assessors reduces observer bias and may lower statistical heterogeneity and increase confidence in the results.

The psychological and financial burden on women with endometriosis and adenomyosis is significant,[43] yet few of the included studies investigated the effect of CHM on health-related quality of life. Given the chronic nature of the condition and lengthy delays in diagnosis, this is an important outcome that warrants greater scrutiny in future CHM research. There is growing recognition that fatigue is a common symptom for both conditions,[44] and this is likely to be included as one of the core outcomes for clinical trials of endometriosis.

Safety of Chinese Herbal Medicine

While CHMs are frequently perceived as safe, they are not without side effects. Evidence from included studies shows that fewer AEs were documented in women who received oral CHM, either alone or in combination with pharmacotherapy, than those who received pharmacotherapy alone. The finding of fewer AEs in women who received the combination of CHM and pharmacotherapy is interesting, given that the pharmacotherapy used was the same in both groups. This may suggest that CHM can mitigate some of the risks with pharmacotherapy; indeed, in clinical practice, it is common for formulas to be modified to reduce the side effects of conventional medications.

Chinese herbal medicine may also have an important role to play in reducing side effects caused by treatment with GnRHa. Symptoms arising from low oestrogen levels, such as hot flushes and night sweats, can cause distress for women with endometriosis, further adding to the burden of the disease. Oral CHM appeared to reduce global symptom severity more than pharmacotherapy did, so further research is needed in this area.

While many studies reported on the safety of CHM, few assessed the severity of these symptoms, and even fewer still attributed causality. This finding is not specific to studies of endometriosis and adenomyosis. There is a clear need for better reporting of AEs in clinical trials of CHM to allow practitioners and patients to make informed choices about their use.

References

1. Flower A, Liu JP, Lewith G, et al. (2012) Chinese herbal medicine for endometriosis. *Cochrane Database Syst Rev* (5): Cd006568.
2. Li Y, Li T, Song S. (2017) Evaluation of efficacy and safety of Dan'efukang soft extract in the treatment of endometriosis: A meta-analysis of 39 randomized controlled trials enrolling 5442 patients. *Evid Based Complement Alternat Med* **2017**: 9767391.
3. Shan J, Cheng W, Zhai DX, et al. (2017) Meta-analysis of Chinese traditional medicine Bushen huoxue prescription for endometriosis treatment. *Evid Based Complement Alternat Med* **2017**: 5416423.
4. 何梅, 周玥, 刘福. (2012) 丹莪妇康煎膏治疗子宫内膜异位症的有效性及安全性评价. *中国医院药学杂志* (7): 528–534.
5. 冉新. (2016) 子宫内膜异位症相关不孕保守性手术后联合中药治疗疗效系统评价. 成都中医药大学.

6. 卫爱民, 沈宇飞. (2014) 散结镇痛胶囊应用于子宫内膜异位症的系统评价. *中国实用医药* (32): 71–72.
7. 周娟, 惠宁. (2010) 散结镇痛胶囊治疗子宫内膜异位症的 Meta 分析. *中国全科医学* **13**(22): 2524–2528.
8. 周玉玲. (2012) 腹腔镜下巧克力囊肿剔除术后中医药治疗的文献系统评价. 广州中医药大学.
9. 宋景艳, 孙振高, 王爱娟, et al. (2017) 中药复方改善子宫内膜异位症相关性不孕症妊娠率的系统评价. *世界中西医结合杂志* **12**(1): 18–22.
10. 崔轶凡, 王庆国. (2010) 中药治疗子宫内膜异位症的 Meta 分析. *中国中医药信息杂志* **17**(4): 25–7.
11. 崔阳阳, 孙伟伟, 赵瑞华. (2014) 中药治疗子宫内膜异位症术后复发的系统评价. *山东中医药大学学报* (6): 529–533.
12. 张丽娜. (2010) 从瘀论治子宫内膜异位症疼痛的系统评价. 黑龙江中医药大学.
13. 张澎, 范郁山, 杨礼泛, et al. (2017) 单纯中药灌肠与西药治疗子宫内膜异位症 Meta 分析. *亚太传统医药* **13**(3): 73–79.
14. 李璐琪, 宫尚群, 范银萍, et al. (2017) 近5年中药灌肠治疗子宫内膜异位症疗效的 Meta 分析. 湖南中医杂志 **33**(7): 149–153.
15. 王娜娜, 赵瑞华, 刘永, et al. (2016) 中药与促性腺激素释放激素激动剂抑制子宫内膜异位症术后复发的网状 meta 分析. *国际中医中药杂志* **38**(12): 1120–1127.
16. 王晓彤, 林海雄. (2016) 腹腔镜术后口服丹术消异方对子宫内膜异位症临床疗效的系统评价与 Meta 分析. *中国实验方剂学杂志* **22**(15): 211–215.
17. 王晓彤, 林海雄, 黄洁明. (2016) 腹腔镜术后联合罗氏内异方对子宫内膜异位症临床疗效的系统评价与 Meta 分析. *时珍国医国药* **27**(5): 1271–1274.
18. 王晓彤, 林海雄, 黄洁明. (2017) 腹腔镜术后配合活血化瘀方药治疗子宫内膜异位症临床疗效的系统评价与 Meta 分析. *中华中医药学刊* **35**(3): 585–588.
19. 田苗. (2014) 中药治疗卵巢巧克力囊肿的 Meta 分析. 黑龙江中医药大学.
20. 练鹏颖, 刘枚芳, 徐景利. (2016) 桂枝茯苓胶囊联合米非司酮治疗子宫内膜异位症随机对照试验的 Meta 分析. *中药新药与临床药理* **27**(4): 564–570.
21. 肖超, 赵静, 覃正文. (2016) 中草药对子宫内膜异位症患者术后生存质量影响的 Meta 分析. *国际妇产科学杂志* **43**(4): 467–470.
22. 邢海燕, 徐丽霞, 梁亚琴, et al. (2017) 中药内服结合保留灌肠治疗内膜异位症的 Meta 分析. *中医药导报* **23**(9): 99–104.

23. 韩萌萌, 高岑, 宋俊生. (2016) 桂枝茯苓丸(胶囊)与激素治疗子宫内膜异位症疗效对比的 Meta 分析. *中国中医急症* **25**(6): 961–964.
24. 顾丽琴, 张一琼. (2014) 中西医结合治疗腹腔镜术后子宫内膜异位症的系统评价. *江西中医药* (8): 34–36.
25. 黄飞翔, 丛慧芳. (2012) 补肾化瘀法治疗子宫内膜异位症系统评价. *吉林中医药* **32**(5): 477–480.
26. 冯欣, 沈庆波, 周丽君, *et al.* (2016) 中西医结合治疗子宫腺肌病的 Meta 分析. *实用中西医结合临床* (8): 45–46.
27. 古子娟, 卢如玲, 袁烁, *et al.* (2018) 散结镇痛胶囊联合曼月乐治疗子宫腺肌病的 Meta 分析. *中国医药导报* **15**(6): 88–93.
28. Kupperman HS, Wetchler BB, Blatt MH. (1959) Contemporary therapy of the menopausal syndrome. *J Am Med Assoc* **171**: 1627–1637.
29. 郑筱萸. (1993) 中药新药临床指导原则. 北京: 中国医药科技出版社.
30. Von Korff M, Dworkin SF, Le Resche L. (1990) Graded chronic pain status: An epidemiologic evaluation. *Pain* **40**(3): 279–291.
31. Cox DJ, Meyer RG. (1978) Behavioral treatment parameters with primary dysmenorrhea. *J Behav Med* **1**(3): 297–310.
32. Ware JJ, Sherbourne C. (1992) The MOS 36-item short-form health survey (SF-36). I. Conceptual framework and item selection. *Med Care* **30**: 473–483.
33. World Health Organization. Division of Mental Health. WHOQOL-BREF: Introduction, administration, scoring and generic version of the assessment: Field trial version. Available from: https://apps.who.int/iris/handle/10665/63529: World Health Organization; 1996.
34. Jones G, Kennedy S, Barnard A, *et al.* (2001) Development of an endometriosis quality-of-life instrument: The Endometriosis Health Profile-30. *Obstet Gynecol* **98**(2): 258–264.
35. Jones G, Jenkinson C, Kennedy S. (2004) Development of the Short Form Endometriosis Health Profile Questionnaire: The EHP-5. *Qual Life Res* **13**(3): 695–704.
36. Cranney A, Welch V, Wells G, *et al.* (2001) Discrimination of changes in osteoporosis outcomes. *J Rheumatol* **28**(2): 413–421.
37. Melzack R. (1975) The McGill Pain Questionnaire: Major properties and scoring methods. *Pain* **1**(3): 277–299.
38. Sinaii N, Plumb K, Cotton L, *et al.* (2008) Differences in characteristics among 1,000 women with endometriosis based on extent of disease. *Fertil Steril* **89**(3): 538–545.
39. Practice Committee of the American Society for Reproductive Medicine. (2008) Treatment of pelvic pain associated with endometriosis. *Fertil Steril* **90**(5): S260–S269.

40. Gerlinger C, Schumacher U, Faustmann T, *et al.* (2010) Defining a minimal clinically important difference for endometriosis-associated pelvic pain measured on a visual analog scale: Analyses of two placebo-controlled, randomized trials. *Health Qual Life Outcomes* **8**: 138.
41. Vercellini P, Vigano P, Somigliana E, *et al.* (2014) Endometriosis: Pathogenesis and treatment. *Nat Rev Endocrinol* **10**(5): 261–275.
42. Hummelshoj L, Prentice A, Groothuis P. (2006) Update on endometriosis. *Womens Health (Lond)* **2**(1): 53–56.
43. Giudice LC. (2010) Clinical practice. Endometriosis. *N Engl J Med* **362**(25): 2389–2398.
44. Schenken R. Endometriosis: Pathogenesis, clinical features, and diagnosis 2019 [cited 2019 28th July]. Available from: https://www.uptodate.com/contents/endometriosis-pathogenesis-clinical-features-and-diagnosis.

References for Included Chinese Herbal Medicine Clinical Studies

Study No.	Reference
H1	Flower A, Lewith GT, Little P. (2011) A feasibility study exploring the role of Chinese herbal medicine in the treatment of endometriosis. *J Altern Complement Med* **17**(8): 691–699.
H2	周琴, 吴燕虹. (2016) "消异汤"治疗子宫内膜异位症保守性术后 30 例临床研究. *江苏中医药* **48**(7): 49–50.
H3	唐杨, 陈莉, 张志花, *et al.* (2013) 安巢驻宫饮联合孕三烯酮治疗子宫内膜异位症后的临床观察. *中国当代医药* **20**(30): 103–104, 106.
H4	王伟, 谈勇, 时燕平, *et al.* (2015) 补肾活血法改善子宫内膜异位症术后患者生存质量随机对照研究. *辽宁中医药大学学报* **17**(9): 69–71.
H5	龚文姣. (2016) 补气活血法对卵巢巧克力囊肿术后复发干预的临床研究. 广西中医药大学.
H6	杨成成. (2013) 赤蒲颗粒治疗子宫内膜异位症(寒凝血瘀证)的II期临床研究. 成都中医药大学.
H7	黄艳辉, 曹立幸, 司徒仪. (2008) 莪棱胶囊治疗气滞血瘀型子宫内膜异位症临床研究. *上海中医药杂志* **42**(3): 46–48.
H8	黄晓晖, 薛素华, 冯宗文, *et al.* (2013) 腹腔镜联合冯氏内异方对I, II期子宫内膜异位症的疗效观察. *世界中西医结合杂志* **8**(3): 252–254, 274.

(*Continued*)

Study No.	Reference
H9	陈捷, 张璇, 陈丽笙, et al. (2010) 腹腔镜配合自拟逐瘀汤治疗血瘀型子宫内膜异位症的临床观察. 成都中医药大学学报 **33**(2): 29–32.
H10	丁仁波, 郭宝枝, 柴秋玲. (2010) 腹腔镜手术联合不同药物治疗子宫内膜异位症伴不孕疗效比较. 广西中医学院学报 **13**(4): 27–28.
H11	王希波, 刘欣, 柳林, et al. (2008) 腹腔镜手术联合中药治疗子宫内膜异位症34例临床观察. 中医杂志 **49**(2): 125–127.
H12	高健, 高亚梅, 王丽萍, et al. (2010) 腹腔镜术后散结镇痛胶囊巩固治疗子宫内膜异位症的疗效分析. 临床军医杂志 **38**(3): 402–404.
H13	吕金香. (2012) 异痛消干预子宫内膜异位症盆腔疼痛的临床观察. 黑龙江省中医研究院.
H14	刘春晖. (2017) 桂枝茯苓丸治疗子宫内膜异位症保守手术后的临床研究. 河北大学.
H15	卢晓男, 徐向荣, 林丽君. (2007) 抗异种玉汤联合GnRH-a治疗重度子宫内膜异位症不孕患者疗效观察. 中国中西医结合杂志 **27**(11): 980–982.
H16	尹瑞春, 董秀华, 李敬, et al. (2010) 散结镇痛胶囊在腹腔镜子宫内膜异位囊肿剥除术后的临床应用. 中国妇幼保健 **25**(30): 4483–4484.
H17	许金榜, 林丹枚, 林巧燕, et al. (2014) 芍药止痛合剂治疗III~IV期子宫内膜异位症临床研究. 中国中医药信息杂志 **21**(04): 26–30.
H18	刘桂兰, 王芳芳, 石晶, et al. (2014) 异痛消治疗子宫内膜异位性不孕的临床研究. 中国中医药现代远程教育 **12**(7): 9–10.
H19	陈玲, 魏爱淳, 李万红, et al. (2014) 益气化瘀法治疗腹腔镜术后盆腔子宫内膜异位症疗效观察. 四川中医 **32**(8): 123–124.
H20	杨红, 齐聪, 曾惠. (2017) 益气活血方治疗复发性卵巢子宫内膜异位囊肿的疗效及对IL-2, IL-6的影响. 中华中医药学刊 **35**(2): 460–462.
H21	多晓玲, 王桂芳. (2017) 中药预处理对子宫内膜异位症的助孕效果观察. 中国临床医生杂志 **45**(12): 95–97.
H22	柳林, 王希波. (2014) 中药预防卵巢子宫内膜异位囊肿术后复发的临床研究. 中国妇幼保健 **29**(34): 5717–5718.
H23	葛慧娟, 曹保利. (2014) 子宫内膜异位症术后应用复方莪术散的疗效观察. 西部中医药 **27**(4): 100–101.
H24	Yang DX, Ma WG, Qu F, et al. (2006) Comparative study on the efficacy of Yiweining and Gestrinone for post-operational treatment of stage III endometriosis. Chin J Integr Med **12**(3): 218–220.

(Continued)

Study No.	Reference
H25	Zhu SM, Liu D, Huang W, *et al*. (2014) Post-laparoscopic oral contraceptive combined with Chinese herbal mixture in treatment of infertility and pain associated with minimal or mild endometriosis: A randomized controlled trial. *BMC Complement Altern Med* **14**: 222.
H26	Lian F, Li XL, Sun ZG, *et al*. (2009) Effect of Quyu Jiedu granule on microenvironment of ova in patients with endometriosis. *Chin J Integr Med* **15**(1): 42–46.
H27	张晓云, 张春雁. (2014) 针药结合预防子宫内膜异位症腹腔镜手术后复发疗效观察. *中国针灸* **34**(2): 139–144.
H28	史淑红, 李佃贵, 孟宪鑫. (2007) 化浊解毒活血法治疗子宫内膜异位症伴痛经 30 例临床观察. *山东医药* **47**(24): 42–43.
H29	蔡晓纯, 陈鉴强. (2017) 清热解毒法治疗子宫内膜异位症不孕临床观察. *实用中医药杂志* **33**(4): 356–358.
H30	陈靓芬, 陈小平, 曾洁华. (2014) 腹腔镜联合药物治疗子宫内膜异位症合并不孕症临床观察. *实用中西医结合临床* **14**(8): 28–30.
H31	陈甦, 吴之婷, 吉丽, *et al*. (2017) 中药人工周期联合地屈孕酮片对宫内膜异位症不孕患者妊娠及血清学的影响. *海南医学* **28**(20): 3318–3321.
H32	高涛, 方晓红, 马景, *et al*. (2018) 月经周期阶段性中药方剂在子宫内膜异位不孕症患者中的应用及对血清免疫因子的影响. *中国临床药理学与治疗学* **23**(6): 672–677.
H33	杨静, 钟伟兰, 梁晓梅. (2016) 当归芍药散治疗子宫内膜异位症合并不孕的临床观察. *深圳中西医结合杂志* **26**(9): 36–37.
H34	付蒙, 吕晓杰. (2017) 地屈孕酮片联合中药人工周期治疗子宫内膜异位症致不孕疗效观察. *中国药业* **26**(11): 44–47.
H35	黄晓燕, 黄筱泓, 束兰娣, *et al*. (2012) 红藤方联合促排卵治疗子宫内膜异位症不孕的临床研究. *浙江中医药大学学报* **36**(12): 1304–1306.
H36	姜洁思. (2012) 消异方对因子宫内膜异位症行 IVF-ET 患者临床症状及妊娠结局影响的临床研究. 山东中医药大学.
H37	李新玲, 连方, 孙振高, *et al*. (2009) 祛瘀解毒中药联合宫腔内人工授精治疗子宫内膜异位症的临床研究. *世界中西医结合杂志* **4**(7): 496–498.
H38	尤娜娜. (2015) 膈下逐瘀汤治疗巧克力囊肿不孕患者腹腔镜术后的疗效评价. 南京中医药大学.

(Continued)

(*Continued*)

Study No.	Reference
H39	陶莉莉, 陈小平, 吴彤, *et al.* (2010) 罗氏内异方联合腹腔镜手术对轻型子宫内膜异位症不孕患者血清 mmp-9, Timp-1 的影响. *江西中医药* **41**(326): 52–54.
H40	黎海芳, 周英. (2014) 罗氏内异方联合腹腔镜治疗中重度子宫内膜异位症不孕临床观察. *陕西中医学院学报* **37**(2): 41–44.
H41	刘海萍, 连方, 郝天羽, *et al.* (2008) 祛瘀解毒颗粒联合IVF-ET治疗子宫内膜异位症不孕疗效观察. *山东医药* **48**(48): 105–106.
H42	孙博, 赵春波, 邵含, *et al.* (2017) 痛愈舒颗粒治子宫内膜异位症性不孕. *长春中医药大学学报* **33**(1): 105–108.
H43	吴雯君, 陈光盛. (2017) 血府逐瘀汤联合亮丙瑞林治疗生育期子宫内膜异位症不孕临床疗效及安全性研究. *中华中医药学刊* **35**(4): 927–930.
H44	王静. (2015) 中西医结合治疗肾虚血瘀型子宫内膜异位症不孕临床疗效观察. 湖南中医药大学.
H45	罗美玲. (2012) 中药联合腹腔镜治疗轻型子宫内膜异位症不孕的临床研究. 广州中医药大学.
H46	张娟, 赵瑞华. (2013) 中药治疗子宫内膜异位症相关不孕症的临床研究. *北京中医药* **32**(11): 855–857.
H47	武颖, 何军琴, 李玛建. (2012) 中药周期序贯疗法对子宫内膜异位症不育患者体外受精胚胎移植的影响. *安徽中医学院学报* **31**(5): 13–16.
H48	张晓芳, 张宜群. (2016) 滋阴补阳中药对子宫内膜异位症合并不孕患者血清性激素水平与妊娠结局的影响研究. *中国性科学* **25**(4): 129–132.
H49	赵成元, 喻琳麟, 王华. (2016) 腹腔镜联合中药定坤丹治疗子宫内膜异位症性不孕症的临床疗效分析. *中国妇幼保健* **31**(4): 796–798.
H50	赵井苓, 李成银, 王娟, *et al.* (2018) 中药周期疗法治疗子宫内膜异位症合并黄体功能不全性不孕症疗效观察. *中医学报* **33**(09): 1750–1755.
H51	应翩. (2013) 中药分阶段治疗子宫内膜异位症临床研究. *中华中医药学刊* **31**(7): 1727–1728.
H52	张文俏. (2010) 补肾祛瘀法治疗子宫内膜异位症的临床免疫学研究. 黑龙江中医药大学.
H53	余陆. (2015) 中药分期治疗肾虚血瘀型复发性卵巢型子宫内膜异位症的临床观察. 安徽中医药大学.
H54	刘洁云. (2017) 琥珀散加减辨治子宫内膜异位症疼痛（血瘀证）的疗效作用机制. *中国实验方剂学杂志* **23**(17): 205–210.

(*Continued*)

Study No.	Reference
H55	陈钧洁. (2015) 补肾化瘀方对肾虚血瘀型子宫内膜异位囊肿腹腔镜术后防治的临床观察. 长春中医药大学.
H56	周华, 齐聪. (2008) 补肾活血法治疗复发性卵巢子宫内膜异位囊肿 30 例临床观察. *中医杂志* **49**(7): 618–621.
H57	周艳, 李强. (2014) 补肾活血化瘀法联合腹腔镜手术治疗子宫内膜异位症的效果观察. *中国医刊* **49**(4): 94–96.
H58	罗梅. (2014) 补肾活血散瘀汤治疗子宫内膜异位症的疗效观察及作用机理初探. 南京中医药大学.
H59	张丽玉. (2017) 补肾祛瘀法联合GnRH-a 治疗子宫内膜异位症（腹腔镜术后）的疗效分析. 福建中医药大学.
H60	程红. (2011) 补肾祛瘀法联合西药防治子宫内膜异位症术后复发的疗效观察. 广州中医药大学.
H61	李孔益, 彭永军, 彭清慧. (2013) 妇科内消胶囊配合介入治疗卵巢子宫内膜异位囊肿临床研究. *新中医* **45**(5): 77–79.
H62	牛丽丽. (2018) 活血散瘀汤治疗子宫内膜异位症患者的临床疗效. *黑龙江医药* **31**(2): 319–321.
H63	康文艳, 王静, 渠媛, *et al.* (2017) 盆腔子宫内膜异位症术后应用补肾化瘀方抑制复发的临床观察. *四川中医* **35**(11): 167–169.
H64	赵亚丽. (2016) 痛经颗粒治疗子宫内膜异位症的临床研究. *医药论坛杂志* **37**(1): 4–6.
H65	苟爱华, 万贵平, 邢玉霞, *et al.* (2013) 温肾消喝汤联合米非司酮治疗子宫内膜异位症的临床疗效观察. *四川中医* **31**(10): 83–86.
H66	邢立明. (2016) 中药补肾化瘀法对子宫内膜异位囊肿术后(肾虚血瘀证)的临床研究. 长春中医药大学.
H67	黄昕寅. (2011) 滋阴补阳序贯法对子宫内膜异位症术后复发干预的临床研究. 南京中医药大学.
H68	赵淑英. (2017) 桂枝茯苓丸联合腹腔镜电凝术对子宫内膜异位症患者术后血清 GSH-Px, Leptin 水平及妊娠率的影响. *中国临床实用医学* **8**(4): 40–42.
H69	康文艳. (2017) 自拟补肾化瘀方用于盆腔子宫内膜异位症保守术后预防复发的临床研究. *山西医药杂志* **46**(18): 2202–2204.
H70	韩蓓. (2016) 鳖甲煎丸联合 GnRHa 预防气滞血瘀型 OEC 术后复发疗效观察. 湖北中医药大学.

(*Continued*)

(Continued)

Study No.	Reference
H71	冯琴琴, 赵洪萍. (2018) 丹莪妇康煎膏联合 GnRH-a 对子宫内膜异位症术后的疗效及预防复发的效果. *天津医药* **46**(5): 540–543.
H72	司徒仪, 梁雪芳, 向东方, *et al.* (1999) 莪棱胶囊治疗子宫内膜异位症65例临床观察. *中医杂志* **40**(11): 680–681.
H73	林芸, 郭久建. (2010) 加味宫外孕 II 号方治疗气滞血瘀型子宫内膜异位症痛经临床观察. *中国优生与遗传杂志* **18**(4): 98–99.
H74	卢燕. (2003) 克痛胶囊治疗子宫内膜异位症的临床研究. 黑龙江中医药大学.
H75	张晓娜. (2012) 木达汤对气滞血瘀型卵巢子宫内膜异位囊肿术后复发的影响. 福建中医药大学.
H76	李佶, 王大增, 张绍芬, *et al.* (2006) 内异片治疗子宫内膜异位症的临床观察. *上海中医药杂志* **40**(7): 51–53.
H77	葛海艳. (2015) 散结镇痛汤联合亮丙瑞林对子宫内膜异位症术后患者疼痛感的影响. *河南中医* **35**(12): 3143–3145.
H78	衣尚国, 刘丽敏. (2018) 消异止痛汤联合孕三烯酮治疗子宫内膜异位症的临床研究. *中国医药指南* **16**(15): 215–216.
H79	刘颖, 陈仁. (2016) 消癥止痛汤治疗气滞血瘀型子宫内膜异位症痛经疗效分析. *新中医* **48**(5): 174–176.
H80	许明会, 江玉. (2014) 消癥方治疗子宫内膜异位症 42 例临床观察. *河南中医* **34**(1): 112–114.
H81	任志珍. (2011) 中药干预盆腔子宫内膜异位症保守术后 1 年复发的临床研究. 北京中医药大学.
H82	杜传清. (2010) 中药治疗对子宫内膜异位症保守术后患者生存质量影响的研究. 中国中医科学院.
H83	张玉兰. (2015) 内异消配合孕三烯酮治疗子宫内膜异位症痛经疗效观察. *山东中医杂志* **34**(5): 363–365.
H84	甄海平. (2012) 加减温经汤对子宫内膜异位症痛经患者生存质量的影响. *河北中医* **34**(3): 379–380.
H85	郑颖惠. (2011) 莪棱胶囊干预子宫内膜异位症内膜粘附作用机制研究. 广州中医药大学.
H86	徐新亚, 张科群. (2018) 自拟益气化瘀方用于巧克力囊肿腹腔镜术后效果. *中国乡村医药* **25**(11): 25–26.
H87	黄魁. (2017) 桂莪棱乌汤对寒凝血瘀型卵巢子宫内膜异位囊肿术后患者的影响. *现代中西医结合杂志* **26**(14): 1555–1557.

(Continued)

Study No.	Reference
H88	赵春梅. (2004) 克痛胶囊治疗子宫内膜异位症的临床评价. 黑龙江中医药大学.
H89	汤艳秋, 吴燕虹. (2015) 温经汤治疗子宫内膜异位症痛经 30 例临床观察. 江苏中医药 **47**(6): 36–37.
H90	王沙沙. (2012) 四逆汤加味治疗子宫内膜异位症临床观察. 南京中医药大学.
H91	胡发龙. (2016) 中西医结合治疗子宫内膜异位症术后 46 例疗效观察. 新中医 **48**(3): 147–149.
H92	苏燕燕. (2018) GnRHa 联合桂枝茯苓胶囊对卵巢巧克力囊肿腹腔镜剥除术后康复及卵巢功能和妊娠结局的影响. 现代中西医结合杂志 **27**(8): 843–846.
H93	杨俊娥. (2010) 内膜异位 I 号方治疗气虚血瘀型子宫内膜异位症的临床研究. 湖北中医药大学.
H94	王秋香. (2016) 内异康复片治疗湿热瘀阻型子宫内膜异位症盆腔疼痛的临床研究. 成都中医药大学.
H95	史杨. (2015) 清热化瘀方治疗子宫内膜异位症临床观察. 广西中医药 **38**(2): 17–18.
H96	徐文娟. (2008) 消积冲剂治疗湿热瘀阻型子宫内膜异位症抗子宫内膜抗体及 CA125 的临床研究. 南京中医药大学.
H97	吴志兵, 张晓甦. (2012) 消积冲剂治疗湿热瘀阻型子宫内膜异位症痛经及对 CA125 的影响. 陕西中医 **33**(7): 771–772.
H98	于清玲, 李忠辉, 王乃平, et al. (2012) 腹腔镜联合中西药治疗子宫内膜异位症的疗效观察. 中国当代医药 **19**(23): 54–55, 57.
H99	李小平, 林舒, 兰巧英. (2011) 疏肝理气化瘀法治疗复发性卵巢子宫内膜异位囊肿临床观察. 光明中医 **26**(7): 1364–1366.
H100	杨波, 张军, 黎海莉, et al. (2006) 中西医结合治疗术后子宫内膜异位症疗效观察. 河北中医 **28**(9): 678–679.
H101	叶青, 孙立兰, 何双. (2016) 活血化瘀补肾中药治疗联合腹腔镜手术治疗子宫内膜异位症不孕患者临床研究. 中国性科学 **25**(6): 139–143.
H102	柴小利, 汪莎. (2010) 补肾化瘀消癥法联合腹腔镜治疗子宫内膜异位症疗效观察. 成都中医药大学学报 **33**(1): 30–31.
H103	陈文滨, 谭彩群. (2007) 子宫内膜异位症术后中西医结合治疗结果分析. 中国基层医药 **14**(12): 2010–2011.

(Continued)

(Continued)

Study No.	Reference
H104	丁仁波. (2018) III~IV 期子宫内膜异位症伴不孕症术后达菲林与中药辅助治疗的疗效观察. *中国妇产科临床杂志* **19**(3): 267–268.
H105	朱崇云, 尹超英, 孙秀丽, et al. (2007) 保守性手术后辅以中药散结治疗子宫内膜异位症临床疗效的观察. *四川医学* **28**(12): 1398–1400.
H106	霍大志, 贺建民. (2013) 散结镇痛胶囊在腹腔镜下卵巢子宫内膜异位囊肿剥除术后临床应用. *浙江中医杂志* **48**(7): 492–493.
H107	陈丽娟. (2010) 散结镇痛胶囊治疗子宫内膜异位症腹腔镜术后疗效观察. *上海中医药杂志* **44**(11): 57–58.
H108	王萍. (2016) 中西医结合预防子宫内膜异位症腹腔镜手术后复发疗效观察. *新中医* **48**(12): 122–123.
H109	蔡竞, 侯秀环. (2012) 中西医结合治疗子宫内膜异位症痛经的临床观察. *实用中西医结合临床* **12**(1): 52–53, 79.
H110	陈丽琴, 吴越慧, 朱聪茶, et al. (2015) 血府逐瘀胶囊在腹腔镜联合 GnRHa 治疗 OEC 中的应用. *中国妇幼健康研究* **26**(3): 511–514.
H111	高德红, 杜绍敏, 朱莉, et al. 桃核承气汤联合达那唑对子宫内膜异位症 CA125 及性激素的影响. *中国生化药物杂志* **36**(4): 115–117.
H112	刘晞, 钟一村. (2016) 丹莪妇康煎膏对子宫内膜异位症患者生活质量及炎症因子水平影响的临床研究. *上海中医药杂志* **50**(11): 52–54.
H113	胡燕燕, 旷红艺. (2018) 丹莪妇康煎膏联合曲普瑞林治疗卵巢巧克力囊肿的临床研究. *现代药物与临床* **33**(9): 2331–2235.
H114	徐芝秀, 马欢杰, 方德利, et al. (2013) 丹莪妇康煎膏治疗子宫内膜异位症的临床效果和安全性分析. *中国妇幼保健* **28**(12): 1880–1881.
H115	沈捷雯, 郑德三, 支毅德. (2014) 丹莪妇康煎膏治疗子宫内膜异位症痛经的疗效分析. *国际中医中药杂志* **36**(11): 994–996.
H116	江雯波, 朱磊. (2015) "五味散"治疗血瘀型子宫腺肌病 30 例临床研究. *江苏中医药* **47**(2): 38–39.
H117	曹颖, 李继康, 曹保利. (2014) 复方莪术散治疗子宫内膜异位症疗效观察. *山东大学学报(医学版)* **52**(S1): 38–39.
H118	廖慧慧, 李芳, 宋红. (2010) 腹腔镜手术联合罗氏内异方治疗轻中度子宫内膜异位症的临床研究. *云南中医中药杂志* **31**(9): 16–18.
H119	张春华, 赖影, 梁雪锋, et al. (2011) 腹腔镜手术联合中西药治疗子宫内膜异位症的疗效观察. *中国医药导报* **8**(36): 97–99.
H120	李姗. (2014) 腹腔镜手术联合中药治疗卵巢型子宫内膜异位症的疗效观察. 河南中医学院.

(Continued)

Study No.	Reference
H121	董建新, 江春花, 白洁. (2017) 活血逐瘀汤联合腹腔镜治疗子宫内膜异位症应用效果及对不良事件预防分析. *辽宁中医药大学学报* **19**(7): 98–100.
H122	任燕梅. (2016) 中西医结合治疗子宫内膜异位症. *长春中医药大学学报* **32**(1): 118–120.
H123	陈雅慧. (2016) 加减温经方治疗子宫内膜异位症痛经 48 例观察. *实用中医药杂志* **32**(6): 541–543.
H124	邝爱华. (2015) 金匮肾气丸对子宫内膜异位症患者术后的促孕效果评价. *中西医结合研究* **7**(3): 123–125.
H125	杨丽娜, 于海燕, 单梅, et al. (2016) 经痛愈舒颗粒治疗子宫内膜异位症术后患者临床研究. *辽宁中医药大学学报* **18**(1): 186–188.
H126	徐群群, 卢敏, 曹阳, et al. (2018) 清热化瘀中药方治疗子宫内膜异位症临床研究. *河北中医* **40**(10): 1452–1457.
H127	萧洁媚, 卜亚丽, 叶敦敏. (2013) 清热解毒活血化瘀中药治疗 III–IV 期子宫内膜异位症不孕患者腹腔镜术后疗效观察. *广州中医药大学学报* **30**(3): 333–336.
H128	杜爱平. (2017) 曲普瑞林+反加疗法联合中药对腹腔镜术后重度子宫内膜异位症患者疼痛感及远期复发率的影响. *现代中西医结合杂志* **26**(17): 1918–1920.
H129	龙金荣. (2012) 手术联合人参皂甙 Rg3 对 III–IV 期子宫内膜异位症的临床对照研究. 山西医科大学.
H130	曹毅君, 徐美炎, 钟云岚. (2016) 疏肝活血化湿法治疗子宫内膜异位症的临床分析. *中国当代医药* **23**(15): 94–96, 102.
H131	刘霞, 肖新春. (2016) 消异方治疗子宫内膜异位症的疗效观察及安全性分析. *天津中医药* **33**(11): 668–671.
H132	林韵. (2016) 宣郁通经汤加减治疗子宫内膜异位症痛经的临床疗效观察. 北京中医药大学.
H133	谢书华. (2016) 血竭安异方治疗子宫内膜异位症临床疗效观察. *中国现代药物应用* **10**(15): 6–8.
H134	汤艳秋. (2010) 异位一号方治疗子宫内膜异位症的临床研究. 苏州大学.
H135	沈萍, 章丽娅, 董丽君. (2014) 益气化瘀法治疗子宫内膜异位症气虚血瘀证的临床研究. *贵阳中医学院学报* **36**(4): 98–100.
H136	马迎红, 黎烈荣. (2015) 益气化瘀方预防子宫内膜异位术后复发的临床研究. *南京中医药大学学报* **31**(3): 291–294.

(Continued)

(Continued)

Study No.	Reference
H137	尉江平, 陈利形. (2013) 中西医结合治疗子宫内膜异位症临床对照研究. *中国中医急症* **22**(1): 122–123.
H138	张慧琴, 赵淑平, 尹亚童. (2010) 中药"异位康"颗粒治疗子宫内膜异位症的研究. *中外妇儿健康·学术版* **18**(11): 63–65.
H139	胡敏, 洪威阳. (2014) 中药分期与单纯西药治疗子宫内膜异位症痛经的效果比较. *中华中医药学刊* **32**(4): 942–944.
H140	钟伟青, 钱红燕. (2016) 中重度子宫内膜异位症患者应用坤泰胶囊联合GnRH-a 疗效及预后分析. *中华中医药学刊* **34**(12): 3069–3072.
H141	陆丽霞, 王军玲. (2016) 逐瘀止痛汤对子宫内膜异位症所致疼痛昏厥及面白的干预效果. *四川中医* **34**(6): 126–128.
H142	赵文霞, 黄骊莉, 严琦, *et al*. (2012) 止痛化癥胶囊增加曲普瑞林治疗子宫腺肌病疗效的临床观察. *黑龙江医药科学* **35**(5): 59–60.
H143	朱婷, 马庆良. (2018) 子宫内膜异位症术后应用葛根与抑那通的临床观察. *中国妇幼健康研究* **29**(6): 785–788.
H144	祝敏捷, 孙莲方, 杨静. (2016) 温经汤治疗子宫内膜异位症的疗效及对机体免疫功能的影响. *现代中西医结合杂志* **25**(2): 148–151.
H145	蔡婷, 姜锐. (2017) 腹腔镜术后辅以散结镇痛汤治疗子宫内膜异位症合并不孕临床研究. *中医药信息* **34**(1): 104–106.
H146	曾荣, 曹保利, 李继坤. (2011) 补肾祛瘀方防治卵巢巧克力囊肿腹腔镜术后复发的观察. *天津医科大学学报* **17**(4): 563–564, 566.
H147	陈婕, 谈勇. (2016) 中药育阴潜阳方干预子宫内膜异位症腹腔镜术后联合促性腺激素释放激动剂治疗的临床研究. *中华中医药杂志* **31**(4): 1516–1519.
H148	朱方红, 蒋莉. (2011) 补肾活血法治疗子宫内膜异位症术后 42 例临床观察. *福建中医药* **42**(1): 32–33.
H149	巫朝霞, 黄敏, 冯虹, *et al*. (2008) 补肾祛瘀法预防中重度子宫内膜异位症腹腔镜保守性手术后复发的临床研究. *新中医* **40**(8): 61–62.
H150	张彩霞, 李力. (2007) 丹莪妇康煎膏辅助治疗卵巢子宫内膜异位囊肿术后 40 例疗效观察. *中国中西医结合杂志* **27**(1): 87–88.
H151	张彩霞. (2007) 丹莪妇康煎膏辅助治疗卵巢子宫内膜异位囊肿术后的临床观察. 湖北中医药大学;湖北中医学院.
H152	王燕萍, 胡满霞. (2007) 丹莪妇康煎膏配合腹腔镜手术治疗子宫内膜异位症疗效分析. *湖北中医杂志* **29**(10): 39.
H153	贾七英, 彭彩桥, 张翠肖. (2014) 腹腔镜联合中药治疗轻型子宫内膜异位症合并不孕症 52 例临床观察. *河北中医* **36**(4): 554–556.

(*Continued*)

Study No.	Reference
H154	陈体平. (2010) 腹腔镜手术结合中医治疗子宫内膜异位的临床观察. *内蒙古中医药* **29**(12): 19–20.
H155	赵红艳, 倪育淳, 周英. (2010) 腹腔镜术辅以化瘀消癥汤治疗子宫内膜异位症合并不孕临床研究. *实用中医药杂志* **26**(7): 450–451.
H156	卢笛, 林艳明, 梁月秀, et al. (2017) 腹腔镜术后联合蠲痛饮治疗子宫内膜异位症的临床研究. *右江民族医学院学报* **39**(6): 485–487, 490.
H157	王萌萌, 杨振宇, 曾涛. (2017) 归芎消癥方治疗中重度子宫内膜异位症的临床研究. *中国临床药学杂志* **26**(5): 288–291.
H158	杨学芳, 周菊英. (2016) 活血化瘀汤联合腹腔镜治疗轻型子宫内膜异位症不孕患者的疗效及对趋化因子和氧化应激因子的影响. *湖北中医杂志* **38**(7): 4–6.
H159	吴述芬. (2013) 活血化瘀中药联合腹腔镜对轻型子宫内膜异位症不孕患者机体氧化应激状态的影响. *江西中医药* **44**(372): 33–35.
H160	万凌屹, 周凌娟, 丁彩飞. (2016) 血府逐瘀汤加减对卵巢子宫内膜异位囊肿术后卵巢功能及妊娠结局的影响. *中华中医药学刊* **34**(1): 173–176.
H161	王倩. (2015) 化瘀消癥汤联合米非司酮预防子宫内膜异位症腹腔镜保守术后复发疗效观察. *新中医* **47**(3): 163–164.
H162	洪佩佩, 张玲璐. (2014) 少腹逐瘀汤加减辅治子宫内膜异位症痛经的疗效观察. *浙江中医杂志* **49**(7): 488–489.
H163	陈沛明. (2013) 血府逐淤汤治疗子宫内膜异位症临床观察. *实用医学杂志* **29**(10): 1712–1713.
H164	郭雅彬, 王芳. (2015) 血府逐瘀胶囊联合孕三烯酮在子宫内膜异位症术后的应用及临床观察. *医学综述* **21**(11): 2060–2061.
H165	刘丽英, 盖赵秀, 姚海东, et al. (2013) 中药化癥汤联合红外线照射预防重症子宫内膜异位症术后复发的疗效观察. *齐齐哈尔医学院学报* **34**(23): 3484–3485.
H166	张春青. (2013) 中药周期调治法防治子宫内膜异位症术后复发的临床观察. *贵阳中医学院学报* **1**(35): 159–160.
H167	张璇, 王小红, 林妍, et al. (2017) 逐瘀汤对血瘀型子宫内膜异位症性不孕的疗效观察. *福建医药杂志* **39**(5): 101–103.
H168	吴莹, 曹保利. (2011) 子宫内膜异位症腹腔镜术后应用复方莪术散的疗效探讨. *吉林中医药* **31**(2): 146–147.
H169	王如英, 周琳. (2004) 活血祛瘀法治疗子宫内膜异位症的临床观察. *中国中西医结合杂志* **24**(3): 258–259.

(*Continued*)

(Continued)

Study No.	Reference
H170	Ding ZR, Lian F. (2015) Traditional Chinese medical herbs staged therapy in infertile women with endometriosis: A clinical study. *Int J Clin Exp Med* **8**(8): 14085–14089.
H171	姚梓平, 秦慧娟, 段丽君, et al. (2018) 补肾调经汤治疗子宫内膜异位症临床研究. *中医学报* **33**(6): 1136–1139.
H172	谢威. (2017) 少腹逐瘀汤联合孕三烯酮对子宫内膜异位症患者雌激素及CA125水平影响研究. *航空航天医学杂志* **28**(1): 102–103.
H173	桂玉然, 马迎红. (2017) 益气化瘀方治疗保守性手术后复发子宫内膜异位症的临床研究. *湖北中医药大学学报* **19**(4): 84–87.
H174	钟晓玲, 王霞灵, 张忠. (2009) 中西医结合治疗子宫内膜异位症的临床研究. *中国医药导报* **6**(24): 65–66.
H175	龚世雄, 姜慧君. (2010) 丹莪妇康煎膏改善子宫内膜异位症患者生存质量的临床研究. *贵阳中医学院学报* **6**(32): 37–39.
H176	边姣燕, 李红萍, 刘虹. (2005) 重度盆腔子宫内膜异位症术后应用桂枝茯苓胶囊与米非司酮的临床观察. *中国妇幼保健* **20**(2): 236–237.
H177	蔡莹莹, 林卫萍, 陈柏莲, et al. (2013) 扶正消异方联合促性腺激素释放激素激动剂预防卵巢子宫内膜异位囊肿术后复发的研究. *中国全科医学* **16**(4): 464–466.
H178	高玉玲, 宋保志. (2008) 175例子宫内膜异位症药物治疗临床观察. *海峡药学* **20**(9): 75–76.
H179	陈亮香. (2013) 中西结合防治子宫内异症术后复发临床分析. *实用预防医学* **20**(5): 587–588.
H180	陈志芳. (2018) 米非司酮联合补肾化瘀汤对卵巢子宫内膜异位症临床疗效及血清学指标的影响. *中国药物经济学* (9): 95–97.
H181	杨丽娜, 从慧芳. (2015) 补肾化瘀中药治疗卵巢子宫内膜异位囊肿术后患者的临床疗效观察. *中医药信息* **32**(6): 82–85.
H182	张会美. (2016) 补肾活血法联合腹腔镜手术治疗子宫内膜异位症不孕的临床观察. 广州中医药大学.
H183	沈旸. (2009) 补肾活血结合外治法治疗盆腔子宫内膜异位症保守术后的临床研究. 南京中医药大学.
H184	黄书慧, 闵淑云, 朱芝玲. (2017) 归芎消异方对卵巢子宫内膜异位症患者术后复发及妊娠情况的影响. *复旦学报·医学版* **44**(1): 42–46.
H185	李欣. (2011) 复方莪术散对子宫内膜异位症患者 VEGF 和 RANTES 表达的影响及临床疗效观察. 天津医科大学.

(Continued)

Study No.	Reference
H186	郝会卿. (2016) 复方莪术散预防子宫内膜异位症术后复发观察. *辽宁中医药大学学报* **18**(8): 214–216.
H187	孟庆芳, 曹保利. (2012) 腹腔镜联合中药辅助治疗子宫内膜异位症合并不孕临床研究. *新中医* **44**(9): 59–60.
H188	高健, 田瑞, 黄立, et al. (2010) 腹腔镜手术联合散结镇痛胶囊治疗子宫内膜异位症的疗效观察. *腹腔镜外科杂志* **15**(5): 376–378.
H189	顺惠芳. (2003) 化瘀消癥法治疗子宫内膜异位症痛经 70 例疗效观察. *新中医* **35**(10): 17–18.
H190	全晓广, 黄敏, 陈雪梅. (2007) 卵巢巧克力囊肿腹腔镜术后中西医结合治疗的临床观察. *医学创新研究* **4**(12): 77–78.
H191	李泽焰, 张洪梅, 李泽平. (2015) 加减当归四逆汤在子宫内膜异位症疼痛中的效果分析. *中国继续医学教育* **7**(15): 1734.
H192	王海燕. (2012) 内异停方观察卵巢子宫内膜异位症保守术后复发及对VEGF 的影响. 南京中医药大学.
H193	王寿芳, 胡晓英. (2012) 暖宫七味丸治疗子宫内膜异位症痛经疗效观察. *浙江中西医结合杂志* **22**(2): 116–117.
H194	李娟. (2007) 舒痛灵汤治疗子宫内膜异位症引起的痛经临床疗效评价. 新疆医科大学.
H195	沈晓婷. (2015) 温肾消癥汤治疗肾虚血瘀型卵巢子宫内膜异位囊肿的疗效观察及作用机理初探. 南京中医药大学.
H196	张慧琴, 马得花, 宋金明, et al. (2011) 异位康冲剂治疗子宫内膜异位症 50 例临床观察. *中医杂志* **52**(1): 27–30.
H197	岳利平. (2018) 中药对子宫内膜异位症及妊娠结局的影响. *光明中医* **33**(3): 373–375.
H198	杜巧梅, 冯惠芳. (2018) 中西医结合治疗子宫内膜异位症疗效观察. *实用中医药杂志* **34**(8): 973–974.
H199	颜望碧, 毛利云. (2010) 子宫内膜异位症腹腔镜手术后辅助散结镇痛胶囊治疗的疗效分析. *中国医师进修杂志* **33**(21): 16–18.
H200	周玉玲, 叶恒君. (2005) 综合疗法治疗复发性子宫内膜异位囊肿 32 例疗效观察. *新中医* **37**(7): 19–20.
H201	Weng Q, Ding ZM, Lv XL, et al. (2015) Chinese medicinal plants for advanced endometriosis after conservative surgery: A prospective, multi-center and controlled trial. *Int J Clin Exp Med* **8**(7): 11307–11311.

(Continued)

(Continued)

Study No.	Reference
H202	李倩. (2016) 补肾调周化瘀法干预卵巢巧克力囊肿术后复发的临床观察. 南京中医药大学.
H203	曹阳, 曹莉莉, 王唯迪, et al. (2017) 良方温经汤治疗子宫内膜异位症浅析. 河北中医 **39**(3): 449–452.
H204	常暖. (1997) 妇痛宁治疗子宫内膜异位症临床和实验研究. 中医杂志 **38**(8): 488–490.
H205	陈星蓓, 章勤. (2015) 章勤治疗子宫内膜异位症所致不孕经验. 浙江中医杂志 **50**(8): 553–554.
H206	崔火仙, 何嘉琳. (2013) 何嘉琳治疗子宫内膜异位症经验介绍. 新中医 **45**(5): 202–203.
H207	笪红英. (2005) 陆启滨从瘀治疗子宫内膜异位症经验. 江西中医药 (2): 13–14.
H208	段丽云, 张丽娟. (2018) 刘瑞芬教授预防子宫内膜异位症术后复发的经验. 云南中医中药杂志 **39**(8): 8–9.
H209	冯乐, 刘思南, 张晓甦. (2016) 张晓甦治疗子宫内膜异位症性痛经的经验. 江苏中医药 **48**(11): 25–27.
H210	付雪, 郭荣. (2013) 郭荣教授治疗巧克力囊肿经验. 湖南中医杂志 **29**(1): 28, 32.
H211	黄世威. (2016) 补肾温阳化瘀法治疗子宫内膜异位症痛经疗效观察. 中国民族民间医药杂志 **25**(21): 109–110.
H212	郭永红. (2009) 李光荣治疗子宫内膜异位症经验. 中国中医药信息杂志 **16**(5): 87–88.
H213	郭永红, 李光荣. (2007) 丹赤饮对子宫内膜异位症患者血清 CA125 和肿瘤坏死因子及性激素水平的影响. 中华中医药杂志 **22**(12): 892–984.
H214	侯建峰. (2007) 高月平治疗子宫内膜异位症经验. 中医杂志 **48**(5): 407, 426.
H215	米齐. (2007) 何嘉琳治疗子宫内膜异位症经验. 中国中医药信息杂志 **14**(1): 83–84.
H216	陈桂玲, 刘笑梅. (2014) 复方术术散在子宫内膜异位症术后的应用. 中国中西医结合外科杂志 **20**(3): 260–261.
H217	林雯雯. (2010) 扶正消异方治疗子宫内膜异位不孕症 24 例. 现代中西医结合杂志 **19**(8): 969–970.
H218	刘蔚霞. (2010) 胡玉荃教授治疗内异症性痛经经验胡玉荃教授治疗内异症性痛经经验. 中医研究 **23**(7): 74–75.

(Continued)

Study No.	Reference
H219	马红艳, 李晓茹, 张黎, et al. (2011) 卓毅教授采用活血化瘀法治疗内异症性不孕症举隅. *中医临床研究* **3**(17): 90–91.
H220	杨敏祥. (2016) 桂茇棱乌汤治疗寒凝血瘀型子宫内膜异位症的临床观察. 北京中医药大学.
H221	尹燕, 曹阳, 张婷婷. (2011) 红藤方治疗术后复发性子宫内膜异位症 41 例的疗效及生存质量评价. *上海中医药大学学报* **25**(1): 36–39.
H222	莫惠玉, 黄素英. (1999) 蔡小荪治疗子宫内膜异位症验案一则. *中医文献杂志* (1): 40.
H223	牛柳霞, 夏亲华. (2016) 夏亲华教授采用补肾活血方治疗子宫内膜异位症经验. *环球中医药* **9**(1): 65–67.
H224	牛向馨. (2011) 平冲化瘀通络法治疗痛经 30 例. *亚太传统医药* **7**(7): 61–62.
H225	牛艳明, 时燕萍. (2016) 时燕萍教授治疗子宫内膜异位症痛经经验. *中医药学报* **44**(2): 139–141.
H226	戚晓菲. (2007) 陈莹教授治疗子宫内膜异位症经验总结. 辽宁中医药大学.
H227	李荣秀. (2008) 活血化瘀法治疗子宫内膜异位症的临床研究及对血液流变学的影响. 云南中医学院.
H228	钱海墨. (2011) 齐聪治疗子宫内膜异位症性不孕经验. *中医杂志* **52**(19): 1689–1691.
H229	孙红, 王祖龙. (2010) 褚玉霞治疗子宫内膜异位症经验. *中医学报* **25**(4): 661–663.
H230	李小平. (2009) 木达汤治疗子宫内膜异位症盆腔痛临床观察. *光明中医* **24**(11): 2102–2104.
H231	王静. (2016) 益肾疏肝方治疗肾虚血瘀型卵巢巧克力囊肿的临床观察. 黑龙江中医药大学.
H232	唐润娟. (2012) 内异痛经汤对子宫内膜异位症痛经症状的影响. *新疆中医药* **30**(2): 16–18.
H233	邬素珍. (2000) 内异丸治疗子宫内膜异位症痛经的临床观察. *中药材* **23**(6): 368–369.
H234	梁瑞宁. (2012) 平冲降逆化瘀通络法治疗痛经(子宫内膜异位症)多中心临床研究. *新中医* **44**(1): 66–68.
H235	韩玉芬, 赵晓莉, 张雪莉. (2015) 少腹逐瘀汤治疗子宫内膜异位症体会. *光明中医* **30**(8): 1762–1763.
H236	周艳艳, 尤昭玲, 冯光荣. (2014) 试析血瘕与子宫内膜异位症. *中医临床研究* **6**(19): 48–449.

(Continued)

(Continued)

Study No.	Reference
H237	黄艳辉, 司徒仪. (2015) 司徒仪教授治疗子宫内膜异位症特色浅析. 湖北中医药大学学报 **17**(3): 95–97.
H238	范丽娟. (2016) 痛愈舒颗粒治疗子宫内膜异位症 EmAb 阳性不孕患者的临床观察. 黑龙江中医药大学.
H239	宿振洁, 金季玲. (2011) 金季玲治疗子宫内膜异位症验案 1 则. 山西中医 **27**(1): 43.
H240	郭纪芬, 张晓甦. (2017) 消积冲剂治疗湿热瘀阻型子宫内膜异位症的疗效研究. 当代医药论丛 **15**(15): 107–109.
H241	杨红, 齐聪, 周华. (2011) 益气活血方治疗卵巢子宫内膜异位囊肿术后复发 118 例. 上海中医药杂志 **45**(8): 39–41.
H242	段燕君. (2005) 折冲饮治疗子宫内膜异位症2则. 中国民间疗法 **13**(2): 48–49.
H243	张利. (2011) 中药分期治疗子宫内膜异位症痛经34例. 江苏中医药 **43**(8): 49–50.
H244	王玉. (2008) 中药干预改善子宫内膜异位症(气滞血瘀型)疼痛及生存质量研究. 云南中医学院.
H245	张娟, 赵瑞华. (2014) 活血补肾周期治疗子宫内膜异位症相关不孕症临床观察. 中国中医药信息杂志 **21**(4): 93–95.
H246	周华, 齐聪. (2008) 齐聪辨治卵巢子宫内膜异位囊肿经验. 上海中医药杂志 **42**(4): 19–20.
H247	潘芳, 肖承悰. (2005) 子宫内膜异位症所致疼痛辨治体会. 中国临床医生 **33**(4): 40–41.
H248	周璐. (2006) 蓬甲饮治疗子宫内膜异位症的临床及实验研究. 北京中医药大学.
H249	商立静. (2016) 自拟方内异灵治疗子宫内膜异位症痛经的临床观察. 黑龙江中医药大学.
H250	陈芷玲. (2003) 清肝引经汤合血府逐瘀汤治疗肺子宫内膜异位症 5 例. 河北中医 **25**(11): 835–836.
H251	卜德艳, 姜丽娟, 赵文方. (2010) 张良英教授辨证论治肺子宫内膜异位症 1 例体会. 云南中医中药杂志 **31**(6): 20–21.
H252	卜德艳, 岳胜难, 姜丽娟. (2012) 张良英教授辨证治疗肺子宫内膜异位症经验初探. 云南中医学院学报 **35**(2): 32–33.
H253	Chu YW. (1996) Treatment of endometriosis and ovarian masses with Fu liu pill. *Journal of Chinese Medicine* (52): 9.

(Continued)

Study No.	Reference
H254	Lin PY, Tsai YT, Lai JN, Yeh CH, Fang RC. (2014) Bian zheng lun zhi as a complementary and alternative treatment for menstrual cramps in women with dysmenorrhea: A prospective clinical observation. *Evid Based Complement Alternat Med* **2014**: 460386.
H255	Park KS. (2018) The efficacy and safety of Korean herbal medicine in a patient with endometrioma of the ovary: A case report. *Explore* 2018: 1–6.
H256	蔡凡, 朱丽萍, 邹振红, et al. (2013) 中药外敷及灌肠治疗复发性子宫内膜异位症35 例. *中国基层医药* **20**(7): 999–1000.
H257	汤艳秋, 徐佳一. (2014) "异位二号方" 灌肠治疗子宫内膜异位症 40 例临床研究. *江苏中医药* **46**(7): 34–35.
H258	万德馨, 张敏鸽, 党群. (2016) 红藤汤灌肠联合外敷治疗子宫内膜异位症保守手术后痛经的临床疗效. *陕西中医* **37**(10): 1289–1290.
H259	樊建霜, 王家员, 孙云. (2015) 活血散瘀灌肠液治疗子宫内膜异位症的效果观察. *中国医药* **10**(5): 686–688.
H260	孙佳慧, 蒋军, 蒋学禄, et al. (2018) 复方大血藤保留灌肠预防 em 术后复发的疗效观察. *浙江临床医学* **20**(8): 1417–1418.
H261	魏美霞, 赵雪娟. (2014) 内异痛经方保留灌肠治疗子宫内膜异位症痛经临床观察. *山西中医* **30**(10): 44–45.
H262	党慧敏, 吴晓玲, 刘艳巧, et al. (2014) 内异消保留灌肠预防子宫内膜异位症术后复发的疗效观察. *陕西中医* **35**(9): 1194–1197.
H263	屈育莉, 刘艳巧, 党慧敏, et al. (2013) 内异消保留灌肠治疗子宫内膜异位症的临床疗效观察. *西安交通大学学报·医学版* **34**(3): 397–399, 402.
H264	吴丹. (2008) 痛愈贴提高子宫内膜异位症患者生活质量的临床研究. 黑龙江中医药大学.
H265	周金花. (2012) 异位痛经灵灌肠治疗子宫内膜异位症痛 46 例. *光明中医* **27**(10): 2009–2010.
H266	韩燕. (2012) 中药保留灌肠对子宫内膜异位症患者血清中 IL-2, IL-10 及瘦素水平影响研究. 泰山医学院.
H267	韩秋丽, 杨宁, 孙宏丽. (2014) 中药灌肠用于卵巢子宫内膜异位囊肿腹腔镜术后的临床研究. *航空航天医学杂志* **25**(7): 918–920.
H268	蔡嘉兴, 高勤, 宋坤玲, et al. (2000) 散结止痛汤灌肠治疗子宫内膜异位症临床研究. *河北中医* **22**(1): 8–9.

(Continued)

(Continued)

Study No.	Reference
H269	王玥, 李进. (2015) 中药红花浸液辅助腹腔镜下手术治疗子宫内膜异位症及对于生育指数的影响. *中医药导报* **21**(15): 79–81.
H270	杨小顾, 严妮子. (2007) 红藤汤保留灌肠治疗子宫内膜异位症疼痛临床分析. *现代中西医结合杂志* **16**(25): 3642–3643.
H271	杜巧梅, 冯惠芳. (2018) 化瘀调经方配合灌肠对子宫内膜异位症患者血管内皮生长因子和肿瘤坏死因子的影响. *陕西中医* **39**(8): 1070–1073.
H272	梁若笳, 蒋军. (2014) 补肾调经活血中药口服结合灌肠对子宫内膜异位症痛经的影响. *中华中医药学刊* **32**(1): 220–222.
H273	廖文英. (2016) 内异方联合灌肠方对 EMT 肾虚血瘀证患者术后复发干预的临床研究. 湖南中医药大学.
H274	柴洪佳, 杨喆, 邹志洁. (2013) 经带宁合中药外用对子宫内膜异位症腹腔镜术后的疗效分析. *深圳中西医结合杂志* **23**(2): 94–97.
H275	张利梅, 翁双燕, 王彩霞, et al. (2016) 卵巢内膜异位囊肿术后多途径干预的临床研究. *中国中医急症* **25**(02): 329–331.
H276	邬素珍, 陈秀廉, 陈伟志, et al. (2006) 内异丸合内异灌肠液联合治疗子宫内膜异位症的临床观察. *中医药学刊* **24**(3): 431–433.
H277	王英, 潘丽贞. (2017) 轻度子宫内膜异位症并不孕腹腔镜术后应用中医分期疗法的临床观察. *广西中医药* **40**(2): 32–34.
H278	范红霞, 王霞灵. (2004) 益气活血方内服与灌肠治疗子宫内膜异位症的临床研究. *天津中医药* **21**(4): 287–289.
H279	王亚校. (2006) 中药保留灌肠配合内服与丹那唑治疗子宫内膜异位症疗效比较. *中国中西医结合杂志* **26**(10): 944–945.
H280	吴晓华, 张翠兰. (2014) 中药口服加外敷治疗子宫内膜异位症术后 32 例. *光明中医* **29**(1): 97–98.
H281	张媛, 刘筱茂, 霍艳宁, et al. (2017) 中药口服联合保留灌肠治疗子宫内膜异位症生存质量及疗效评价. *环球中医药* **10**(7): 712–715.
H282	杨松淞, 张晓华. (2013) 中药周期加灌肠综合防治卵巢子宫内膜异位囊肿术后复发临床观察. *新中医* **45**(2): 74–76.
H283	陈碧晖, 刘奇志, 柴洪佳, et al. (2012) 补肾活血化瘀中药三联疗法在子宫内膜异位症合并不孕患者腹腔镜术后的应用. *实用医学杂志* **28**(21): 3651–3653.
H284	白艳华. (2003) 金季玲教授治疗子宫内膜异位症经验举隅. *天津中医学院学报* **22**(3): 51–52.

(*Continued*)

Study No.	Reference
H285	邓小雨, 张彦辉, 雷磊. (2014) 雷磊治疗子宫内膜异位症经验. *湖南中医杂志* **30**(5): 26–27.
H286	孙帅, 沈慰, 翟东霞, *et al.* (2014) 化瘀解毒组方治疗子宫内膜异位症 58 例疗效观察. *中医杂志* **55**(19): 1668–1671.
H287	宋艳华. (2004) 益气补肾化瘀法治疗子宫内膜异位症的临床及实验研究. 第二军医大学.
H288	高磊, 陈燕, 禚洪波. (2001) 内异助孕丸配合中药灌肠治疗子宫内膜异位症合并不孕17例. *河北中医* **23**(8): 590.
H289	王肖, 尤昭玲. (2014) 浅析尤昭玲教授对子宫内膜异位症的认识及中医治疗特色. *中华中医药杂志* **29**(8): 2457–2460.
H290	王英. (2016) 秦振华学术思想与临床经验总结及分期疗法对不同类型内异症不孕的临床研究. 福建中医药大学.
H291	宋艳华, 俞瑾, 俞超芹. (2005) 俞氏内异方结合中药灌肠外敷治疗子宫内膜异位症 36 例临床观察. *中国中西医结合杂志* **25**(8): 748–749.
H292	安艳. (2014) 痛经汤对寒凝血瘀型子宫腺肌病痛经的临床研究. 南京中医药大学.
H293	白亚鹭, 张丽琴. (2018) 中药治疗早期子宫腺肌症的临床研究. *中国医药指南* **16**(11): 234–235.
H294	曹瑾琼. (2018) 中西医结合治疗气滞血瘀型子宫腺肌病伴痛经疗效观察. *中国民族民间医药杂志* **27**(6): 65–67.
H295	曹丽蓉. (2006) 中西医结合治疗子宫腺肌病临床观察. 湖北中医学院.
H296	曾薇薇, 殷岫绮. (2014) "化瘀凉血方"治疗子宫腺肌病 32 例临床研究. *江苏中医药* **46**(1): 32–34.
H297	曾艺文, 刘耀崇. (2018) 乌梅汤合宣郁通经汤加减治疗子宫腺肌症痛经的临床观察. *中医药导报* **24**(5): 92–94.
H298	陈志芳. (2018) 左炔诺孕酮宫内释放系统联合桂枝茯苓胶囊治疗子宫腺肌症的临床效果. *河南医学研究* **27**(16): 2969–2970.
H299	董泗霞. (2012) 化瘀消癥方联合米非司酮治疗围绝经期子宫腺肌病的临床观察. 山东中医药大学.
H300	杜嫦燕, 柴洪佳, 黎汉文, *et al.* (2010) 化瘀消结方治疗子宫腺肌病介入术后的疗效观察. *国际中医中药杂志* **32**(4): 326–327.
H301	段素社 邢风琴, 张素健, *et al.* (2006) 自拟溯源追本汤治疗子宫腺肌病 166 例临床观察. *现代中西医结合杂志* **15**(24): 3350–3351.

(*Continued*)

(Continued)

Study No.	Reference
H302	冯丽娜, 洪莉. (2017) 桂枝茯苓胶囊联合左炔诺孕酮宫内节育系统治疗子宫腺肌症的疗效观察. *现代药物与临床* **32**(8): 1516–1519.
H303	付虹, 张丽萍. (2018) 米非司酮联合宫瘤消胶囊治疗子宫腺肌症的临床效果观察. *中国医药* **13**(3): 440–442.
H304	傅宝君, 孙淑玉, 丁婷婷. (2008) 腺肌丸治疗瘀热互结型子宫腺肌病痛经70例临床研究. *上海中医药杂志* **42**(8): 53–54.
H305	葛江风, 詹尧平. (2017) 小剂量米非司酮配合中药治疗子宫腺肌病的临床观察. *中国基层医药* **24**(8): 1161–1164.
H306	郭英, 廖英. (2010) 桂枝茯苓丸加味治疗子宫腺肌病的近期临床观察. *中国中医药科技* **17**(4): 348–349.
H307	韩迎娣. (2008) 补肾活血化瘀法治疗肾虚血瘀型子宫腺肌病的临床研究. 福建中医学院.
H308	何菊. (2018) 中药周期治疗子宫腺肌病的临床效果观察. *中国中医药科技* **25**(3): 453–454.
H309	胡珊. (2015) 桂枝茯苓丸联合妈富隆治疗气滞血瘀型子宫腺肌病的疗效观察. 湖北中医药大学.
H310	黄艳辉, 肖静, 刘立群. (2015) 温阳化瘀散结汤治疗血虚寒凝型子宫腺肌病临床观察. *广州中医药大学学报* **32**(5): 834–837, 842.
H311	李能霞, 王国俊, 翟建霞, et al. (2016) 达菲林加曼月乐联合葛根二仙汤治疗子宫腺肌病临床研究. *新中医* **48**(8): 167–169.
H312	梁荣丽, 罗宋. (2011) 左炔诺孕酮宫内释放系统联合桂枝茯苓胶囊治疗子宫腺肌病的疗效观察. *华西医学* **26**(1): 72–74.
H313	刘芳, 巨瑛, 杨红晔, et al. (2016) 桂枝茯苓丸联合西药治疗子宫腺肌病继发性痛经患者的临床疗效及对血清 IL-6, PGE2 及 et 的影响. *陕西中医* **37**(10): 1279–1280.
H314	刘秀峰. (2012) 决津煎合失笑散加味治疗寒凝血瘀型子宫腺肌病痛经 35 例. *福建中医药大学学报* **22**(1): 54–56.
H315	楼月芳, 杨小芳. (2012) 行气祛瘀汤治疗子宫腺肌病的临床疗效观察. *中国现代医生* **50**(19): 83–84, 86.
H316	马幼菊, 马晓莉. (2014) 散结镇痛胶囊联合曼月乐治疗子宫腺肌病疗效观察. *医学研究与教育* **31**(4): 16–19.
H317	牛晶娟. (2017) 桂枝茯苓胶囊联合孕三烯酮治疗子宫腺肌症的临床研究. *现代药物与临床* **32**(5): 835–839.

(Continued)

Study No.	Reference
H318	邵艳社. (2015) 西黄胶囊联合曼月乐治疗气滞血瘀型弥漫性子宫腺肌病的临床研究. 天津中医药大学.
H319	邵永红, 王芸. (2013) 散结镇痛胶囊联合曼月乐治疗子宫腺肌病临床效果及安全性评价. *实用药物与临床* **16**(11): 1038–1041.
H320	石东涛, 白睿. (2016) 桂枝茯苓胶囊联合左炔诺孕酮宫内释放系统治疗子宫腺肌病临床研究. *海南医学院学报* **22**(22): 2772–2774.
H321	石利香. (2018) 补肾活血散瘀汤治疗肾虚血瘀型子宫腺肌症的临床观察. *光明中医* **33**(8): 1112–1113, 1141.
H322	石少琦. (2016) 滋肾疏肝汤对子宫腺肌病伴不孕患者 IVF-ET 早期妊娠的影响. 河南中医药大学.
H323	司小丽, 苏宝珍, 杨梅枝. (2018) 桂枝茯苓胶囊联合左炔诺孕酮宫内节育系统对子宫腺肌症患者子宫内膜厚度及激素水平的影响. *中国医院用药评价与分析* **18**(8): 1055–1057.
H324	苏健, 田李军. (2013) 从脾论治子宫腺肌病继发痛经的临床观察. *四川中医* **31**(6): 115–116.
H325	王红新. (2007) 消癥化腺方合止痛化腺方分期治疗子宫腺肌病的临床研究. 山东中医药大学.
H326	王金香, 王爱丽, 梁虹. (2017) 桃红四物汤治疗子宫腺肌症痛经的临床疗效观察. *世界中医药* **12**(8): 1771–1773, 1777.
H327	王楠, 章根琴. (2017) 止痛化癥胶囊联合孕三烯酮胶囊治疗子宫腺肌病临床观察. *新中医* **49**(6): 77–79.
H328	王霞. (2016) 助阳化瘀消癥汤配合曼月乐治疗子宫腺肌症疗效观察. *山西中医* **32**(7): 27–28.
H329	魏竞男, 王爱丽, 陈彦, et al. (2017) 黄芪健脾益气汤治疗子宫腺肌病气虚血瘀证的临床研究. *中医药导报* **23**(23): 91–93.
H330	吾慧瑛, 孙心林, 林莉. (2010) 复方金笑汤联合米非司酮治疗子宫腺肌病的临床观察. *中国民间疗法* **18**(6): 51–52.
H331	吴丹. (2017) 补肾活血汤治疗肾虚血瘀型子宫腺肌病月经过多的临床观察. 黑龙江中医药大学.
H332	吴伟平. (2015) 曼月乐联合散结镇痛胶囊治疗子宫腺肌病临床对比分析. *中国医师杂志* **17**(6): 936–938.
H333	肖菊梅, 张翰儒. (2017) 少腹逐瘀胶囊治疗寒凝血瘀型子宫腺肌病临床研究. *新中医* **49**(11): 75–77.

(Continued)

(*Continued*)

Study No.	Reference
H334	许浪萍, 潘群玉, 陈艳丹. (2018) 活血祛瘀补肾序贯疗法联合GnRH-a,曼月乐治疗子宫腺肌病疗效探析. *四川中医* **36**(7): 154–156.
H335	杨舫, 帕里扎提, 王清. (2017) 益坤抑痛平治疗子宫腺肌病痛经的疗效及安全性评价. *中日友好医院学报* **31**(4): 214–217.
H336	杨君, 任艳芳, 华芳芳. (2009) 改良式手术联合散结镇痛胶囊治疗子宫腺肌症的临床研究. *医学信息内,外科版* **22**(6): 501–503.
H337	杨培丽, 祝鑫瑜, 章新根. (2016) 自拟少腹逐瘀汤联合西药治疗子宫腺肌病痛经疗效及对血清 CA125, TNF-α, IL-8 水平影响. *现代中西医结合杂志* **25**(29): 3233–3236.
H338	张英芝, 劳佩维, 沈柯炜. (2017) 孕三烯酮胶囊联合丹黄祛瘀胶囊治疗子宫肌腺病的临床研究. *中国临床药理学杂志* **33**(10): 880–883.
H339	叶青, 艾白媛. (2008) 活血消癥胶囊与化瘀止痛胶囊分期治疗子宫腺肌病临床研究. *中国中医急症* **17**(2): 179–181.
H340	元凤霞. (2014) 炔雌醇环丙孕酮片联合散结镇痛胶囊治疗子宫腺肌病的疗效观察. *现代药物与临床* **29**(6): 668–671.
H341	张立新. (2017) 中西医联合治疗子宫腺肌症痛经评价. *光明中医* **32**(11): 1640–1641.
H342	张丽华. (2015) 玄丹散结汤联合曼月乐治疗气滞血瘀型子宫腺肌病的临床研究. 南京中医药大学.
H343	张妙玉, 覃秋萍, 欧幸甘. (2017) 葛根二仙汤与达菲林加曼月乐联用治疗子宫腺肌病的临床观察. *中国民族民间医药杂志* **26**(5): 132–134.
H344	张玉锋, 张炜, 张宝丽, *et al.* (2018) 活血逐瘀汤治疗子宫腺肌症临床研究. *新中医* **50**(4): 121–124.
H345	赵越秀. (2012) 散结镇痛胶囊对子宫腺肌症患者 ca125 表达的影响. *浙江中医杂志* **47**(9): 650.
H346	郑颖. (2016) 中药消异方对子宫腺肌症患者疼痛症状及子宫内膜容受性的改善. 山东中医药大学.
H347	曹文丽. (2010) 散结镇痛胶囊治疗子宫腺肌病合并不孕症临床观察. *中国乡村医药* **17**(12): 40–41.
H348	成臣, 桂涛, 黄美华, *et al.* (2014) 补肾活血散瘀汤治疗肾虚血瘀型子宫腺肌症的临床观察. *中国中西医结合杂志* **34**(11): 1302–1305.
H349	孔庆兰, 林涛, 迟玉丽, *et al.* (2014) 祛瘀消异汤治疗子宫腺肌病的临床疗效分析. *临床合理用药杂志* **7**(21): 121–123.

(*Continued*)

Study No.	Reference
H350	李杰兰, 马卫军. (2011) 左炔诺孕酮宫内缓释系统联合桂枝茯苓治疗子宫腺肌病 50 例. *中国生育健康杂志* **22**(5): 304–305.
H351	陶艳玲, 徐鑫, 甄学慧. (2013) 曼月乐联合散结镇痛胶囊治疗子宫腺肌病的临床评价. *中国妇幼保健* **28**(19): 3204–3206.
H352	徐敏霞, 赵灵琴. (2018) 补肾祛瘀方治疗肾虚血瘀型子宫腺肌症的效果观察. *现代实用医学* **30**(2): 223–225.
H353	陈静, 胡国华. (2016) 胡国华治疗子宫腺肌病痛经经验. *世界中西医结合杂志* **11**(11): 1481–1483, 1488.
H354	陈倩. (2008) 丹昆散结饮治疗子宫腺肌病(痰瘀互结证)的临床疗效观察. 北京中医药大学.
H355	杜欢欢. (2012) 朱颖治疗子宫腺肌症验案1则. *江西中医药* **43**(6): 12.
H356	冯士华. (2010) 中药散瘀止痛方治疗子宫腺肌症 69 例分析. *中国误诊学杂志* **10**(28): 6968.
H357	姜彦, 应翩, 任辉, *et al.* (2010) 张萍青治疗子宫腺肌症经验. *辽宁中医药大学学报* **12**(1): 114–115.
H358	李爱芳. (2012) 下瘀血汤合四逆散加味治疗子宫腺肌病疗效观察. *中国中医药信息杂志* **19**(4): 76–77.
H359	李坤寅, 方庆霞. (2009) 化瘀止痛方对子宫腺肌病痛经患者 PGF2α, PGE2, OT 影响的临床研究. *新中医* **41**(2): 63–65.
H360	李敏, 刘金星. (2009) 化瘀消癥汤治疗子宫腺肌病 48 例. *河南中医* **29**(4): 383–384.
H361	李晓曦. (2013) 加味琥珀散治疗子宫腺肌症所致气滞血瘀型痛经的临床观察. *中国农村卫生* (01Z): 122–123.
H362	李艳霞. (2017) 理气活血法治疗气滞血瘀型子宫腺肌症的临床观察. 黑龙江中医药大学.
H363	李元琪. (2018) 罗颂平运用膏方治疗子宫腺肌症经验. *安徽中医药大学学报* **37**(1): 26–67.
H364	梁杰, 时燕萍. (2017) 时燕萍教授治疗子宫腺肌病经验. *浙江中医药大学学报* **41**(4): 304–306.
H365	刘宇新, 满玉晶, 侯丽辉. (2008) 琥珀散治愈子宫腺肌病 1 例. *辽宁中医药大学学报* **10**(12): 118.
H366	马云松, 朱磊, 李红梅. (2011) 中药治疗子宫腺肌病 30 例临床观察. *黑龙江中医药* **40**(1): 12–13.

(*Continued*)

(Continued)

Study No.	Reference
H367	梅本华. (2009) 自拟血竭方治疗子宫腺肌症 40 例. *中医药临床杂志* **21**(3): 237–238.
H368	牛艳明. (2016) 内异停方联合温化止痛方序贯治疗子宫腺肌病痛经的临床疗效观察及对 TSGF 的影响. 南京中医药大学.
H369	钱菁, 赵海英. (2012) 夏桂成诊治子宫腺肌病痛经的临床经验. *江苏中医药* **44**(12): 11–12.
H370	睢从璐, 佟庆, 张芸娜, *et al.* (2014) 金哲应用川夏宁坤汤治疗子宫腺肌病 1 例. *北京中医药* **33**(2): 146–147.
H371	孙海媛, 贾成祥. (2016) 门成福治疗子宫腺肌病经验述要. *中华中医药杂志* **31**(10): 4045–4047.
H372	孙先航, 赵可宁. (2017) 夏桂成教授治疗子宫腺肌病痛经的临床经验. *浙江中医药大学学报* **41**(9): 734–737.
H373	唐明华, 徐亚琳, 王采文. (2012) 王采文教授治疗子宫内膜异位症痛经的经验. *世界中西医结合杂志* **7**(10): 841–842.
H374	王宝金, 李根霞. (2012) 丹莪妇康煎膏治疗子宫腺肌病患者的临床效果观察. *中国妇幼保健* **27**(26): 4150–4151.
H375	王清. (2005) "抑痛平"治疗子宫腺肌症痛经 35 例临床观察. *中国康复理论与实践* **11**(8): 651–652.
H376	王帅, 凌静, 曾玉燕, *et al.* (2015) 李坤寅治疗子宫腺肌病经验撷粹. *中国中医基础医学杂志* **21**(3): 358–359, 364.
H377	袁亚敏, 丁春桃. (2007) 魏绍斌主任医师治疗子宫腺肌病经验. *四川中医* **25**(6): 4–5.
H378	赵文丽, 高月平. (2017) 高月平教授从肝肾论治子宫腺肌病继发痛经经验. *四川中医* **35**(7): 10–12.
H379	周丽娟, 潘丽贞. (2016) 麻黄附子细辛汤加减治疗子宫腺肌病痛经 38 例. *实用中医药杂志* **32**(1): 24–25.
H380	孔珏莹, 曾薇薇, 高雅琦, *et al.* (2018) 化瘀散结灌肠液治疗热灼血瘀型子宫腺肌病的临床观察. *上海中医药杂志* **52**(6): 44–46, 55.
H381	于胜男, 刘彦, 王瑞云, *et al.* (2017) 中药灌肠联合超声聚焦治疗子宫腺肌瘤30例临床观察. *中国民族民间医药杂志* **26**(19): 108–109.
H382	张励. (2018) 少腹逐瘀汤直肠灌注治疗子宫腺肌症疗效观察. *山西中医* **34**(4): 44, 53.
H383	刘红. (2014) 折冲饮加减保留灌肠治疗肾虚血瘀型子宫腺肌病的临床观察. 黑龙江中医药大学.

(Continued)

Study No.	Reference
H384	徐文娟. (2008) 益气散结剂保留灌肠治疗子宫内膜异位症的临床研究. 南京中医药大学.
H385	杨胜霞. (2010) 脐疗法配合琥珀散加减治疗子宫腺肌病的临床观察. 黑龙江中医药大学.
H386	林燕. (2010) 中医综合疗法(二期疗法)治疗子宫腺肌病的临床研究. 成都中医药大学.
H387	魏少奔. (2014) 中医综合疗法治疗子宫腺肌病的临床研究. 成都中医药大学.
H388	边文会, 杜惠兰, 陈惠娟, et al. (2008) 补肾温阳化瘀法对子宫内膜异位症患者痛经影响的临床研究. *临床医药实践杂志* **1**(13): 370–373.
H389	曹芸. (2017) 散结镇痛胶囊对子宫内膜异位症及子宫腺肌病痛经治疗效果观察. *首都食品与医药* **24**(12): 79–80.
H390	陈静, 叶妮, 郭慧宁, et al. (2017) 痛经宁治疗气滞血瘀型子宫内膜异位症及子宫腺肌病痛经的临床观察. *上海中医药杂志* **51**(S1):127–129, 132.
H391	刘研. (2010) 异痛消胶囊治疗子宫内膜异位症盆腔疼痛的临床研究. 黑龙江省中医研究院.
H392	倪晓君, 鲍兰频. (2011) 化瘀止痛汤联合米非司酮治疗子宫内膜异位症痛经的疗效观察. *中国现代医生* **49**(33): 42–43, 66.
H393	施灵美, 邹雪平, 王凌燕. (2017) 诺雷德针联合散结镇痛胶囊治疗子宫内膜异位症的临床疗效观察. *中国生化药物杂志* **37**(7): 104–105, 108.
H394	刘建新. (2011) 散结镇痛胶囊治疗子宫内膜异位症的临床研究. 湖北中医药大学.
H395	齐丹. (2009) 滋阴补阳序贯合并化瘀法联合 GnRH-a 对 EMS 术后复发影响的研究. 南京中医药大学.
H396	骆春, 谢正华. (2015) 骆氏痰瘀同治法治疗子宫内膜异位性疾病 40 例临床观察. *世界临床药物* **36**(5): 349–352.
H397	徐巧燕, 傅宝君. (2014) 内异胶囊治疗子宫内膜异位症痛经临床观察. *实用中医药杂志* **30**(2): 98–99.
H398	郑玮琳. (2016) 痛经文献分析及益气化瘀法治疗子宫内膜异位症痛经临床研究. 广州中医药大学.
H399	艾莉. (2002) 消异饮治疗子宫内膜异位症的临床与实验研究. 北京中医药大学.
H400	蔡琼. (2007) 消癥汤治疗子宫内膜异位症的临床观察及对 EMAb, CA125, IL–8 的影响. 云南中医学院.

(Continued)

(Continued)

Study No.	Reference
H401	曾倩, 陈艳, 李艳锦, et al. (2011) 攻补合治法治疗顽固性痛经 45 例疗效观察. 辽宁中医杂志 **38**(1): 13–14.
H402	戴育兰. (2006) 补肾调周化瘀法治疗 EMT 的临床研究. 南京中医药大学.
H403	戴泽琦, 赵瑞华. (2017) 赵瑞华治疗子宫内膜异位症相关不孕症经验. 世界中西医结合杂志 **12**(7): 921–924.
H404	范培, 梁瑞宁. (2010) 梁瑞宁治疗子宫内膜异位症的临床经验. 湖北中医杂志 **32**(5): 33–34.
H405	李田田. (2016) 活血消异方治疗子宫内膜异位症的临床观察及实验研究. 中国中医科学院.
H406	史梅莹. (2010) 葫芦巴丸加减治疗子宫内膜异位症腺肌病痛经及盆腔痛临床研究. 北京中医药大学.
H407	郭永红. (2004) 活血散结法治疗子宫内膜异位症在临床及其相关细胞因子作用的机理研究. 中国中医科学院;中国中医研究院.
H408	王誉燃, 黎小斌, 陈秋霞. (2018) 黎小斌治疗卵巢巧克力囊肿. 长春中医药大学学报 **34**(2): 261–263.
H409	徐彩. (2009) 中医治疗子宫内膜异位症,子宫腺肌症的临床研究. 北京中医药大学.
H410	杨琪. (2017) 温肾化瘀法治疗肾虚血瘀型子宫内膜异位性疾病的临床观察. 北京中医药大学.
H411	张春花. (2018) 增损葫芦巴丸治疗子宫内膜异位症所致痛经疗效观察. 西部中医药 **31**(5): 84–86.
H412	张绚丽. (2013) 化瘀止痛法治疗子宫内膜异位症盆腔疼痛,子宫腺肌病痛经的临床观察. 北京中医药大学.
H413	赵翠英, 金季玲. (2008) 金季玲治疗子宫内膜异位症经验. 江西中医药 **39**(6): 26–27.
H414	司徒仪, 沈碧琼, 梁雪芳, et al. (1998) 子宫内膜异位症瘀证本质及活血化瘀疗效机理探讨. 北京中医 **17**(3): 11–13.
H415	Tanaka T. (2003) A novel anti-dysmenorrhea therapy with cyclic administration of two Japanese herbal medicines. Clin Exp Obstet Gynecol **30**(2–3): 95–98.
H416	孙怀玲. (2010) 祛瘀镇痛合剂治疗子宫内膜异位引发痛经的临床及实验研究. 四川中医 **28**(4): 87–89.
H417	王丽, 阴慧琴. (2009) 中药保留灌肠与口服序贯治疗子宫内膜异位症 36 例. 山西中医学院学报 **10**(1): 30–31.

Study No.	Reference
H418	曾雅云. (2018) GnRH-a 联合左归丸治疗肾阴亏虚型子宫内膜异位症的骨量观察. 福建中医药大学.
H419	陈香. (2016) GnRH-a 联合清心消癥汤与联合反加疗法治疗子宫内膜异位症术后的疗效评估. 南京中医药大学.
H420	吴俞虹. (2016) 补肾祛瘀法防治肾虚血瘀型内异症术后 GnRH-a 治疗副反应的研究. 福建中医药大学.
H421	胡诗寒. (2016) 仙子益真改善 EMS 术后 GnRHa 致低雌激素症状的临床观察. 广州中医药大学.
H422	黄金平. (2015) 二仙汤治疗内异症术后 GnRH-a 致绝经相关症状的临床研究. 广州中医药大学.
H423	刘长青, 秦爱新, 姜芳芳, et al. (2014) 促性腺激素释放激素激动剂联合坤泰胶囊治疗中重度子宫内膜异位症的临床观察. *中国中西医结合杂志* **34**(11): 1288–1291.
H424	王帅男. (2017) 左归丸对子宫内膜异位症应用 GnRH-a 后肾阴虚证型骨量变化的临床观察. 福建中医药大学.
H425	夏爱军, 韩克, 翁时秋. (2014) 益肾宁坤方治疗醋酸亮丙瑞林所致围绝经期症状的临床研究. *环球中医药* **7**(10): 792–794.
H426	杨脂, 叶平. (2017) 知柏地黄汤加减治疗诺雷得所致围绝经期症状观察. *浙江中医杂志* **52**(5): 329–330.
H427	朱利. (2016) 滋肾宁心汤治疗应用 GnRH-a 患者类绝经期症状的临床疗效观察. 南京中医药大学.
H428	马晓燕. (2016) 滋肾疏肝活血汤防治卵巢子宫内膜异位症术后应用 GnRH-a 类药物副反应的临床研究. 新疆医科大学.
H429	王梦梦. (2017) 左归丸对子宫内膜异位症术后 GnRH-a 副作用的治疗及生存质量的影响. 新疆医科大学.
H430	Chen JM, Gao HY, Ding Y, et al. (2015) Efficacy and safety investigation of Kuntai capsule for the add-back therapy of gonadotropin-releasing hormone agonist administration to endometriosis patients: A randomized, double-blind, blank- and tibolone-controlled study. *Chin Med J* **128**(4): 427–432.
H431	陈香, 时燕萍. (2017) 清心消癥汤联合 GnRH-a 对中重度子宫内膜异位症保守性手术治疗后的观察分析. *中医药信息* **34**(6): 69–73.

(*Continued*)

Study No.	Reference
H432	杨扬, 龚护民, 袁少洋. (2018) 小金丸联合戈舍瑞林治疗子宫内膜异位症的临床研究. *现代药物与临床* **33**(9): 2326–2330.
H433	叶喜阳, 邓宇傲, 马利国, *et al.* (2010) 仙灵骨葆胶囊植物雌激素活性的临床观察. *福建医科大学学报* **44**(2): 137–139, 145.
H434	黄丹丹. (2014) 中药联合 GnRH-a 防治卵巢子宫内膜异位症术后复发的临床研究. 新疆医科大学.

6

Pharmacological Actions of Frequently Used Herbs

OVERVIEW

This section reviews the available experimental evidence for the possible biological activities and mechanisms of the 10 most frequently used Chinese herbs from randomised controlled trials in Chapter 5.

Introduction

Several systematic reviews of the potential effects of Chinese herbal medicine (CHM) for endometriosis symptoms have revealed some promising results (see Chapter 5). The evidence from clinical studies included in Chapter 5 has also shown benefits of CHM in increasing the chance of a cure and reducing the risk of endometriosis recurrence, albeit with some limitations in study quality. If such treatments are to play an increasingly greater role in the clinical management of endometriosis, it will be important to examine how CHMs exert their clinical effects. This chapter reviews experimental evidence for a selection of the most frequently used herbs in clinical trials, with data gathered from studies that used *in vitro* experimental cells and *in vivo* animal models.

The pathological processes and mechanisms of endometriosis are complicated and have been described in Chapter 1. Ectopic growth of endometrium in the pelvic cavity induces an inflammatory response and pelvic pain. Invasion and adhesion of endometrial tissue, immune dysfunction, angiogenesis, and changes in hormones are the main mechanical factors that contribute to the development of endometriosis.

Animal models of human endometriosis are vital experimental tools to investigate and assess the therapeutic effects of herbs and/or compounds, as well as their underlying mechanisms. Various animal models of endometriosis have been well established.[1] Among these, surgically induced auto-transplant of endometrial or uterine tissue outside the uterus is most commonly used.[2]

Methods

The herbs reviewed were *chi shao* 赤芍, *chuan xiong* 川芎, *dan shen* 丹参, *dang gui* 当归, *e zhu* 莪术, *gan cao* 甘草, *san leng* 三棱, *tao ren* 桃仁, *xiang fu* 香附, and *yan hu suo* 延胡索. A review of common formulas, such as *Shao fu zhu yu tang* 少腹逐瘀汤 and *Gui zhi fu ling jiao nang* 桂枝茯苓胶囊, is also included. Extracts and isolated compounds from each herb have demonstrated vast pharmacological effects. In particular, herbs and compounds with anti-inflammatory, anti-hyperalgesic, and immunomodulatory properties are generally beneficial for the whole body and the reproductive system specifically.

Experimental studies of herbs and/or herb compounds that investigated the mechanism of action relevant to endometriosis were selected. Relevant actions included attenuating endometriosis-associated inflammatory response, preventing apoptosis, inhibiting proliferation, blocking invasion and adhesion of endometrial tissue, preventing retrograde menstruation, suppressing angiogenesis, alleviating pelvic pain, enhancing immunomodulatory function, and modulating hormone production.

The constituent compounds of selected herbs were determined by examining herbal monographs, high-quality reviews of CHM, *materia medica*, and other materials found through PubMed. To identify pre-clinical studies, a literature search of PubMed, Google Scholar, and PubMed Central was undertaken. Search terms included the Chinese *pinyin* and scientific name(s) for each herb, as well as the main compounds contained in the plant. These were combined with terms for endometriosis, inflammation, endometrium proliferation, invasion, adherence, angiogenesis, analgesia, immunity, oestrogen, progesterone, and endometriosis rodent models.

Experimental Studies on *Chi Shao* 赤芍

Chi shao 赤芍 (red peony root) is sourced from *Paeonia lactiflora* Pall or *Paeonia veitchii* Lynch. The majority of their constituents are classified into flavonoids, monoterpene glycosides, and polyphenols. Paeoniflorin is the most abundant (over 72%); other compounds such as paeonol, albiflorin, pentagalloylglucose lactiflorin, benzoylpaeonifloriin, daucosterol, d-catechin, and oxypaeoniflorin are key components of *chi shao*. Pharmacological activities include anti-inflammatory, antioxidant, antiviral, antibacterial, antifungal, antitumor, anti-arthritis, anticoagulant, antiplatelet, and immunomodulatory activities.[3]

Anti-endometriosis Actions

Endometriosis-associated inflammation is a key component in the development of endometriosis. Various cytokines, growth and angiogenic factors, and adhesion molecules enhance the invasion, adhesion, angiogenesis, and/or proliferation of ectopic endometrial tissues in the pelvis. These factors include tumour necrosis factor alpha (TNF-α), interleukin (IL)-1, IL-6, IL-8, monocyte chemotactic protein-1 (MCP-1), matrix metalloproteinases (MMPs), vascular endothelial growth factor (VEGF), transforming growth factor beta (TGF-β), inter-cellular adhesion molecule-1 (ICAM-1), and tissue inhibitors of MMPs (TIMPs). Other inflammatory mediators, such as locally produced prostaglandin F2-α and cyclooxygenase (COX)-2, are involved in promoting oestrogen production, endometrial cell proliferation, and endometriosis-associated pain.[4] Conventional drug treatments for endometriosis act through suppressing the endometriosis-associated inflammatory response.

Numerous studies have shown that *chi shao* and its compounds demonstrated potential anti-inflammatory activity through modulating inflammatory cytokines and inflammatory responses, as well as regulating expression of cytokine mRNA and/or cell signalling proteins.[3] The inhibitory effect of paeoniflorin on IL-1β, IL-2, IL-12, TNF-α, interferon gamma (IFN-γ), c-jun, and c-fos was reported through regulation of the mitogen-activated protein kinase (MAPK) pathway in phytohaemagglutinin-stimulated peripheral blood mononuclear cells.[5] Paeoniflorin has also been investigated in a rat model of endometriosis (endometriosis of cold coagulation and Blood stasis, ECB) that mimics the Chinese medicine syndrome observed in humans. The ECB model was established through the combined approach of endometrial auto-transplantation and ice-water immersion, although the authors did not describe whether endometrial tissue growth differs as a result of ice-water immersion. Treatment with paeoniflorin could reduce the volume of the ectopic endometrial lesion. Paeoniflorin also resulted in different degrees of atrophy in the ectopic endometrial tissue, clearance of inflammatory cells, significantly fewer mesenchymal cells, fewer blood vessels, and less fibrosis. Further mechanism studies indicated that the effects of paeoniflorin on ECB rats could be due to regulation of the metabolic expression of multiple metabolic pathways.[6]

Analgesic Actions

Paeoniflorin has particularly attracted attention for its antinociceptive activities. Paeoniflorin demonstrated dose-related antinociception as mediated by the activation of kappa-opioid receptors in the formalin-induced nociceptive behaviour of mice,[7] by the adenosine A(1) receptor in visceral hyperalgesia as induced by separation of neonates from maternal rats,[8] and by an interaction with N-methyl-D-aspartate receptors on the excitatory amino acid agonist- and morphine-induced nociceptive behaviour in mice.[9] Another monoterpene glycoside, albiflorin, also showed antinociceptive activity by reducing activation of calcium/calmodium-dependent protein kinase II (CaMKII) and c-Jun N-terminal kinases (c-JNK) in the hypothalamus of albiflorin-treated mice.[10]

Hormone Regulation

Using an industry standard approach of recombinant yeast-based assay to screen endocrine activity, *chi shao* was found to exert strong anti-oestrogenic activity compared to the known active standard of tamoxifen.[11]

Immunomodulatory Actions

There is plenty of evidence to show that *chi shao* and its compounds demonstrate potential immunomodulatory activity.[3] Total glycosides of paeony (TGP) is a water/ethanol extract that is prepared from the dried root without the bark of *P. lactiflora* Pall that contains over 90% paeoniflorin. TGP was reported to have dual immunomodulatory effects depending on the activity of immuno-responses on lymphocyte proliferation, T helper (Th)/trophobloast stem (Ts) lymphocyte differentiation, pro-inflammatory cytokine production, and production of IgM-antibodies.[12]

Experimental Studies on *Chuan Xiong* 川芎

Chuan xiong 川芎 (*Ligusticum chuanxiong* Hort, LC), which belongs to the *Umbelliferae* family, is used for pain conditions as well as for various cardiovascular and cerebrovascular diseases. More than 200 compounds have been isolated and identified from *L. chuanxiong*; these include volatile oils, phenols and organic acids, alkaloids, phthalides, and polysaccharides. Ferulic acid (FA), ligustilide, tetramethylpyrazine (TMP, also known as ligustrazine (LZ)), and senkyunolide A are the main active constituents of *L. chuanxiong*. Pharmacological activities include anti-inflammation, antioxidation, and antidiabetic effects, as well as effects on cardiovascular and cerebrovascular diseases, among others.[13,14]

Anti-endometriosis Actions

Evidence from several studies suggests that LC and its wide range of compounds exert great anti-inflammatory effects in various tissues and diseases *in vitro* and *in vivo* through the suppression of inflammatory responses and inflammatory cytokines, including interleukins, TNF-α, MCP-1, MMPs, vascular cell adhesion protein (VCAM)-1, ICAM-1, TIMP-1, COX-1, COX-2, and prostaglandin E2 (PGE2).[13,14]

Foshou san formula is composed of three main compounds, FA, LZ, and tetrahydropalmatine (THP), which are sourced from LC, *Angelica sinensis*, and *Corydalis yanhusuo*. *Foshou san* formula has demonstrated powerful anti-endometriosis activity. The combination of FA, LZ, and THP showed anti-inflammatory and anti-angiogenesis actions on endometriosis.[15]

More recently, the effects of the combination of FA, LZ, and THP on invasion, metastasis, and epithelial–mesenchymal transformation in endometriosis rats have been investigated.[16] The combination inhibited ectopic endometrial tissue growth and ameliorated the pathological changes in the ectopic endometrium, resulting in a thinner ectopic endometrium, looser arrangement of cells, a less pseudoglandular appearance, and fewer blood vessels and inflammatory cells. Further mechanism studies found that FA, LZ, and THP could restrain invasion and metastasis by downregulating expressions of MMP-2 and MMP-9 and upregulating TIMP-1, indicating that anti-endometriosis activity could be related to the regulation of transformation of epithelial cells into mesenchymal cells.[16] The in-depth study further showed that ligustrazine demonstrated binding activity with B-cell lymphoma 2 (Bcl-2), Bax, caspase-9, caspase-3, and poly (ADP-ribose) polymerase in molecular docking. The pro-apoptotic mechanism of the elevated shrink rate of ectopic endometrium with the combination of FA, LZ, and THP might be through the Bcl-2 pathway.[17]

Analgesic Actions

The ethanol extract of LC was observed to exert analgesic effects, increase the reaction time for nociception on the mouse hot-plate responses, and produce a longer latency and fewer writhes in the acetic acid–induced writhing test.[18] It also effectively relieved dysmenorrhoea and prolonged the incubation period caused by oxytocin in mice. Comparative analgesic effect of LC indicated that ethanol extract of LC decoction had a greater advantage of analgesic effect than crude LC decoction in mice.[18] The combination of LC and *Radix angelica* at the ratio of 1.5:1 produced the greatest effect on uterine tissue, with results showing a reduction in writhing time, an increase in the concentration of nitric oxide (NO), and a reduction in the concentration of calcium ions (Ca^{2+}).[19]

TMP showed antinociceptive effects with elevation of the thermal nociception threshold and prolongation of the withdrawal latency of the ipsilateral hind paw after noxious heating;[20] this effect was achieved through inhibition of the high voltage–gated calcium current and tetrodotoxin resistant–sodium current of the dorsal root ganglion neuron in rats.

The volatile oil was reported to improve the mouse hot plated-induced pain threshold and reduce the acetic acid-induced writhing reaction.[21] It also provided synergistic analgesia when used with ibuprofen through transdermal drug delivery, shown by promoting ibuprofen absorption and enhancing the inhibitory actions of ibuprofen on dysmenorrhoea pain in mice.[22]

Hormone Regulation

In endometriosis rats, the combination of FA, LZ, and THP not only reduced the volume of ectopic endometrial tissue and diminished the growth of endometriosis, but also decreased the oestradiol (E2) level in serum in accordance with the suppressed expression of gonadotropin-releasing hormone (GnRH), follicle-stimulating hormone, and luteinising hormone (LH). Further mechanism studies showed that FA, LZ, and THP decreased the expression of oestrogen receptors (ER), heat-shock protein 90, and COX-2, enhanced the ability of peritoneal macrophages to undergo phagocytosis in rats with endometriosis, and upregulated the expression of kinase IκBα, which in turn downregulated the expression of IL-1β and TNF-α. These data indicated that the anti-endometriosis effect of FA, LZ, and THP might be associated with the downregulation of the hypothalamic–pituitary–ovarian axis, the oestrogen response element pathway, and peritoneal macrophages.[23]

Immunomodulatory Actions

The compounds phthalides, senkyunolide A, and ligustilide showed immunomodulatory effects in mouse aortic endothelial cells. CD137 expression was inhibited by suppressing the expression of activating protein (AP)-1 and the AKT/nuclear factor kappa beta (NF-κB) signalling pathway.[24]

Experimental Studies on *Dan Shen* 丹参

Dan shen 丹参 is derived from the dried root of *Salvia miltiorrhiza* Bunge (SM). Based on their structural characteristics, the principal bioactive constituents can be classified into two groups. A lipid-soluble lipophilic group (known as tanshinones) includes tanshinone I, tanshinone IIA, tanshinone IIB, cryptotanshinone, and dihydrotanshinone. A water-soluble polyphenolic group (known as salvianolic acids/depsides) includes salvianolic acid B (Sal B), salvianolic acid A (Sal A), and danshensu. Pharmacological activities include anti-inflammatory, antioxidant, antineuropathic pain, antidiabetes, anticancer, antifibrotic, antihepatocytic, and neuroprotective actions.[25]

Anti-endometriosis Actions

Remarkable anti-inflammatory effects have been reported with *S. miltiorrhiza* and its compounds in a wide range of tissues *in vitro* and *in vivo*.[25] It has been reported that *S. miltiorrhiza* and tanshinones could repress pro-inflammatory cytokines, such as IL-1β, IL-6, IL-8, TNF-α, and NO, and promote anti-inflammatory cytokines, such as TGF-s, IL-4, and IL-10.[26,27] Indeed, in the rat model of endometriosis, the extract of *S. miltiorrhiza* was observed to markedly decrease the levels of both cancer antigen 125 (CA-125) and pro-inflammatory cytokines, such as IL-18 and TNF-α, and increase the level of IL-13 in the peritoneal fluid. The anti-endometriosis effect was attributed to tanshinone IIA, a compound that has been shown to have anti-apoptotic properties.[28]

Both *S. miltiorrhiza* extract and tanshinone IIA have also been observed to suppress MMP-9 expression through the AP-1/MAPK signalling pathway and inhibit invasion and growth of human breast cancer cells[29] by regulating adhesion molecules such as ICAM-1 and VCAM-1.[30] Furthermore, in ectopic endometrial stromal cells (EESCs), tanshinone IIA could induce apoptosis, attenuate cell viability, and suppress cell migration and the invasion of EESCs. A mechanistic study revealed that tanshinone IIA significantly inhibited the expression of 14-3-3ζ in EESCs, and the overexpression of 14-3-3ζ could restore cell viability, migration, and invasion in tanshinone IIA-treated EESCs,[31] indicating that 14-3-3ζ may mediate the actions of tanshinone IIA.

In addition to anti-inflammatory, anti-invasion, and anti-adhesion actions, *S. miltiorrhiza* and tanshinone IIA could also suppress angiogenesis by inhibiting the VEGF/ VEGFR2/hypoxia inducible factor-1α (HIF-1α) signalling pathway[32] as well as the matrix invasion and modification of MMP-2/TIMP-2 secretion.[33] The finding was confirmed in cultured stromal cells; *S. miltiorrhiza* inhibited proliferation of ectopic stromal cells by inhibiting expression of protein and MMP-9 mRNA.[34]

Analgesic Actions

The analgesic effect of root extracts of *S. miltiorrhiza* were seen with inhibition of the discharges of visceral pain by acting directly on the peripheral nerve trunk via the central nervous system.[35] Furthermore, the aqueous seed extract from *S. leriifolia* demonstrated antinociceptive activity in the hot-plate test, which was inhibited by pretreatment with naloxone, indicating that antinociceptive effects might be mediated by opioid receptors.[36]

Hormone Regulation

Tanshinone IIA was reported to prevent and treat oestrogen/androgen-induced benign prostatic hyperplasia in the prostate epithelial cells and stromal cells of rats. These effects occurred by suppressing expression of ERα, androgen receptors (AR), cyclin B1, and cyclin D1 and proliferating cell nuclear antigen (PCNA).[37]

Immunomodulatory Actions

It was observed that water-soluble polysaccharides from *S. officinalis* exhibited the highest mitogenic and comitogenic activities through the comitogenic thymocyte test, indicating that it possessed immunomodulatory activity.[38] This finding was further confirmed *in vivo*. A polysaccharide from *S. miltiorrhiza* significantly improved immune function in gastric cancer rats through stimulating proliferation of splenocytes, promoting production of anti-inflammatory cytokines (IL-2, IL-4, and IL-10), repressing secretion of pro-inflammatory cytokine (IL-6 and TNF-α), augmenting the killing activity of natural killer (NK) cells and cytotoxic T lymphocytes, and enhancing the phagocytotic function of macrophages, suggesting that A polysaccharide could serve as an effective immunomodulator.[39]

Experimental Studies on *Dang Gui* 当归

Dang gui 当归, sourced from *Angelica sinensis* (Oliv.) Diels, consists of over 70 compounds. FA, Z-ligustilide, n-butylidenephthalide, butyl-phthalide, and polysaccharides are considered the main active components in *A. sinensis*. These compounds have diverse biological activities, including anti-inflammatory, anti-arthrosclerosis, antioxidant, antithrombotic, antiplatelet, antihepatotoxic, cardioprotective, and immunomodulatory activities.[40]

Anti-endometriosis Actions

The anti-inflammatory and anti-angiogenesis activity of ligustilide produces actions against endometriosis. Strong anti-inflammatory activities were seen with ligustilide, which inhibited the lipopolysaccharide (LPS)-induced production of NO, PGE2, TNF-α, and nitric oxide synthase (NOS) in macrophages.[41] From a mechanistic perspective, ligustilide could abolish the activation of AP-1, nuclear factor kappa B (NF-κB), and IκBα, and also inhibit the phosphorylation of IκB kinase (IKK), MAPKs, and the intracellular reactive oxygen species (ROS) level.[41]

A volatile oil of *A. sinensis* (VOAS) and n-butylidenephthalide (BP) were both reported to exert anti-angiogenic effects *in vitro* and *in vivo*. VOAS inhibited the migration, proliferation, and formation of capillary-like tubes in human umbilical vein endothelial cells.[42] BP suppressed endothelial sprouting in an *ex vivo* mouse aortic ring model and prevented the development of zebrafish sub-intestinal vessels *in vivo* by suppressing cell cycle progression and inducing apoptosis via the activation of p38 and the extracellular signal-regulated kinase (ERK)1/2 pathway.[42] The anti-endometriosis effect of FA on rats with endometriosis has been reported in the combined use of FA, LZ, and THP (see 'Experimental studies on *chuan xiong*').

Analgesic Actions

A water extract of *A. sinensis* possessed significant analgesic activity by decreasing the frequency of acetic acid-induced wringing reactions and increasing the pain threshold in the hot-plate procedure in mice.[43] Moreover, FA was found to reverse the reserpine-induced decrease in nociceptive threshold in both mechanical allodynia and thermal hyperalgesia through modulation of the monoaminergic system.[44] Additionally, the volatile oil constituents, such as butylidenephthalide, ligustilide, and butylphthalide, were found to be capable of relaxing rat uterine contractions that were induced by the non-specific antispasmodics prostaglandin F2α, oxytocin, and acetylcholine.[45]

Hormone Regulation

A. sinensis exhibited anti-progestogenic-like activity in a dose-response manner in the progesterone response element–driven luciferase reporter gene bioassay.[46]

Immunomodulatory Actions

A number of studies have shown that *A. sinensis* and its compounds exhibit potential immunomodulatory activities *in vitro* and *in vivo* by activating non-specific immunity, including proliferation of total spleen cells, activation of macrophages and NK cells, and specific immunity, such as activation of helper T (Th) cells and B cells.[47] *A. sinensis* also regulated the expression of Th1- and Th2-related cytokines.

Experimental Studies on *E Zhu* 莪术

E zhu 莪术 (*Curcumae Rhizoma*) is derived from the dry rhizomes of *Curcuma kwangsiensis* S. G. Lee et C. F. Liang, *Curcuma phaeocaulis* Val. and *Curcuma wenyujin* Y. H. Chen et C. Ling. The chemical constituents from *Curcumae Rhizoma* are primarily sesquiterpenes (such as the main constituents of essential oils) and diarylheptanoids (also known as curcumin components, such as curcumin, demethoxycurcumin, and bisdemethoxycurcumin); other compounds include alkaloids and polysaccharides. Among them, curcumin, a natural panacea and one of the few albeit most well-known star molecules, has captured worldwide attention. Pharmacological activities of *Curcumae Rhizoma* include antioxidant, antiviral, antimicrobial, antitumor, antithrombosis, antiplatelet aggregation, and hepatoprotective activities, among others.[48,49]

Anti-endometriosis Actions

Plenty of evidence has shown that *e zhu* and its compounds demonstrate powerful anti-endometriosis activities by impeding the growth of the ectopic endometrium, attenuating lesion volumes, and altering cellular organisation of ectopic lesions through anti-inflammation, anti-invasion, and anti-adhesion actions, as well as anti-angiogenesis properties in endometrial lesions.

It was reported that the extract of *C. phaeocaulis* and *C. wenyujin* showed anti-inflammation activities by inhibiting paw swelling through the suppression of COX-2 activity and inhibition of carrageenan-induced paw oedema volume by reducing the levels of TNF-α and IL-6, respectively.[50,51]

Curcumin has strong anti-inflammatory actions. It has been observed that curcumin not only significantly suppressed TNF-α-induced secretion of IL-6, IL-8, MCP-1, and the activation and transcription of NF-κB in human ectopic endometriotic stromal cells,[52] but also remarkably attenuated the expression of TNF-α by increasing Iκ-B expression and decreasing the nuclear translocation of NF-κB in endometriotic mice.[53,54]

The effects of curcumin on adhesion molecules and MMPs that are involved in cell invasion and adhesion have been investigated. An *in vitro* study showed that the expressions of ICAM-1 and VCAM-1 were inhibited by curcumin in human ovarian endometriotic stromal cells.[52] *In vivo*, curcumin decreased serum MMP-2 and MMP-9[55] and downregulated the expression of MMP-3 in endometriotic mice.[53] Curcumin also upregulated the expression of TIMP-2, downregulated the expression of membrane type 1 matrix metalloproteinase (MT1MMP), and suppressed the expression and activation of MMP-2 in the BALB/c mice endometriosis model.[56]

In vivo and *in vitro* studies have assessed the anti-angiogenic activity of curcumin. In an *in vitro* study, curcumin reduced cell proliferation, inhibited growth of human ectopic and eutopic stromal cells, and suppressed VEGF secretion in human endometriotic stromal cell cultures.[57] Curcumin decreased microvessel density (MVD) in ectopic endometrium in rodent models of endometriosis and the expression of VEGF in serum and ectopic endometrium.[58] Curcumin was also found to reduce the implant size of ectopic endometrial tissue and cell proliferation of ectopic endometrial epithelial cells by suppressing PCNA.[59]

Analgesic Actions

In the animal model of pelvic inflammation established by injecting phenol mucilage into the right side of the uterus of rats, the extract of *C. wenyujin* demonstrated very strong anti-inflammatory and antinociceptive effects. It exerted significant inhibitions of the ear oedema and cotton pellet-induced granuloma formation, as well as remarkable reductions of carrageenan-induced paw oedema volume and acetic acid-induced writhing response with a concomitant decrease in levels of TNF-α and IL-6.[51]

Hormone Regulation

In isolated endometriotic stromal and epithelial cells, curcumin demonstrated suppressed proliferation of cells and reduced oestradiol production, thus impeding the growth and development of tissue.[60]

Immunomodulatory Actions

Studies have shown curcumin to have powerful immunomodulatory activity by interacting with not only immune cellular components, such as macrophages, dendritic cells, and B and T lymphocytes, but also with molecular components associated with inflammation, such as chemokines, cytokines, and various transcription factors.[61]

Experimental Studies on *Gan Cao* 甘草

Gan cao 甘草 (licorice) from *Glycyrrhiza glabra* L, *Glycyrrhiza inflata* Bat., and *Glycyrrhiza uralensis* Fisch. has been traditionally used to treat coughs, influenza, gastric ulcers, and liver damage and for detoxification. Four hundred compounds have been isolated, of which the main bioactive constituents are more than 20 types of triterpene saponins and more than 300 types of flavonoids. These compounds exhibit extensive pharmacological properties, such as anti-inflammatory, anti-allergic, antioxidative, antiviral, anticarcinogenic, antithrombotic, anti-ulceric, immunoregulatory, hepatoprotective, and cardioprotective effects.[62,63]

Anti-endometriosis Actions

The anti-inflammatory activity of licorice is well documented due to its use in treatment of inflammation-related diseases throughout Chinese medicine (CM) history. The extract of licorice and its compounds, such as triterpenes and flavonoids, showed anti-inflammatory properties by decreasing pro-inflammatory cytokines and inflammatory mediators.[63] Glycyhrritinic acid has also exhibited anti-inflammatory properties in different animal models. Inhibition of glucocorticoid metabolism was observed, which enhanced their effects on inflammation. Other derivatives, such as glycyrrhizin, glyderinine, lichochalocone A, and isoliquiritigenin, have been also reported to exert anti-inflammatory effects through different pathways.[62,64]

Specifically, treatment with the hexane/ethanol extract of G. uralensis in mice suppressed inflammatory cytokine production and expression of CD31, CD45, HIF-1α, COX-2, and iNOS, reduced cell proliferation, induced cell cycle arrest or apoptosis, and inhibited expression of adhesive and angiogenic molecules, such as ICAM-1, VCAM-1, MMP-9, and VEGF-A in mice.[65]

In addition to the actions of the crude extract, glycyrrhizic acid was observed to inhibit tumour growth and angiogenesis in mice by impeding angiogenic activities, such as invasion, migration, and tube formation in endothelial cells through targeting the ERK pathway.[66] Additionally, isoliquiritin apioside (ISLA), a compound from G. uralensis, also effectively suppressed the migration and invasion of HT1080 cells and decreased the production of placental growth factor, MMP-9, and VEGF by impairing the hypoxia inducible factor 1 alpha (HIF1α) pathway. ISLA also inhibited tube formation in human umbilical vein endothelial cells (HUVECs).[67]

In LPS-stimulated mouse endometrial epithelial cells (MEEC), glycyrrhizin remarkably inhibited LPS-induced IL-1β, TNF-α, PGE_2, and NO production and attenuated the expression of LPS-induced iNOS, COX-2, NF-κB, and toll-like receptor (TLR)4 activation, thus indicating that the inhibitory effect of glycyrrhizin on the

LPS-induced inflammatory response could be mediated by suppressing the TLR4 signalling pathway in MEEC.[68] The root extract of *G. glabra* showed similar anti-endometriosis effects as the GnRHa diphereline in a rat model of endometriosis, with a remarkable reduction of the mean area, hemosiderin-laden macrophage counts, and histopathologic grades of endometrial implants.[69]

Analgesic Actions

Isoliquiritigenin from *G. glabra* demonstrated inhibitory effects on spontaneous contractions of isolated rat uterus and acetylcholine-, KCl-, and oxytocin-induced uterus contractions, displaying its analgesic and uterine-relaxing effects *in vitro*. *In vivo*, isoliquiritigenin also exhibited effectiveness in reducing pain in the acetic acid-induced writhing response and hot-plate tests through involvement of Ca^{2+} channels, NOS, and COX in non-pregnant mice at the Institute of Cancer Research.[70]

Hormone Regulation

G. uralensis inhibited progesterone activity in a dose-response manner.[46] Anti-oestrogenic activity of high concentrations of glycyrrhizin in rabbits was also observed, which is consistent with antagonism at ERs.[71]

Immunomodulatory Actions

The immunomodulatory activities of licorice have been attributed to its bioactive ingredients, which include glycyrrhizin, glycyrrhetinic acid, licochalcone A, isoliquiritigenin (ISL), and polysaccharides. Both glycyrrhetinic acid and glycyrrhizin induced interferon activity and enhanced NK cell activity. Lichochalocone A inhibited T cell proliferation and cytokine production. ISL could decrease the production of NF-κB, COX-2, iNOS, and interferon regulatory factor 3 activation via the toll-interleukin-1 receptor domain-containing adapter inducing interferon-beta (TRIF)-dependent signalling pathway of TLRs.[64,72]

Experimental Studies on *San Leng* 三棱

San leng 三棱, the rhizome from *Sparganium stoloniferum* Buch.-Ham (*Sparganiaceae* family) and also known as *Sparganii Rhizoma* (RS), is commonly used to promote blood circulation and remove blood stasis in CM. The major compounds in *S. stoloniferum* are phenylpropanoids, volatile oil, flavonoids, alkaloids, isocoumarins, sucrose esters, and stilbenoid derivatives. Pharmacological activities include anti-inflammatory, antithrombotic, antiplatelet, analgesic, anti-angiogenesis, and anti-oestrogenic effects.[73,74]

Anti-endometriosis Actions

It was reported that an isocoumarin compound from *S. stoloniferum*, Sparstolonin B (SsnB), exerted strong anti-inflammatory effects. SsnB could be a selective TLR2 and TLR4 antagonist to block inflammatory signalling triggered by TLR2 and TLR4 in mouse peritoneal and human macrophages.[75] SsnB also inhibited LPS-induced inflammation in HUVECs shown by attenuated LPS-induced expression of MCP-1, IL-1β, ICAM-1 and, VCAM-1, as well as decreased adhesion of monocytes to LPS-activated HUVECs through the suppression of LPS-induced phosphorylation of ERK1/2 and Akt.[76] Furthermore, SsnB was found to inhibit angiogenesis *in vitro* by inhibiting tube formation in human endothelial cells and the migration of HUVECs, as well as in *ex vivo* by reducing the length and branching number of blood vessels in the chick chorioallantoic membrane.[77]

In addition to the pure compound, a *San leng wan* (SLW) formula consisting of *Rhizoma sparganii* (*san leng*) and *Rhizoma curcumae* (*e zhu*) has been shown to exert anti-inflammatory activities by significantly inhibiting the glacial acetic acid-induced increase in mice blood capillary permeability, xylene-induced swelling in mice ears, carrageenan-induced oedema in rat paws, and cotton pellet-induced chronic granuloma in rats.[78] SLW also showed anti-angiogenesis actions in a rat model by decreasing MVD and suppressing expressions of TNF-α and VEGF in the ectopic endometrium.[79]

Analgesic Actions

SLW demonstrated a significant analgesic effect by increasing the pain threshold of mice in the hot-plate test and decreasing the number of acetic acid-induced writhings through the inhibition of PGE2.[78]

Hormone Regulation

In an *in vitro* model of eutopic primary cultured endometrial cells of endometriosis and hysteromyoma, SLW could inhibit the secretion of oestradiol by suppressing the expression of steroidogenic factor-1 and 17-beta-hydroxysteroid dehydrogenase 1, and potentiating the expression of chicken ovalbumin upstream-transcription factor and 17-beta-hydroxysteroid dehydrogenase 2.[80] The inhibition of the secretion of E2 by SLW was further confirmed in eutopic endometrial cells.[81]

Experimental Studies on *Tao Ren* 桃仁

Tao ren 桃仁 (the fruit kernel of peach; *Prunus persica* (L.) Batsch and *Prunus davidiana* (Carr.) Franch), which belongs to the *Rosaceae* family, is well known for the treatment of hemiplegia, constipation, chronic rhinitis, cough, asthma, dysmenorrhoea, arthritis, and diarrhoea. Various compounds have been isolated from *Prunus* seeds, including amygdalin, cyanogenic glycosides, prunasin, emulsin, glycerides, and sterols. Pharmacological activities include anticancer, antidiabetic, anti-inflammatory, anti-asthmatic, anti-atherosclerotic, and antioxidant effects.[82,83]

Anti-endometriosis Actions

The acute anti-inflammatory effects of nectarine kernel alcoholic extract (NAE) were examined using the carrageenan-induced rat hind paw oedema test. Treatment with NAE significantly reduced paw oedema in both the early and late phases compared with indomethacin, which only reduced paw oedema during the late phase of inflammation.[83]

It has been reported that amygdalin, a bioactive compound from *P. persica*, possesses various activities that might combat endometriosis. Amygdalin showed powerful inhibitory effects on the levels of cytokines and on inflammation through the suppression of NF-κB, NOD-, LRR-, and pyrin domain-containing protein 3 signalling-pathways and consequently reducing the expression of inflammatory cytokines IL-1β, IL-6, and TNF-α. It demonstrated actions to induce apoptosis, inhibit cell proliferation, and inhibit adhesion of various cancer cells through the Akt/mammalian target of rapamycin pathway. It also showed antifibrotic activity via suppression of the TGFβ/connective tissue growth factor pathway.[84]

Indeed, compared to leuprolide acetate, a synthetic GnRHa, amygdalin was found to be superior in reducing implant volumes and preventing recurrent growth of the ectopic endometrium.[85] An attenuation of experimental endometriosis in rats was also observed with the combined treatment of amygdalin and atorvastatin. Concurrent reductions in levels of TNF-α, IL-6, MMP-2, and MMP-9 in the peritoneal fluid were also seen, as was decreased malondialdehyde (MDA) content (a marker of lipid peroxidation) and increased levels of glutathione, catalase, glutathione peroxidase, and superoxide dismutase in endometrial implants. These findings suggest that anti-inflammatory, anti-angiogenesis, and antioxidant activities might be responsible for anti-endometriosis effects.[86]

In addition to the actions of the individual herb, actions relevant to endometriosis have been shown when *tao ren* was used as part of a multi-herb formula. The herbal formula *Taoren-Quyu* decoction, composed of *P. persica*, *S. miltiorrhiza*, *A. sinensis*, and *Leonurus artemisia*, has been used to treat endometriosis for many years. In rats, *Taoren-Quyu* decoction exerted strong anti-endometriosis activity by significantly reducing the volume of endometriosis cysts, inhibiting the formation of endometriosis-like lesions, decreasing the serum levels of CA125, endometrial antibodies, and E2, decreasing expression of MVD, VEGF, and angiopoietin, suppressing levels of TNF-α and IL-18, and increasing IL-13 levels in the peritoneal fluids. The mechanism of these various actions might be associated with enhancing apoptosis of ectopic endometrial cells, anti-angiogenesis actions,[87] and anti-inflammatory activity.[88]

Analgesic Action

An antinociceptive effect on thermally induced pain was reported with NAE; antinociceptive actions were seen with both the hot-plate model in rats and acetic acid-induced writhing reflex in mice.[83] Administration of NAE prolonged reaction times on the hot-plate test and was comparable to the standard drug, tramadol. Meanwhile, NAE was also found to reduce the writhing response induced by acetic acid to a similar level as the standard drug, indomethacin. The antinociceptive effects were attributed to the total polyphenolic and flavonoid components of NAE.[83]

Hormone Regulation

Using an industry standard approach of recombinant yeast-based assay to screen endocrine activity, *Prunus* seed was found to exert strong anti-oestrogenic activity compared with the known active standard, tamoxifen.[11]

Immunomodulatory Actions

Amygdalin was reported to suppress inflammatory responses and promote the immunomodulation function of regulatory T cells that are critical for the regulation of T cell-mediated immune responses.[89]

Experimental Studies on *Xiang Fu* 香附

Xiang fu 香附, sourced from *Cyperus rotundus* L, contains various chemical constituents such as essential oils (α-longipinane, α-cyperone, β-caryophyllene oxide, β-selinene, and cyperene), flavonoids (flavans, flavones, flavanonols, isoflavane, anthocyanidins, and catechins), tannins, and alkaloids. Pharmacological properties include anti-inflammatory, antioxidant, antipruritic, antidiarrheal, antiemetic, antihelminthic, antihistamine, antihyperglycemic, antihypertensive, antimalarial, anti-obesity, antiplatelet, analgesic, cardioprotective, cytoprotective, cytotoxic, gastroprotective, hepatoprotective, and neuroprotective activities.[90,91]

Anti-endometriosis Actions

The beneficial effect of *C. rotundus* in endometriosis was attributed to its bioactive compounds, such as α-cyperone and β-caryophyllene oxide (CPO).[92] It was found that α-cyperone inhibited PGE2 production and suppressed LPS-induced expression of COX-2 and IL-6 by downregulating the NF-κB pathway. CPO was also reported to potentiate TNF-α-induced apoptosis and inhibit proliferation, invasion, and angiogenesis by decreasing TNF-α-induced increases in the expression of COX-2, cyclin D1, c-myc, MMP-9, ICAM-1, and VEGF. These pro-apoptotic, antiproliferative, anti-invasive, and anti-angiogenic effects of CPO might be associated with the suppression of the NF-κB pathway.[93] Indeed, in a rat model of endometriosis, CPO suppressed the growth of endometriotic implants and induced apoptosis in the cyst luminal epithelium and in blood vessel endothelial cells.[94]

Analgesic Actions

C. rotundus has been used as pain relief in folk medicine. The hydromethanol extract of *C. rotundus* was examined against chemical and heat-induced nociception. The hydromethanol extract showed a marked inhibition on thermal-induced hyperalgesia in the hot-plate test, an increase in the tail withdrawal–reflex time in the tail-immersion test, and a decrease in paw-licking behaviour in both the early and late phases of the formalin-induced paw-licking test. This shows actions on both the neurogenic and inflammatory responses, respectively, indicating that the hydromethanol extract exhibited a rapid, long-lasting central and peripheral antinociceptive effect.[95]

Moreover, the volatile oils rich in the leaves and seeds of *C. rotundus* also inhibited neurogenic and inflammatory pain in rats.[96] This was illustrated by a reduction in paw oedema, comparable to indomethacin, in carrageenan-induced rat paw oedema, attenuated swelling in the formaldehyde-injected rat hind paw, and reduction in formalin-induced neurogenic and inflammatory pain in both the early and late phases.

Hormone Regulation

The methanolic tuber extract of *C. rotundus* showed similar anti-oestrogenic effects as tamoxifen in reducing the thickness of the endometrial lining and caused no proliferation in endometrial epithelial cells.[97] More direct evidence for amentoflavone, a bioactive compound of *C. rotundus*, showed a marked reduction in plasma oestradiol and progesterone levels, inhibition of tumour-like proliferation in rats with uterine fibroids, and promotion of apoptosis in uterine fibroid cells.[98]

Experimental Studies on *Yan Hu Suo* 延胡索

Yan hu suo 延胡索 (*Corydalis yanhusuo* W.T. Wang) is traditionally used in China for drug addiction and pain relief. The main bioactive components that have been isolated from *C. yanhusuo* are berberine, dehydrocorydaline, palmatine, protopine, and tetrahydropalmatine (THP). Pharmacological activities include anti-inflammatory, analgesic, anti-angiogenesis, and anti-tumour effects.[99]

Anti-endometriosis Actions

The therapeutic value of *C. yanhusuo* in endometriosis was attributed to its anti-inflammatory, anti-invasive, anti-adhesive, and anti-angiogenesis properties. *In vitro*, protopine demonstrated a significant decrease in LPS-induced production of TNF-α, IL-1β, IL-6, and MCP-1, suppressed secretion of NO and PGE2 by downregulating iNOS and COX-2 expression, and inhibited the activity of NF-kB. In a carrageenan-induced inflammatory mouse model, protopine treatment significantly suppressed carrageenan-induced paw oedema, indicating that protopine could attenuate carrageenan- and LPS-induced inflammation through modulation of MAPKs/NF-κB signalling cascades.[100] Moreover, protopine showed anti-invasion and anti-adhesive effects in MDA-MB-231 cells, illustrated by remarkably reducing the expression of ICAM-1, epidermal growth factor receptor, and αv-integrin, β1-integrin, and β5-integrin, which are part of a group of major cell surface adhesion molecules.[101] Similarly, the extract of C. yanhusuo was also reported to inhibit the proliferation, migration, and invasion of MDA-MB-231 cells and suppress the expression and activity of MMP-9 *in vitro*.[102] Additionally, THP was reported to not only suppress LPS-induced overexpression of ICAM-1 and E-selectin in HUVECs,[103] but also reduce monocytes from binding to the endothelium through the downregulation of ICAM-1 and VCAM-1 in endothelial cells.[104] In particular, treatment with THP in a rat model of endometriosis resulted in a reduction of lesion size.[105] Finally, the anti-endometriosis effect of THP on rats with endometriosis has been reported in the combined use of FA, LZ, and THP (see 'Experimental studies on *chuan xiong*').

Analgesic Actions

The antinociceptive responses of C. yanhusuo to acute, inflammatory, and neuropathic pains have been systematically evaluated with four standardised pain assays.[99] In the tail-flick test, where responses to acute thermal stimuli are recorded, C. yanhusuo increased the latency of tail flicking. In the formalin-paw assay, C. yanhusuo significantly reduced the time that mice spent licking their paw in both the acute neurogenic pain phase (early phase) and the inflammatory pain phase (late phase). Two other tests were conducted: the *von Frey* filament to measure mechanical allodynia and the hot-box assays to measure thermal hyperalgesia. In these tests, *C. yanhusuo* was seen to significantly increase paw withdrawal thresholds and mouse hind paw withdrawal latencies, respectively, in mice with spinal nerve ligation. These data indicated that *C. yanhusuo* was effective in suppressing nociceptive responses to chemically induced inflammatory pain, thermally induced acute pain, and injury-induced neuropathic pain; acute and neuropathic pains were mediated through antagonism of dopamine D2 receptors.[99] In particular, treatment with THP in a rat model of endometriosis led to remarkable improvement in response to noxious thermal stimulus (accompanied by a reduction in all mediators involved in central sensitisation), histone deacetylase 2 in the dorsal root ganglia, tyrosine kinase receptor A, and calcitonin gene-related peptide in ectopic endometrium. These findings indicate that THP could generalise hyperalgesia in endometriosis rats.[105]

Hormone Regulation

Two methods of regulating hormones have gained attention for the treatment of endometriosis: 1) anti-oestrogen agents, such as tamoxifen, that inhibit oestrogens from binding to ERs and 2) aromatase inhibitors that block biosynthesis of oestrogens from androgens and reduce serum levels of oestrogens. Aromatase is an enzyme for oestrogen biosynthesis that converts testosterone to oestradiol or androstenedione to oestrone.[106] The tertiary and quaternary protoberberine alkaloids isolated from the dichloromethane extract of *C. yanhusuo* have been reported to possess potent aromatase-inhibiting activities.[107]

Experimental Studies on Herbal Formulas

Shao Fu Zhu Yu Tang 少腹逐瘀汤

Shao fu zhu yu tang (Shao fu zhu yu decoction, SZD), the core formula for the treatment of endometriosis containing 10 commonly used herbs (*chi shao* 赤芍, *dang gui* 当归, *chuan xiong* 川芎, *xiao hui xiang* 小茴香, *gan jiang* 干姜, *yan hu suo* 延胡索, *rou gui* 肉桂,

mo yao 没药, *pu huang* 蒲黄, and *wu ling zhi* 五灵脂), was extensively investigated to determine its ability to prevent and/or relieve endometriosis-associated symptoms, both *in vitro* and *in vivo*. SZD was reported to inhibit adhesions of ectopic endometrium and growth of endometrial cells by significantly reducing the expressions of VEGF and TNF-α in rats with endometriosis.[108] In addition, it could significantly attenuate lesion volume, reduce the size of ectopic lesions, and alter the cellular organisation of ectopic lesions in rats with endometriosis by facilitating cell apoptosis. Other actions included inhibiting cell proliferation and expressions of MVD, HIF-1α, and CD34 in the ectopic endometrium. These findings indicate that SZD may be effective in preventing the recurrence of endometriosis.[109]

Furthermore, SZD formula has been reported to inhibit the isolated uterine smooth muscle contraction induced by oxytocin *in vitro*.[110] *In vivo*, SZD formula exerted significant analgesic activities on acetic acid-induced abdominal contraction, formalin-induced paw licking, and oxytocin-induced writhing response in oestrogen-treated mice through the suppression of PGE2 and NO production.[111] Several molecular mechanisms by which SZD might treat dysmenorrhoea in endometriosis were proposed:

- suppressed expression of neurotransmitter receptor neurokinin 1, oestrogen receptor G-protein-coupled-receptor 2 (GPER2), MAPK, and signal transducer and activator of transcription 1 (STAT1);
- reduced levels of IL-6 and TNF-α in the ectopic uterine cavity tissue;
- reduction in inflammatory pain through the GPER2/MAPK/STAT1 axis.[112]

Gui Zhi Fu Ling Wan 桂枝茯苓丸

Gui zhi fu ling wan (GFW), composed of five herbal plants (*gui zhi, fu ling, tao ren, mu dan pi,* and *chi shao*), has been found to attenuate endometriosis in rats by inducing endometriotic cell apoptosis and suppressing cell proliferation and metastasis of endometriotic cells through the downregulation of apoptosis-inhibiting factor Bcl-2 and upregulation of apoptosis-promoting factor Bax.[113] Moreover, the anti-endometriosis effect of GFW on ECB model rats has been examined. After oral administration of GFW, the volume of ectopic endometrial tissue in GFW-treated rats was significantly smaller. The abnormalities of ectopic endometrial tissue improved: there was a reduction in epithelial cells at the cavity surface and fewer interstitial cells and blood vessels.[114]

Further investigation of the anti-adhesive and anti-angiogenesis effects of GFW in the rat model of endometriosis revealed that GFW reduced the mRNA expression of ICAM-1 and MCP-1 of ectopic endometrium in rats,[115] remarkably suppressed the expression of PCNA and platelet endothelial cell adhesion molecule-1 (also known as CD31) in the ectopic endometrial tissue, and decreased the expression of HIF-1α and VEGF in the peritoneal fluid of rats.[116]

In rat models of endometriosis, the immunomodulatory activity of GFW reduced the volume of lesions and increased the percentage of immunocytes, including NK cells and CD^{+3}, CD^{+4}, and CD^{+4}/CD^{+8} cells, suggesting that the suppression of endometriotic implants by GFW could be through modulation of the immune function.[117]

Summary of the Pharmacological Actions of the Common Herbs

Each of these 10 herbs has attracted research attention in experimental models that are of relevance to endometriosis. Powerful anti-endometriosis effects were observed for all herbs through impeding the growth of the ectopic endometrium; attenuating lesion volumes by reducing inflammation; cell proliferation, cell invasion, and adhesion; and anti-angiogenesis properties in endometrial lesions.

Analgesic actions were observed for all herbs. In particular, *chi shao, chuan xiong, dang gui, e zhu, gan cao, tao ren, xiang fu*, and *yan hu suo* exerted very strong antinociceptive activities through the suppression of mediators involved in inflammatory and neuropathic pain. Hormone regulation was observed in all herbs, with strong actions observed for *chuan xiong, san leng,* and *yan hu suo* through antagonising ER, reducing oestradiol production, and inhibiting aromatase activity. Immunomodulatory actions were observed for most herbs, apart from *san leng, xiang fu,* and *yan hu suo.* Immunomodulatory effects occurred by enhancing the production of immune stimulators and inhibiting the production of an immune suppressor.

Notably, two main formulas used to treat endometriosis, *Shao fu zhu yu tang* 少腹逐瘀汤 and *Gui zhi fu ling* 桂枝茯苓 preparations, contain most of the 10 herbs reviewed in this chapter and have been observed to significantly relieve endometriosis-associated symptoms *in vitro* and *in vivo* via the mechanisms described above. These *in vitro* and *in vivo* studies examined herb actions specific to endometriosis and provide potential explanations of the clinical benefits of these common herbs. The findings highlight that CHMs have multiple components that can act on multiple pathways relevant to endometriosis, which reflects the ability of CM to synergistically address multiple targets.

References

1. Bruner-Tran K, Mokshagundam S, Herington J, *et al.* (2018) Rodent models of experimental endometriosis: Identifying mechanisms of disease and therapeutic targets. *Curr Womens Health Rev* **14**(2): 173–188.
2. Vernon MW, Wilson EA. (1985) Studies on the surgical induction of endometriosis in the rat. *Fertil Steril* **44**(5): 684–694.
3. Parker S, May B, Zhang C, *et al.* (2016) A pharmacological review of bioactive constituents of *Paeonia lactiflora* Pallas and *Paeonia veitchii* Lynch. *Phytother Res* **30**(9): 1445–1473.
4. Bina F, Soleymani S, Toliat T, *et al.* (2019) Plant-derived medicines for treatment of endometriosis: A comprehensive review of molecular mechanisms. *Pharmacol Res* **139**: 76–90.
5. Huang X, Su S, Duan JA, *et al.* (2016) Effects and mechanisms of Shaofu-Zhuyu decoction and its major bioactive component for Cold-Stagnation and Blood-Stasis primary dysmenorrhea rats. *J Ethnopharmacol* **186**: 234–243.

6. Wu X, Sun X, Zhao C, et al. (2019) Exploring the pharmacological effects and potential targets of paeoniflorin on the endometriosis of cold coagulation and blood stasis model rats by ultra-performance liquid chromatography tandem mass spectrometry with a pattern recognition approach. *Chem Sci* **9**(36): 20796–20805.
7. Tsai HY, Lin YT, Tsai CH, et al. (2001) Effects of paeoniflorin on the formalin-induced nociceptive behaviour in mice. *J Ethnopharmacol* **75**(2–3): 267–271.
8. Zhang XJ, Chen HL, Li Z, et al. (2009) Analgesic effect of paeoniflorin in rats with neonatal maternal separation-induced visceral hyperalgesia is mediated through adenosine A(1) receptor by inhibiting the extracellular signal-regulated protein kinase (ERK) pathway. *Pharmacol Biochem Behav* **94**(1): 88–97.
9. Chen YF, Lee MM, Fang HL, et al. (2016) Paeoniflorin inhibits excitatory amino acid agonist-and high-dose morphine-induced nociceptive behavior in mice via modulation of N-methyl-D-aspartate receptors. *BMC Complement Altern Med* **16**: 240.
10. Zhang Y, Sun D, Meng Q, et al. (2016) Calcium channels contribute to albiflorin-mediated antinociceptive effects in mouse model. *Neurosci Lett* **628**: 105–109.
11. Tempest HG, Homa ST, Routledge EJ, et al. (2008) Plants used in Chinese medicine for the treatment of male infertility possess antioxidant and anti-oestrogenic activity. *Syst Biol Reprod Med* **54**(4–5): 185–195.
12. He DY, Dai SM. (2011) Anti-inflammatory and immunomodulatory effects of *Paeonia lactiflora* Pall., a traditional chinese herbal medicine. *Front Pharmacol* **2**: 10.
13. Chen Z, Zhang C, Gao F, et al. (2018) A systematic review on the rhizome of *Ligusticum chuanxiong* Hort. (Chuanxiong). *Food Chem Toxicol* **119**: 309–325.
14. Ran X, Ma L, Peng C, et al. (2011) *Ligusticum chuanxiong* Hort: A review of chemistry and pharmacology. *Pharm Biol* **49**(11): 1180–1189.
15. Wang X, Yang Y, Chen G, et al. (2011) Inhibitory effects of *Jiawei Foshou San* on angiogenesis of endometriosis in rats model and its mechanism. *Chin Pharmacol Bull* **27**: 350–354.
16. Chen Y, Wei J, Zhang Y, et al. (2018) Anti-endometriosis mechanism of *Jiawei Foshou San* based on network pharmacology. *Front Pharmacol* **9**: 811.

17. Wei J, Zhao B, Zhang C, et al. (2019) Jiawei Foshou San induces apoptosis in ectopic endometrium based on systems pharmacology, molecular docking, and experimental evidence. *Evid Based Complement Alternat Med* **2019**: 2360367.
18. Gao D, Xu L. (2010) Comparative analgesic effect of Ligusticum chuanxiong pieces and its products in mice. *Pharmacogn Mag* **6**(22): 132–134.
19. Wang H, Tang Y, Guo J, et al. (2010) [Antidysmenorrheic effects of Radix angelica and Rhizoma Chuanxiong with different proportions and preparation methods on dysmenorrhea model mice]. *Zhongguo Zhong Yao Za Zhi* **35**(7): 892–895.
20. Bie BH, Chen Y, Zhao ZQ. (2006) Ligustrazine inhibits high voltage-gated Ca(2+) and TTX-resistant Na(+) channels of primary sensory neuron and thermal nociception in the rat: A study on peripheral mechanism. *Neurosci Bull* **22**(2): 79–84.
21. Peng C, Xie X, Wang L, et al. (2009) Pharmacodynamic action and mechanism of volatile oil from *Rhizoma Ligustici Chuanxiong Hort.* on treating headache. *Phytomedicine* **16**(1): 25–34.
22. Chen J, Jiang QD, Wu YM, et al. (2015) Potential of essential oils as penetration enhancers for transdermal administration of ibuprofen to treat dysmenorrhoea. *Molecules* **20**(10): 18219–18236.
23. Tang Q, Shang F, Wang X, et al. (2014) Combination use of ferulic acid, ligustrazine and tetrahydropalmatine inhibits the growth of ectopic endometrial tissue: A multi-target therapy for endometriosis rats. *J Ethnopharmacol* **151**(3): 1218–1225.
24. Lei W, Deng YF, Hu XY, et al. (2019) Phthalides, senkyunolide A and ligustilide, show immunomodulatory effect in improving atherosclerosis, through inhibiting AP-1 and NF-kappaB expression. *Biomed Pharmacother* **117**: 109074.
25. Su CY, Ming QL, Rahman K, et al. (2015) *Salvia miltiorrhiza*: Traditional medicinal uses, chemistry, and pharmacology. *Chin J Nat Med* **13**(3): 163–182.
26. Ma S, Zhang D, Lou H, et al. (2016) Evaluation of the anti-inflammatory activities of tanshinones isolated from *Salvia miltiorrhiza* var. alba roots in THP-1 macrophages. *J Ethnopharmacol* **188**: 193–199.
27. Moon S, Shin S, Kim S, et al. (2011) Role of *Salvia miltiorrhiza* for modulation of Th2-derived cytokines in the resolution of inflammation. *Immune Netw* **11**(5): 288–298.

28. Zhou ZH, Weng Q, Zhou JH, et al. (2012) Extracts of Salvia miltiorrhiza Bunge on the cytokines of rat endometriosis models. Afr J Tradit Complement Altern Med **9**(3): 303–314.
29. Kim JM, Noh EM, Song HK, et al. (2017) Salvia miltiorrhiza extract inhibits TPA-induced MMP-9 expression and invasion through the MAPK/AP-1 signaling pathway in human breast cancer MCF-7 cells. Oncol Lett **14**(3): 3594–3600.
30. Nizamutdinova IT, Lee GW, Lee JS, et al. (2008) Tanshinone I suppresses growth and invasion of human breast cancer cells, MDA-MB-231, through regulation of adhesion molecules. Carcinogenesis **29**(10): 1885–1892.
31. Wan L, Zou Y, Wan LH, et al. (2015) Tanshinone IIA inhibits the proliferation, migration and invasion of ectopic endometrial stromal cells of adenomyosis via 14-3-3zeta downregulation. Arch Gynecol Obstet **292**(6): 1301–1309.
32. Xing Y, Tu J, Zheng L, et al. (2015) Anti-angiogenic effect of tanshinone IIA involves inhibition of the VEGF/VEGFR2 pathway in vascular endothelial cells. Oncol Rep **33**(1): 163–170.
33. Tsai MY, Yang RC, Wu HT, et al. (2011) Anti-angiogenic effect of Tanshinone IIA involves inhibition of matrix invasion and modification of MMP-2/TIMP-2 secretion in vascular endothelial cells. Cancer Lett **310**(2): 198–206.
34. Lu M, Li Y, Zeng R, et al. (2016) Effect of Salviae miltiorrhizae on stromal cells MMP-9 m RNA and protein expression of endometriosis. Journal of New Chinese Medicine **48**(4): 278–280.
35. Liu C, Shi W, Sun L, et al. (1990) Effects of radix Salviae miltiorrhizae on visceral pain discharges in the posterior nucleus of the thalamus in cats. Zhongguo Zhong Yao Za Zhi **15**: 112–115.
36. Hosseinzadeh H, Haddadkhodaparast MH, Arash AR. (2003) Antinociceptive, antiinflammatory and acute toxicity effects of Salvia leriifolia Benth seed extract in mice and rats. Phytother Res **17**(4): 422–425.
37. Wang C, Du X, Yang R, et al. (2015) The prevention and treatment effects of tanshinone IIA on oestrogen/androgen-induced benign prostatic hyperplasia in rats. J Steroid Biochem Mol Biol **145**: 28–37.
38. Capek P, Hribalova V. (2004) Water-soluble polysaccharides from Salvia officinalis L. possessing immunomodulatory activity. Phytochemistry **65**(13): 1983–92.

39. Wang N, Yang J, Lu J, et al. (2014) A polysaccharide from *Salvia miltiorrhiza* Bunge improves immune function in gastric cancer rats. *Carbohydr Polym* **111**: 47–55.
40. Wei WL, Zeng R, Gu CM, et al. (2016) *Angelica sinensis* in China-A review of botanical profile, ethnopharmacology, phytochemistry and chemical analysis. *J Ethnopharmacol* **190**: 116–141.
41. Su YW, Chiou WF, Chao SH, et al. (2011) Ligustilide prevents LPS-induced iNOS expression in RAW 264.7 macrophages by preventing ROS production and down-regulating the MAPK, NF-kappaB and AP-1 signaling pathways. *Int Immunopharmacol* **11**(9): 1166–1172.
42. Yeh JC, Cindrova-Davies T, Belleri M, et al. (2011) The natural compound n-butylidenephthalide derived from the volatile oil of *Radix Angelica sinensis* inhibits angiogenesis in vitro and in vivo. *Angiogenesis* **14**(2): 187–197.
43. Song M. LQ, He C. (2009) Identification and analgetic effect of *Angelica sinensis* extract. *Journal of Xianning University* **23**: 194–196.
44. Xu Y, Zhang L, Shao T, et al. (2013) Ferulic acid increases pain threshold and ameliorates depression-like behaviors in reserpine-treated mice: Behavioral and neurobiological analyses. *Metab Brain Dis* **28**(4): 571–583.
45. Ko WC. (1980) A newly isolated antispasmodic — butylidenephthalide. *Jpn J Pharmacol* **30**(1): 85–91.
46. Ahmed HM, Yeh JY, Tang YC, et al. (2014) Molecular screening of Chinese medicinal plants for progestogenic and anti-progestogenic activity. *J Biosci* **39**(3): 453–461.
47. Chen XP, Li W, Xiao XF, et al. (2013) Phytochemical and pharmacological studies on Radix *Angelica sinensis*. *Chin J Nat Med* **11**(6): 577–587.
48. Sun W, Wang S, Zhao W, et al. (2017) Chemical constituents and biological research on plants in the genus Curcuma. *Crit Rev Food Sci Nutr* **57**(7): 1451–1523.
49. Zhou Y, Xie M, Song Y, et al. (2016) Two traditional Chinese medicines *Curcumae Radix* and *Curcumae Rhizoma*: An ethnopharmacology, phytochemistry, and pharmacology review. *Evid Based Complement Alternat Med* **2016**: 4973128.
50. Tohda C, Nakayama N, Hatanaka F, et al. (2006) Comparison of anti-inflammatory activities of six *Curcuma* rhizomes: A possible curcuminoid-independent pathway mediated by *Curcuma phaeocaulis* extract. *Evid Based Complement Alternat Med* **3**(2): 255–260.

51. Zhou J, Qu F, Zhang H, et al. (2010) Comparison of anti-inflammatory and anti-nocicetive activities of *Cucuma wenyujin* Y.H. Chen et C. Ling and *Scutellaria baicalensis* Georgi. *Afr J Tradit Complement Altern Med* **7**(4): 339–349.
52. Kim KH, Lee EN, Park JK, et al. (2012) Curcumin attenuates TNF-alpha-induced expression of intercellular adhesion molecule-1, vascular cell adhesion molecule-1 and proinflammatory cytokines in human endometriotic stromal cells. *Phytother Res* **26**(7): 1037–1047.
53. Jana S, Paul S, Swarnakar S. (2012) Curcumin as anti-endometriotic agent: Implication of MMP-3 and intrinsic apoptotic pathway. *Biochem Pharmacol* **83**(6): 797–804.
54. Swarnakar S, Paul S. (2009) Curcumin arrests endometriosis by down-regulation of matrix metalloproteinase-9 activity. *Indian J Biochem Biophys* **46**(1): 59–65.
55. Jana S, Chakravarty B, Chaudhury K. (2014) Letrozole and curcumin loaded-PLGA nanoparticles: A therapeutic strategy for endometriosis. *J Nanomedicine Biotherapeutic Discov* **4**(1): 1–10.
56. Jana S, Rudra DS, Paul S, et al. (2012) Curcumin delays endometriosis development by inhibiting MMP-2 activity. *Indian J Biochem Biophys* **49**(5): 342–348.
57. Cao H, Wei YX, Zhou Q, et al. (2017) Inhibitory effect of curcumin in human endometriosis endometrial cells via downregulation of vascular endothelial growth factor. *Mol Med Rep* **16**(4): 5611–5617.
58. Zhang Y, Cao H, Hu YY, et al. (2011) Inhibitory effect of curcumin on angiogenesis in ectopic endometrium of rats with experimental endometriosis. *Int J Mol Med* **27**(1): 87–94.
59. Kizilay G, Uz YH, Seren G, et al. (2017) In vivo effects of curcumin and deferoxamine in experimental endometriosis. *Adv Clin Exp Med* **26**(2): 207–213.
60. Zhang Y, Cao H, Yu Z, et al. (2013) Curcumin inhibits endometriosis endometrial cells by reducing estradiol production. *Iran J Reprod Med* **11**(5): 415–422.
61. Catanzaro M, Corsini E, Rosini M, et al. (2018) Immunomodulators inspired by nature: A review on curcumin and echinacea. *Molecules* **23**(11): 2778.
62. Hosseinzadeh H, Nassiri-Asl M. (2015) Pharmacological effects of *Glycyrrhiza* spp. and its bioactive constituents: Update and review. *Phytother Res* **29**(12): 1868–1886.

63. Yang R, Yuan BC, Ma YS, *et al.* (2017) The anti-inflammatory activity of licorice, a widely used Chinese herb. *Pharm Biol* **55**(1): 5–18.
64. Asl MN, Hosseinzadeh H. (2008) Review of pharmacological effects of *Glycyrrhiza* sp. and its bioactive compounds. *Phytother Res* **22**(6): 709–724.
65. Park SY, Kwon SJ, Lim SS, *et al.* (2016) Licoricidin, an active compound in the hexane/ethanol extract of Glycyrrhiza uralensis, inhibits lung metastasis of 4T1 murine mammary carcinoma cells. *Int J Mol Sci* **17**(6): 934.
66. Kim KJ, Choi JS, Kim KW, *et al.* (2013) The anti-angiogenic activities of glycyrrhizic acid in tumor progression. *Phytother Res* **27**(6): 841–846.
67. Kim A, Ma JY. (2018) Isoliquiritin apioside suppresses in vitro invasiveness and angiogenesis of cancer cells and endothelial cells. *Front Pharmacol* **9**: 1455.
68. Wang XR, Hao HG, Chu L. (2017) Glycyrrhizin inhibits LPS-induced inflammatory mediator production in endometrial epithelial cells. *Microb Pathog* **109**: 110–113.
69. Namavar Jahromi B, Farrokhnia F, Tanideh N, *et al.* (2019) Comparing the effects of *Glycyrrhiza glabra* root extract, a cyclooxygenase-2 Inhibitor (celecoxib) and a gonadotropin-releasing hormone analog (diphereline) in a rat model of endometriosis. *Int J Fertil Steril* **13**(1): 45–50.
70. Shi Y, Wu D, Sun Z, *et al.* (2012) Analgesic and uterine relaxant effects of isoliquiritigenin, a flavone from *Glycyrrhiza glabra*. *Phytother Res* **26**(9): 1410–1417.
71. Tamaya T, Sato S, Okada HH. (1986) Possible mechanism of steroid action of the plant herb extracts glycyrrhizin, glycyrrhetinic acid, and paeoniflorin: Inhibition by plant herb extracts of steroid protein binding in the rabbit. *Am J Obstet Gynecol* **155**(5): 1134–1139.
72. Peng F, Du Q, Peng C, *et al.* (2015) A review: The pharmacology of isoliquiritigenin. *Phytother Res* **29**(7): 969–977.
73. Sun J, Wang S, Wei YH. (2011) Reproductive toxicity of Rhizoma Sparganii (*Sparganium stoloniferum* Buch.-Ham.) in mice: Mechanisms of anti-angiogenesis and anti-estrogen pharmacologic activities. *J Ethnopharmacol* **137**(3): 1498–1503.
74. Zong Q, Xiong Y, Deng K. (2018) Two new sucrose esters from the rhizome of *Sparganium stoloniferum* Buch.-Ham. *Nat Prod Res* **32**(14): 1632–1638.

75. Liang Q, Wu Q, Jiang J, *et al.* (2011) Characterization of sparstolonin B, a Chinese herb-derived compound, as a selective Toll-like receptor antagonist with potent anti-inflammatory properties. *J Biol Chem* **286**(30): 26470–26479.
76. Liang Q, Yu F, Cui X, *et al.* (2013) Sparstolonin B suppresses lipopolysaccharide-induced inflammation in human umbilical vein endothelial cells. *Arch Pharm Res* **36**(7): 890–896.
77. Bateman HR, Liang Q, Fan D, *et al.* (2013) Sparstolonin B inhibits proangiogenic functions and blocks cell cycle progression in endothelial cells. *PLoS One* **8**(8): e70500.
78. Qin C, Xu X, Zhu H. (2008) The studies on the anti-inflammatory and analgesia effects of SLW. *Pharmacology and Clinics of Chinese Materia Medica* (5): 7–10.
79. Chen Y, Xu XY, Ye L, *et al.* (2008) [Inhibitory effects of Sanleng pellet on angiogenesis of endometriosis in rats]. *Zhongguo Zhong Yao Za Zhi* **33**(3): 303–307.
80. Li A, Xu XY, Wang H, *et al.* (2008) [Study on inhibitory effect of medicated serum of SLW on estrogen production by human endometrial cells of endometriosis]. *Zhongguo Zhong Yao Za Zhi* **33**(6): 686–690.
81. Zhang Y, Zhang Y, Wang W. (2009) Effects of Jiawei sanleng wan on estrogen secretion and angiogenesis of human endometriumof endometriosis. *Chinese Journal of Biochemical Drugs* **28**(11): 831–836.
82. Aziz S, Rahman H. (2013) Biological activities of *Prunus persica* L. Batch. *J Med Plants Res* **7**: 947–951.
83. Elshamy AI, Abdallah HMI, El Gendy AEG, *et al.* (2019) Evaluation of anti-inflammatory, antinociceptive, and antipyretic activities of *Prunus persica* var. *nucipersica* (nectarine) kernel. *Planta Med* **85**(11–12): 1016–1023.
84. Liczbinski P, Bukowska B. (2018) Molecular mechanism of amygdalin action in vitro: Review of the latest research. *Immunopharmacol Immunotoxicol* **40**(3): 212–218.
85. Dogru HY, Isguder CK, Arici A, *et al.* (2017) Effect of amygdalin on the treatment and recurrence of endometriosis in an experimental rat study. *Period Biol* **119**(3): 173–180.
86. Hu F, Hu Y, Peng F. (2019) Synergistic and protective effect of atorvastatin and amygdalin against histopathological and biochemical alterations in Sprague-Dawley rats with experimental endometriosis. *AMB Express* **9**(1): 37.

87. Liu HZ, Han XX, Liu J, et al. (2017) Effect of Taoren quyu decoction on human endometrial cells and its anti-endometriosis activity in rats. *Asian Pac J Trop Med* **10**(7): 696–700.
88. Jin Y, Zheng J. (2019) Effect of Taoren-Quyu decoction on endometriosis in rats. *Tropical Journal of Pharmaceutical Research* **18**(5): 1057–1060.
89. Jiagang D, Li C, Wang H, et al. (2011) Amygdalin mediates relieved atherosclerosis in apolipoprotein E deficient mice through the induction of regulatory T cells. *Biochem Biophys Res Commun* **411**(3): 523–529.
90. Kamala A, Middha SK, Karigar CS. (2018) Plants in traditional medicine with special reference to *Cyperus rotundus* L.: A review. *3 Biotech* **8**(7): 309.
91. Peerzada AM, Ali HH, Naeem M, et al. (2015) *Cyperus rotundus* L.: Traditional uses, phytochemistry, and pharmacological activities. *J Ethnopharmacol* **174**: 540–560.
92. Jung SH, Kim SJ, Jun BG, et al. (2013) alpha-Cyperone, isolated from the rhizomes of *Cyperus rotundus*, inhibits LPS-induced COX-2 expression and PGE2 production through the negative regulation of NFkappaB signalling in RAW 264.7 cells. *J Ethnopharmacol* **147**(1): 208–214.
93. Kim C, Cho SK, Kim KD, et al. (2014) beta-Caryophyllene oxide potentiates TNFalpha-induced apoptosis and inhibits invasion through down-modulation of NF-kappaB-regulated gene products. *Apoptosis* **19**(4): 708–718.
94. Abbas MA, Taha MO, Zihlif MA, et al. (2013) beta-Caryophyllene causes regression of endometrial implants in a rat model of endometriosis without affecting fertility. *Eur J Pharmacol* **702**(1–3): 12–9.
95. Imam MZ, Sumi CD. (2014) Evaluation of antinociceptive activity of hydromethanol extract of *Cyperus rotundus* in mice. *BMC Complement Altern Med* **14**: 83.
96. Biradar S, Kangralkar V, Mandavkar Y, et al. (2010) Anti-inflammatory, anti-arthritic, analgesic and anticonvulsant activity of Cyperus essential oils. *Int J Pharm Pharm Sci* **2**: 112–115.
97. Busman H, Yanwirasti, Jamsari, et al. (2016) Antiestrogenic effect of tuber extract of *Cyperus rotundus* L. on the endometrial thickness of mice (*Mus musculus* L.). *World Journal of Pharmaceutical and Life Sciences* **2**(6): 341–347.

98. Ju Y, Xiao B. (2016) Chemical constituents of Cyperus rotundus L. and the inhibitory effects on uterine fibroids. *Afri Health Sci* **16**(4): 1000–1006.
99. Wang L, Zhang Y, Wang Z, *et al.* (2016) The antinociceptive properties of the Corydalis *yanhusuo* extract. *PLoS One* **11**(9): e0162875.
100. Alam MB, Ju MK, Kwon YG, *et al.* (2019) Protopine attenuates inflammation stimulated by carrageenan and LPS via the MAPK/NF-kappaB pathway. *Food Chem Toxicol* **131**: 110583.
101. He K, Gao JL. (2014) Protopine inhibits heterotypic cell adhesion in MDA-MB-231 cells through down-regulation of multi-adhesive factors. *Afr J Tradit Complement Altern Med* **11**(2): 415–424.
102. Gao JL, Shi JM, He K, *et al.* (2008) Yanhusuo extract inhibits metastasis of breast cancer cells by modulating mitogen-activated protein kinase signaling pathways. *Oncol Rep* **20**(4): 819–824.
103. Zhang ZM, Jiang B, Zheng XX. (2005) [Effect of l-tetrahydropalmatine on expression of adhesion molecules induced by lipopolysaccharides in human umbilical vein endothelium cell]. *Zhongguo Zhong Yao Za Zhi* **30**(11): 861–864.
104. Yang BR, Yu N, Deng YH, *et al.* (2015) L-tetrahydropalamatine inhibits tumor necrosis factor-alpha-induced monocyte-endothelial cell adhesion through downregulation of intercellular adhesion molecule-1 and vascular cell adhesion molecule-1 involving suppression of nuclear factor-kappa B signaling pathway. *Chin J Integr Med* **21**(5): 361–368.
105. Zhao T, Liu X, Zhen X, *et al.* (2011) Levo-tetrahydropalmatine retards the growth of ectopic endometrial implants and alleviates generalized hyperalgesia in experimentally induced endometriosis in rats. *Reprod Sci* **18**(1): 28–45.
106. Ferrero S, Remorgida V, Maganza C, *et al.* (2014) Aromatase and endometriosis: Estrogens play a role. *Ann N Y Acad Sci* **1317**: 17–23.
107. Shi J, Zhang X, Ma Z, *et al.* (2010) Characterization of aromatase binding agents from the dichloromethane extract of *Corydalis yanhusuo* using ultrafiltration and liquid chromatography tandem mass spectrometry. *Molecules* **15**(5): 3556–3566.
108. Liu J, He K, Li Q. (2012) Influences of Shaofu Zhuyu Wan on expressions of TNF-α and VEGF in rats with endometriosis. *Journal of Beijing University of Traditional Chinese Medicine* **35**(6): 391–393, 435.
109. Zhu G, Jiang C, Yan X, *et al.* (2018) Shaofu Zhuyu Decoction regresses endometriotic lesions in a rat model. *Evid Based Complement Alternat Med* **2018**: 3927096.

110. Su S, Hua Y, Duan JA, et al. (2010) Inhibitory effects of active fraction and its main components of Shaofu zhuyu decoction on uterus contraction. *Am J Chin Med* **38**(4): 777–787.
111. Ma H, Su S, Duan J, et al. (2011) Evaluation of the analgesic activities of the crude aqueous extract and fractions of Shao Fu Zhu Yu decoction. *Pharm Biol* **49**(2): 137–145.
112. Cui Y, Wu J, Cai W, et al. (2018) Molecular mechanism of Shaofu Zhuyu decoction in treating endometriosis dysmenorrhea based on GPER2/MAPK/STAT1 axis. *China Journal of Chinese Materia Medica* **43**(16): 3362–3367.
113. Hu C, Wang Z, Pang Z, et al. (2014) Guizhi Fuling capsule, an ancient Chinese formula, attenuates endometriosis in rats via induction of apoptosis. *Climacteric* **17**(4): 410–416.
114. Wu X, Zhao C, Zhang A, et al. (2018) High-throughput metabolomics used to identify potential therapeutic targets of Guizhi Fuling Wan against endometriosis of cold coagulation and blood stasis. *Chem Sci* **8**: 19238–19250.
115. Cai X, Hu C, Hu T, et al. (2011) Effects of Guizhi Fuling capsule on the expression of MCP-1 and ICAM-1 mRNA of ectopic endometrium in rats with endometriotics. *Chinese Journal of Experimental Traditional Medical Formulae* **17**(15): 202–205.
116. Wan G, Zhang Z, Tang W. (2014) Anti-angiogenesis effects and mechanism of Guizhi Fuling Wan on endometriosis in a rat model. *Chinese Journal of Experimental Traditional Medical Formulae* **20**(1): 161–165.
117. Ji X, Gao J, Cai X, et al. (2011) Immunological regulation of Chinese herb Guizhi Fuling capsule on rat endometriosis model. *J Ethnopharmacol* **134**(3): 624–629.

7

Clinical Evidence for Acupuncture and Related Therapies

OVERVIEW

Acupuncture and related therapies provide an additional treatment option for women with endometriosis. Several acupuncture therapies have been tested in clinical trials, and a selection of studies are summarised in this chapter. Acupuncture and moxibustion were tested in 15 clinical studies and may be beneficial for reducing pain associated with endometriosis.

Introduction

Acupuncture is part of a family of techniques that stimulate acupuncture points to correct imbalances of energy and restore health to the body. Methods of stimulating acupuncture points include:

- Acupuncture: insertion of an acupuncture needle into acupuncture points;
- Moxibustion: burning of a herb (usually *ai ye*, 艾叶, *Artemesia vulgaris* L.) close to or on the skin to induce a warming sensation;
- Warm needle: a method of combining acupuncture with moxibustion;
- Electroacupuncture: electrical stimulation of the needle following insertion.

Previous Systematic Reviews

Four published systematic reviews (SRs) have evaluated the effect of acupuncture therapies on endometriosis. One SR included eight randomised controlled trials (RCTs), all of which compared acupuncture with various Chinese medicine (CM) treatments.[1] The results of this comparison are difficult to determine, particularly when the effect of CM has not been established.

The second SR included 13 RCTs, four of which evaluated the effectiveness of acupuncture compared with pharmacotherapy on the effective rate (a global measure of symptom severity) and dysmenorrhoea symptom scores.[2] This SR found the effective rate of acupuncture for endometriosis to be superior to pharmacotherapy, but the results were similar between groups for dysmenorrhoea symptom scores. The methodological quality of the included studies ranged from moderate (for the effective rate) to high (for the dysmenorrhoea symptom score). Two of the studies included in the SR by Xiao et al. (2017)[2] that reported on dysmenorrhoea symptom scores are included in this chapter.

A systematic review by Xu et al. (2017)[3] evaluated acupuncture for pelvic pain due to endometriosis. Ten studies were included, and meta-analysis showed that acupuncture resulted in a greater reduction in pain than controls, which included sham acupuncture, medications, and Chinese herbal medicine (CHM). Acupuncture also improved the clinical effective rate, a global assessment of symptoms, and provided a greater reduction in cancer antigen (CA)-125. The review did not report on the safety of acupuncture for pelvic pain due to endometriosis.

Finally, a Cochrane SR published in 2011 of acupuncture for endometriosis included one RCT that compared acupuncture with CHM.[4] The review found that acupuncture reduced dysmenorrhoea severity based on the criteria from the 1993 *Guideline for Clinical Research on New Chinese Herbal Medicine Drugs* (中药新药临床研究指导原则; 'the 1993 Guideline'),[5] and the effective rate was higher with acupuncture than with CHM. The clinical importance of this finding is unclear when the efficacy of CHM is uncertain.

Identification of Clinical Studies

A total of 37,518 citations were found after searching the English and Chinese language biomedical databases. Full-text review of 3,008 citations found that 2,994 articles were not eligible for inclusion (Figure 7.1). In total, 11 RCTS, three controlled clinical trials (CCTs), and one non-controlled study met the inclusion criteria. Twelve focused on women with endometriosis, while the remaining studies evaluated acupuncture therapies in women with adenomyosis. The interventions tested in the studies included manual acupuncture alone or with other interventions, such as moxibustion and electroacupuncture, and moxibustion alone or applied to acupuncture needles (warm needle). Two additional RCTs were identified for interventions not commonly practised outside of China, but they will not be presented here. Studies are presented according to diagnosis (endometriosis or adenomyosis) and are indicated by the letter 'A' followed by a number (e.g., A1). The references for studies can be found at the end of this chapter.

Endometriosis

The majority of included studies (13 of the 15 studies) focused on the potential role of acupuncture therapies for women with endometriosis, with most studies testing acupuncture alone or combined with other related therapies.

Acupuncture

Eleven studies evaluated the effects of manual acupuncture alone or in combination with other related therapies. Eight were RCTs (A1–A8), two were CCTs (A9, A10), and one was a non-controlled study (A11).

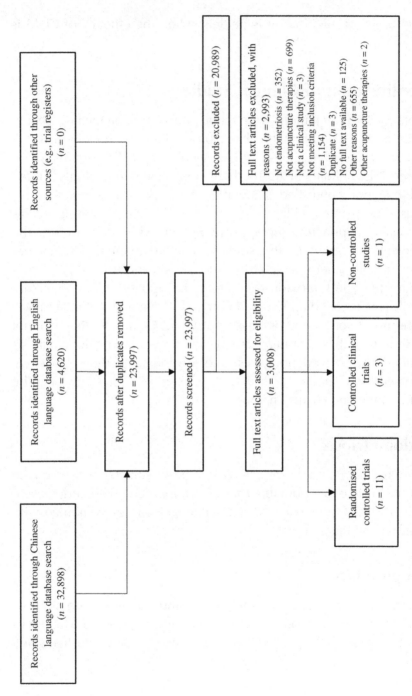

Figure 7.1. Flowchart of study selection process: Acupuncture and related therapies.

Randomised Controlled Trials of Acupuncture for Endometriosis

Acupuncture was evaluated in eight RCTs involving 590 participants (A1–A8). Five studies were conducted in mainland China, while other studies were conducted in Brazil, Austria, and the United States (US). Two studies involved three arms: one study tested two acupuncture groups and one control group (A2) and the other included a catgut embedding group (excluded from analysis), a warm needle group, and a gestrinone control group (A1). The interventions used in the study that tested two acupuncture groups were considered sufficiently similar that results could be merged for analysis. One study included four arms: acupuncture, CHM, acupuncture plus CHM, and a control group (A4). Only the results for the comparison of acupuncture versus gestrinone will be presented here.

All but one RCT included participants aged 18 years or over; Wayne et al. (2008; A8) included women between 13 and 22 years. Among other studies, the average age of women ranged from 30.5 years to 36.3 years. Women had lived with endometriosis for between three months and 7.2 years. The duration of treatment varied from five weeks to three months, and the follow-up period ranged from two to six months. Three studies used laparoscopy for diagnosis (A4, A7, A8). Two determined the stage of endometriosis according to the revised American Society for Reproductive Medicine (rASRM) criteria (A4, A7); one study included women with stage II–III endometriosis (A4) and the other included women with stage II–IV endometriosis. Participants in one study underwent surgery on enrolment in the study (A4). Two RCTs reported CM syndromes: one study included women with Blood stasis (A3), while the other used *qi* and Blood stasis, Kidney deficiency and Blood stasis, and phlegm and Blood stasis as syndromes to guide treatment (A4).

Acupuncture interventions included acupuncture alone (A2, A4–A7) or combined with moxibustion (A4), moxibustion and ear electroacupuncture (A8), or warm needle (A1). Acupuncture points were predominantly located on the Conception Vessel, Liver, Spleen, Stomach, and Bladder meridians. The most frequently used points

Table 7.1. Frequently Used Points in Acupuncture Randomised Controlled Trials

Acupuncture Point	Frequency of Use
SP6 Sanyinjiao 三阴交	7
CV3 Zhongji 中极	6
CV4 Guanyuan 关元	5
SP10 Xuehai 血海	4
BL32 Ciliao 次髎	3
ST36 Zusanli 足三里	3
LR3 Taichong 太冲	2
LI4 Hegu 合谷	2
BL23 Shenshu 肾俞	2
CV6 Qihai 气海	2
EX-CA1 Zigong 子宫	2

were SP6 Sanyinjiao 三阴交, CV3 Zhongji 中极, CV4 Guanyuan 关元, and SP10 Xuehai 血海 (Table 7.1).

One study used different points seven days before and after menstruation (A1), one used acupuncture needling followed by moxa on ginger applied to CV4 Guanyuan 关元 (A4), and one study needled 8–12 points on the Extraordinary and Divergent meridians, followed by moxa on the back shu 俞 and sacral areas and electroacupuncture to reactive ear points (A8). In addition to the main points of SP10 Xuehai 血海, SP6 Sanyinjiao 三阴交, and CV4 Guanyuan 关元, one study described additional acupuncture points that were selected according to CM syndromes (A4): CV8 Shenque 神阙, ST36 Zusanli 足三里, and CV6 Qihai 气海 were used for qi deficiency and Blood stasis, KI3 Taixi 太溪 and KI6 Zhaohai 照海 were used for Kidney deficiency and Blood stasis, and ST40 Fenglong 丰隆 and SP9 Yinlingquan 阴陵泉 were used for phlegm and Blood stasis.

Comparisons included sham acupuncture (four studies; A3, A6–A8) and hormone therapy (HT) (four studies; A1, A2, A4, A5). Only one study used an integrative medicine approach of combining acupuncture therapy with usual care (A7). Hormone therapy included gestrinone (A4), danazol (A2, A5), and gonadotropin-releasing hormone agonists (GnRH-a) (A1).

Due to differences in the interventions, comparators, and outcome measures used, it was not possible to pool results for meta-analysis. Three studies reported on health-related quality of life using the Endometriosis Health Profile (EHP)-30 item questionnaire[6] (A3, A6, A8). Baseline data in one study (A6) was imbalanced and a second study (A8) analysed results using the Wilcoxon rank sum test due to the small sample size (suggesting that data were not normally distributed); as such, it was not considered appropriate to conduct meta-analysis with these results. One study (A5) focused on the side effects of acupuncture and reported outcomes other than those pre-specified as part of this review.

Risk of bias assessments

All eight acupuncture RCTs were described as being randomised, but only four reported sufficient detail to make a judgement about the potential risk of bias for sequence generation (A1, A2, A4, A6) and only two studies reported sufficient detail for allocation concealment (A1, A6). One RCT allocated participants according to the visit order and was assessed as having high risk of bias for sequence generation (A2). Studies that used appropriate methods for group allocation were evaluated as posing low risk of bias for sequence generation (A1, A4, A6), while those did not report details of sequence generation or allocation concealment were assessed as having unclear risk of bias. Four studies reported that blinding was achieved by using a sham acupuncture intervention (low risk of bias; A3, A6–A8). Four studies were judged as having unclear risk as blinding of study personnel was not feasible, while the remaining four studies did not blind study personnel (high risk; A1–A4). Two studies described the methods used to blind outcome assessors and were assessed as having low risk of bias (A6, A8), three provided insufficient information (A3, A5, A7), and the remaining three (A1, A2, A4) were judged as having high risk as the method of blinding outcome assessors was not reported.

Three studies indicated that there were no dropouts (A1, A2, A5) and one study had few dropouts for reasons unlikely to relate to the intervention (A6); these four studies were assessed as having low risk of bias. Remaining studies were judged as having unclear risk due to the following reasons: one study reported in two theses reported inconsistent numbers of withdrawals (A3), two studies reported small numbers of dropouts such that it was difficult to determine the impact on results (A7, A8), and one reported that none of the 100 participants dropped out (A4), which seemed unlikely given that treatment was provided for more than six months. Only one study had registered the trial in a clinical trial register and reporting of pre-specified outcomes could be verified, posing low risk of bias (A6). One study (A3) reported multiple outcomes in two theses, but as it was not possible to determine which study planned to report which outcomes, the study was judged as having high risk. The methodological quality of the included studies was limited by poor reporting (Table 7.2).

Outcomes

The most frequently reported outcomes were endometriosis-related pain, including dysmenorrhoea, pelvic pain, and dyspareunia, and health-related quality of life. A 10 cm visual analogue scale (VAS) was the most common scale to evaluate pain, and the EHP-30 was

Table 7.2. Risk of Bias of Randomised Controlled Trials: Acupuncture

Risk of Bias Domain	Low Risk n (%)	Unclear Risk n (%)	High Risk n (%)
Sequence generation	3 (37.5)	4 (50)	1 (12.5)
Allocation concealment	2 (25)	6 (75)	0 (0)
Blinding of participants	3 (37.5)	2 (25)	3 (37.5)
Blinding of personnel*	0 (0)	4 (50)	4 (50)
Blinding of outcome assessors	2 (25)	3 (37.5)	3 (37.5)
Incomplete outcome data	4 (50)	4 (50)	0 (0)
Selective outcome reporting	1 (12.5)	6 (75)	1 (12.5)

*Blinding of personnel (acupuncturists) is difficult for manual therapy studies.

used for quality of life. In addition, one study each assessed the recurrence rate and the size of ovarian cysts. None of the studies reported on pregnancy outcomes, uterine volume, menstrual volume, fatigue, or outcomes relating to the side effects of GnRHa. Some studies had incomplete documentation of results; these results were excluded from further analysis.

Dysmenorrhoea

Three studies assessed dysmenorrhoea using a VAS or the scale from the 1993 Guideline (A1–A3). Results are presented according to comparisons.

Acupuncture versus sham acupuncture

One study measured dysmenorrhoea using a VAS and the scale from the 1993 Guideline at the end of treatment (A3). Both results showed that acupuncture could reduce dysmenorrhoea; dysmenorrhoea VAS scores were 2.4 cm lower at the end of treatment (59 women, [95% confidence intervals (CI) −2.80, −2.00]) and scores on the 1993 Guideline were 4.15 points lower (59 women, [−5.99, −2.31]) with acupuncture compared to sham acupuncture.

Acupuncture versus hormone therapy

One study that compared acupuncture with danazol measured the number of women with dysmenorrhoea at the end of treatment (A2). The results showed that the chance of having dysmenorrhoea after treatment was not statistically different between women who received acupuncture and those who received danazol (75 women, risk ratio [RR] 0.66 [0.35, 1.25]).

Warm needle acupuncture versus hormone therapy

One RCT assessed dysmenorrhoea using the 1993 Guideline (A1). When warm needle acupuncture was compared with goserelin, there was no significant difference between groups, either at the end of treatment (57 women, mean difference [MD] 1.27 points [−0.11, 2.65]) or at follow-up assessment (57 women, MD 0.53 points [−1.03, 2.09]).

Pelvic pain

Pelvic pain was reported in three studies (A6–A8) and assessed using a VAS or a numeric analogue scale (NAS), scored 0–10. One study reported data incompletely (A7) such that analysis was not possible. As differences in the comparisons prevented a meta-analysis from being conducted, results for individual studies are reported below.

Acupuncture versus sham acupuncture

Results from individual studies showed that women who received acupuncture had, on average, pelvic pain VAS scores that were 2.65 cm lower at the end of treatment than women who received sham acupuncture (42 women, [−3.40, −1.90]; A6) and VAS scores that were 3.53 cm lower at follow-up after two months (42 women, [−4.40, −2.66]; A6).

Acupuncture plus moxibustion and electroacupuncture versus placebo acupuncture

One small study that tested the combination of acupuncture, moxibustion, and electroacupuncture documented the change in pelvic pain NAS scores from baseline to the end of treatment (A8). The combination of acupuncture therapies did not result in a statistically different change in pelvic pain compared with placebo acupuncture. This was found after eight weeks of treatment (14 women, MD −0.50 points [−3.28, 2.28]) and six months of follow up (14 women, MD −0.80 points [−4.66, 3.06]).

Dyspareunia

Two studies examined dyspareunia (A2, A6). One study assessed dyspareunia using a 10 cm VAS (A6), while the other documented the number of women with dyspareunia at the end of treatment (A2).

Acupuncture versus sham acupuncture

One RCT with 42 participants measured dyspareunia using a 10 cm VAS (A6). Acupuncture resulted in a greater reduction in dyspareunia scores at the end of treatment (MD −2.88 cm [−3.83, −1.93]) and at follow-up (MD −3.86 [−4.77, −2.95]) compared to sham acupuncture.

Acupuncture versus hormone therapy

One study that compared acupuncture with danazol measured the number of women with dyspareunia at the end of treatment (A2). Treatment with acupuncture did not reduce women's chances of having dyspareunia at the end of treatment more than danazol did (26 women, RR 1.07 [0.57, 2.00]).

Recurrence

Recurrence of ovarian cysts after surgery was reported in one RCT (A4). The risk of recurrence was not significantly different between acupuncture plus moxibustion and gestrinone after three months of treatment (20 women, RR 1.00 [0.07, 15.26]) and at follow-up (60 women, RR 0.11 [0.01, 1.98]).

Ovarian cyst size

One RCT measured the effect of acupuncture on the diameter of ovarian cysts (A3), and results showed that the mean diameter was smaller with acupuncture than with sham acupuncture (MD −3.88 mm [−7.06, −0.70]). While this was a statistically significant finding, it is unclear whether a reduction of approximately four millimetres is clinically important.

Quality of life

Health-related quality of life was assessed in six RCTs (A1, A3, A4, A6–A8). Outcome measures included the EHP-30 and −5 item versions, the Medical Outcome Study 36-Item Short-Form Health Survey (SF-36),[7] and the Pediatric Quality of Life Inventory (PedsQL™).[8]

Acupuncture versus sham acupuncture

Two studies that compared acupuncture with sham acupuncture measured health-related quality of life with the EHP-30 (A3, A6). Due to baseline imbalance in one domain for one study (A6), meta-analysis was considered inappropriate. Results for individual studies are reported.

One study of 42 women (A6) found acupuncture to be superior in reducing total scores on the EHP-30 (MD −25.59 points [−32.28, −18.90]), as well as scores for the following additional modules:

- Work: MD −12.45 points [−21.15, −3.75];
- Sexual relationships: MD −28.91 points [−36.47, −21.35];
- Feelings about the medical profession: (MD −23.45 points [−32.57, −14.33]);
- Feelings about treatment (MD −32.77 points [−39.45, −26.09]);
- Feelings about infertility (MD −29.23 points [−51.95, −6.51]).

No difference was seen between groups in terms of relationship with children (MD −6.95 [−17.53, 3.63]), although this may be due to baseline imbalance.

The second study that measured quality of life with the EHP-30 included 59 women (A3). Acupuncture was found to reduce EHP-30 scores in the domains of:

- Pain: MD −15.36 points [−19.34, −11.38];
- Control and powerlessness: MD −8.79 points [−14.14, −3.44];
- Social support: MD −13.48 points [−18.50, −8.46];
- Emotional wellbeing: MD −5.58 points [−9.75, −1.41];
- Self-image: MD −7.05 points [−13.42, −0.68]);

Acupuncture also reduced scores for the following additional EHP-30 modules:

- Work: MD −14.41 points [−21.63, −7.19];
- Relationship with children: MD −10.26 points [−16.69, −3.83];
- Sexual relationships: MD −11.83 points [−18.30, −5.36];
- Feelings about the medical profession: MD −11.35 points [−17.31, −5.39];
- Feelings about treatment: MD −8.99 points [−14.43, −3.55];
- Feelings about infertility: MD −9.85 points [−16.77, −2.93]).

Acupuncture plus moxibustion versus gestrinone

One study dichotomised results for the EHP-5, with a score of 33 or lower categorised as a poor responder to treatment (A4). The chance of being a poor responder was not statistically different between acupuncture plus moxibustion and gestrinone when assessed at the end of treatment (60 women, RR 0.50 [0.05, 5.22]) or at follow-up (60 women, RR 0.11 [0.01, 1.98]).

Acupuncture plus moxibustion and electroacupuncture versus placebo acupuncture

One RCT of 14 women that tested the combination of acupuncture, moxibustion, and ear electroacupuncture measured health-related quality of life using the EHP-30 (A8). At the end of treatment, the change score from baseline was not statistically different between the combination of acupuncture, moxibustion, and ear electroacupuncture and placebo acupuncture for the EHP-30 in terms of:

- Total score: MD −19.70 points [−39.71, 0.31];
- Pain: MD −20.50 points [−41.84, 0.84];
- Control and powerlessness: MD −21.70 points [−52.55, 9.15];
- Social support: MD −5.90 points [−26.90, 15.10];
- Emotional wellbeing: MD −19.40 points [−40.86, 2.06];
- Self-image: MD −31.40 points [−63.25, 0.45].

At six-month follow-up, the total change in EHP-30 score was lower among women who received acupuncture therapies than those who received placebo acupuncture (MD −20.90 points [−38.06, −3.74]), but no differences were seen in the other domains of:

- Pain: MD 8.60 points [−6.70, 23.90];
- Control and powerlessness: MD 26.20 points [−5.28, 57.68]);
- Social support: MD 9.30 points [−14.92, 33.52]);
- Emotional wellbeing: MD 12.70 points [−6.96, 32.36]);
- Self-image: MD −32.60 points [−65.83, 0.63]).

Wayne et al. (2008; A8) also assessed health-related quality of life with the PedsQL™, which contains four domains — physical, emotional wellbeing, social support, and school — that are scored 0–100, with higher scores indicating better quality of life. There were no statistically significant differences between groups at the end of treatment for the physical (14 women, MD 9.10 points [−8.49, 26.69]), emotional wellbeing (14 women, MD 22.20 points [−1.17, 45.57]), social support (14 women, MD 10.00 points [−7.44, 27.44]), and school domains (14 women, MD 10.50 points [−15.98, 36.98]). However, at follow-up assessment, women who received the combination of acupuncture, moxibustion, and ear electroacupuncture scored higher than women who received placebo acupuncture — indicating better quality of life — on the physical (14 women, MD 19.90 points [9.90, 29.90]) and social support domains (14 women, MD 14.30 points [0.24, 28.36]). No such benefits were seen at follow-up on the emotional wellbeing (14 women, MD 15.70 points [−1.67, 33.07]) or school domains (14 women, MD 6.70 points [−10.25, 23.65]).

Warm needle acupuncture versus hormone therapy

One RCT, involving 59 women, evaluated quality of life using the SF-36 (A1). Analysis of results showed that the vitality score was higher at the end of treatment (MD 10.41 points [4.17, 16.65]) — indicating better quality of life — in women who received warm needle acupuncture compared with goserelin. Conversely, end of treatment scores for the emotional role function and social function domains were worse in people who received warm needle acupuncture (MD −23.13 points [−35.92, −10.34] and MD −5.08 points [−9.35, −0.81], respectively). There were no statistically significant differences between groups for the other domains of physical function (MD −1.58 points [−6.58, 3.42]), role physical (MD 6.56 points [−4.98, 18.10]), bodily pain (MD −6.78 points [−16.48, 2.92]), general health (MD −1.85 points [−7.28, 3.58]), and mental health (MD 1.86 points [−1.10, 4.82]).

Assessment using Grading of Recommendations Assessment, Development and Evaluation

The strength and quality ('certainty') of the evidence for clinically important questions was assessed using the Grading of Recommendations Assessment, Development and Evaluation (GRADE) framework (see Chapter 4). After consultation with clinical experts in endometriosis and discussion with the research team, consensus was reached on items for inclusion in summary-of-findings tables. The consensus was that critical questions relate to endometriosis and test the interventions of acupuncture and moxibustion compared with sham acupuncture (including placebo acupuncture) or HT. As such, the possible comparisons for summary-of-findings tables were:

- Acupuncture versus sham acupuncture;
- Acupuncture versus HT;
- Acupuncture plus HT versus sham acupuncture;
- Acupuncture plus HT versus sham acupuncture plus HT;
- Acupuncture plus HT versus HT;

- Moxibustion versus sham.
- Moxibustion versus HT.
- Moxibustion plus HT versus sham plus HT.
- Moxibustion plus HT versus HT.

While there are established methods and techniques for sham acupuncture, no such methods and techniques exist for moxibustion. Thus, we were unable to prepare summary-of-findings tables for comparisons involving moxibustion and sham moxibustion. Further, there were no studies that tested the comparisons of acupuncture plus HT versus HT or acupuncture plus HT versus sham acupuncture.

Outcomes selected for inclusion in summary-of-findings tables were dysmenorrhoea, pelvic pain and dyspareunia (all measured with a VAS), recurrence, live birth rate, quality of life measured with the EHP-30, and adverse events. Findings relating to acupuncture are presented here (see the 'Moxibustion' section for GRADE results for studies of moxibustion).

Acupuncture versus sham acupuncture

Two studies that compared acupuncture with sham acupuncture reported on the clinically important outcomes we selected (A3, A6). Low certainty evidence showed that acupuncture was superior to sham acupuncture in improving dysmenorrhoea VAS scores, while moderate certainty evidence indicated that acupuncture was superior in terms of pelvic pain and dyspareunia VAS scores (Table 7.3). Both studies also documented total and domain scores for the EHP-30 (see results in section 'Quality of Life'); findings from the study by Zhang (A3) were judged as low certainty evidence, while findings from De Sousa *et al.* (2016; A6) were considered moderate certainty evidence. Neither study reported on safety.

Acupuncture versus hormone therapy

Two RCTs compared acupuncture with HT (A2, A5). Neither study reported on clinical outcomes, but both reported on safety. Six adverse events (AEs) in the acupuncture groups were three cases of

Table 7.3. GRADE: Acupuncture versus Sham Acupuncture

Outcome	Absolute Effect		Relative Effect (95% CI) No. of Participants & Studies	Certainty of the Evidence (GRADE)
	With Acupuncture	With Placebo/Sham		
Dysmenorrhoea VAS Treatment duration: 3 m	2.2 cm Average difference: 2.4 cm lower (95% CI: 2.8 to 2.2 cm lower)	4.6 cm	MD −2.40 (−2.80 to −2.00) Based on data from 59 patients in 1 study	⊕⊕☐☐ LOW[a,b]
Pelvic pain VAS Treatment duration: 5 w	2.85 cm Average difference: 2.65 cm lower (95% CI: 3.4 to 1.9 cm lower)	5.5 cm	MD −2.65 (−3.40 to −1.90) Based on data from 42 patients in 1 study	⊕⊕⊕☐ MODERATE[b]
Dyspareunia VAS Treatment duration: 5 w	2.35 cm Average difference: 2.88 cm lower (95% CI: 3.83 to 1.93 cm lower)	5.23 cm	MD −2.88 (−3.83 to −1.93) Based on data from 42 patients in 1 study	⊕⊕⊕☐ MODERATE[b]

Abbreviations: CI, confidence intervals; m, months; MD mean difference; VAS, visual analogue scale; w, weeks.
[a]High risk of bias due to lack of blinding of personnel and selective outcome reporting; downgraded one level.
[b]Small sample size; downgraded one level.
References
Dysmenorrhoea VAS: A3.
Pelvic pain VAS: A6.
Dyspareunia VAS: A6.

weight gain, two cases of acne, and one case of breast pain. More AEs were documented with HT: 14 cases of weight gain, 11 cases of acne, 10 cases of hyperthermia, eight cases of irregular vaginal bleeding, eight cases of abnormal liver function, seven cases of nausea and vomiting, and five cases of breast pain.

Controlled Clinical Trials of Acupuncture for Endometriosis

Two CCTs of acupuncture for women with endometriosis were included (A9, A10). In total, 122 participants with an average age of between 33 and 36 years were enrolled. Both studies were conducted in mainland China and provided treatment for six months with a follow-up after one year. One study documented the CM syndrome of *qi* deficiency and Blood stasis (A10).

Each study used different interventions. One study used manual acupuncture on the points CV6 *Qihai* 气海, SP8 *Diji* 地机, SP6 *Sanyinjiao* 三阴交, LI4 *Hegu* 合谷, LR3 *Taichong* 太冲, CV4 *Guanyuan* 关元, and CV3 *Zhongji* 中极; electroacupuncture was also used on EX-CA1 *Zigong* 子宫 (A9). The other study applied acupuncture to SP10 *Xuehai* 血海, SP6 *Sanyinjiao* 三阴交, LR2 *Xingjian* 行间, and LR3 *Taichong* 太冲 and used warm needle on CV6 *Qihai* 气海, CV4 *Guanyuan* 关元, CV3 *Zhongji* 中极, and EX-CA1 *Zigong* 子宫 (A10). Both studies compared acupuncture with mifepristone.

Due to differences in the interventions, results are presented separately for each study. One CCT compared the effect of acupuncture plus electroacupuncture against mifepristone for dysmenorrhoea using the VAS (A9). The result showed no significant difference between the two groups (72 women, MD −0.84 cm [−1.72, 0.04]).

Both studies reported the recurrence rate, but as it was not clear whether the cases reported in one study (A9) were true cases of recurrence, these results were not analysed. Results from the second study showed no difference between acupuncture plus warm acupuncture and mifepristone in reducing the chance of endometriosis recurrence at one year in women who met the criteria for 'cured' at the end of treatment (50 women, RR 0.56 [0.22, 1.43]).

The size of ovarian cysts was smaller in women who received warm needle acupuncture than in those who received mifepristone (50 women, MD −0.93 [−1.20, −0.66]; A10).

Non-controlled Studies of Acupuncture for Endometriosis

Only one case report was eligible to be included in the review of non-controlled studies (A11). The study was conducted in the US and provided 9–15 acupuncture treatments to two adolescent girls with endometriosis-related chronic pelvic pain lasting more than one year. One girl — who continued to experience pelvic pain after two laparoscopies with surgical ablation of endometriosis, continuous use of oral contraceptives, and treatment with HT and non-steroidal anti-inflammatory drugs — was diagnosed with the CM syndromes *yang ming* 陽明/*shao yang* 少陽 pattern, *qi* and Blood stagnation with Blood stasis, Spleen and Kidney deficiency, and *qi* stagnation turning to heat. Acupuncture was applied to CV4 *Guanyuan* 关元, CV6 *Qihai* 气海, ST28 *Shuidao* 水道, ST36 *Zusanli* 足三里, SP6 *Sanyinjiao* 三阴交, SP10 *Xuehai* 血海, KI3 *Taixi* 太溪, GB43 *Xiaxi* 侠溪, PC6 *Neiguan* 内关, and BL23 *Shenshu* 肾俞, as well as points on the Conception Vessel meridian, while moxibustion was applied to ST36 *Zusanli* 足三里, SP6 *Sanyinjiao* 三阴交, and BL23 *Shenshu* 肾俞.

The second girl, whose CM syndrome diagnosis was *qi* and *yang* deficiency, also received acupuncture plus moxibustion but to different points. Acupuncture was applied to SP10 *Xuehai* 血海, SP6 *Sanyinjiao* 三阴交, CV4 *Guanyuan* 关元, CV6 *Qihai* 气海, LU7 *Lieque* 列缺, KI3 *Taixi* 太溪, and PC6 *Neiguan* 内关, as well as points on the *Chong* 衝 and *Ren* 任 meridians. Moxibustion also was used on SP6 *Sanyinjiao* 三阴交 and abdominal points.

Safety of Acupuncture for Endometriosis

Six of the 11 acupuncture studies described AEs (A1, A2, A4, A5, A8, A9). One RCT (A5) and one CCT (A9) reported that no AEs occurred in either group. Adverse events with acupuncture were three cases of weight gain, two cases of acne, and one case of breast pain (A2). Three cases of skin burn were reported with warm needle acupuncture (A1), while nine minor and expected AEs, such as light-headedness, bruising, and burns, were reported with the combination of acupuncture, moxibustion, and ear electroacupuncture (A8).

More AEs were observed in control groups than in treatment groups, and no AEs were reported with sham acupuncture. Adverse events with HT were 14 cases of weight gain, 14 cases of abnormal liver function, 11 cases of acne, 10 cases of hyperthermia, eight cases of irregular vaginal bleeding, seven cases of dry mouth and hot flushes, seven cases of nausea and vomiting, and five cases of breast pain.

Moxibustion

Two RCTs, involving 202 women, evaluated moxibustion alone or as integrative medicine with HT to treat endometriosis (A12, A13). No CCTs or non-controlled studies of moxibustion were included. Both studies were conducted in mainland China; one was a three-arm study that compared moxibustion alone and with gestrinone to gestrinone alone in 90 post-operative patients with stage III–IV endometriosis as determined by the rASRM (A12). Results for the two treatment groups were analysed separately.

The mean age of participants ranged from 33.26 to 35.8 years. Treatment was provided for three (A13) or six months (A12), and one study conducted follow-up assessment 18–27 months after the end of treatment. Participants in one study (A12) were diagnosed with the CM syndrome of Blood stasis. This study applied moxibustion to CV4 *Guanyuan* 关元, CV6 *Qihai* 气海, EX-CA1 *Zigong* 子宫, BL32 *Ciliao* 次髎, SP10 *Xuehai* 血海, SP8 *Diji* 地机, and SP6 *Sanyinjiao* 三阴交.

The second study, which did not document CM syndromes, included 90 women whose mean age was 35.8 years in the moxibustion group and 33.5 years in the mifepristone group. Herbal moxibustion was applied to the points GV14 *Dazhui* 大椎 and GV4 *Mingmen* 命门 on alternate days for three months. Herbal moxibustion involved piercing small holes in a medicinal cake made from *Si ni tang* 四逆汤 (made from 30 g each of *fu zi* 附子, *gan jiang* 干姜, and *gan cao* 甘草) and burning a 1 cm wide and 1.5 cm high moxa cone on top of the *Si ni tang* 四逆汤 cake.

Risk of Bias Assessment

Both RCTs were described as randomised, but only one reported using a random number table for sequence generation (low risk of bias; A13). This study did not specify the method of allocation concealment (unclear risk). The second study was judged to pose unclear risk for both sequence generation and allocation concealment due to insufficient information. Neither study mentioned that participants and study personnel were blind to group allocation (high risk). One study reported that the outcome assessor was blind to group allocation, but no further information was provided (A12); this study was evaluated as having unclear risk of bias. The other study did not mention blinding of outcome assessors (high risk).

One RCT reported that data were available for all participants (low risk; A13). In the other study, the reasons for participant withdrawal were described for some but not all women (unclear risk). No trial registrations or published protocols were identified for either RCTs, so both were assessed as having unclear risk of bias. The methodological quality of the included studies was limited.

Outcomes

The results of RCTs could not be pooled for meta-analysis because different outcomes were reported. Results are presented for individual studies. One RCT of 52 women measured dysmenorrhoea with a verbal rating scale (VRS; A12). There was no significant difference between moxibustion and gestrinone (MD −0.50 points [−1.02, 0.02]); however, dysmenorrhoea VRS scores were lower among women who received the combination of moxibustion and gestrinone than in women who received gestrinone alone (MD −0.59 points [−1.03, −0.15]).

The same study also evaluated the potential for moxibustion to reduce the recurrence of pain or cysts. Women who received moxibustion alone had a higher chance of recurrence than women who received gestrinone (RR 4.32 [1.01, 18.43]), but the chance of recurrence when moxibustion was combined with gestrinone was not greater than with gestrinone alone (RR 0.52 [0.05, 5.39]).

Findings from the second RCT showed that herbal moxibustion resulted in a smaller ovarian cyst maximum diameter after three months of treatment compared to mifepristone (90 women, MD −1.21 cm [−1.46, −0.96]; A13).

Assessment Using Grading of Recommendations Assessment, Development and Evaluation

Following the process described in Chapter 4, two summary-of-findings assessments were developed for the comparisons of moxibustion versus HT and moxibustion plus HT versus HT.

Moxibustion versus hormone therapy

Although two studies compared moxibustion with HT (A12, A13), only one reported on the selected clinically important outcomes (A12). Results showed that the chance of recurrence of pain and cysts was higher with moxibustion than with HT (Table 7.4). While the evidence was judged to be of low certainty — limiting confidence in the results — practitioners should consider the appropriateness of moxibustion on a case-by-case basis given the potential risks. Adverse events with moxibustion were two cases of hirsuitism and/or acne and one case of irregular vaginal bleeding. More AEs were reported with gestrinone: 13 cases of weight gain, eight cases of

Table 7.4. GRADE: Moxibustion versus Hormone Therapy

Outcome	Absolute Effect		Relative Effect (95% CI) No. of Participants & Studies	Certainty of the Evidence (GRADE)
	With Moxibustion	With HT		
Recurrence of pain and cysts Treatment duration: 6 m	30 per 100 Difference: 23 more per 100 patients (95% CI: 0 to 100 more per 100 patients)	7 per 100	RR 4.32 (1.01 to 18.43) Based on data from 52 patients in 1 study	⊕⊕◯◯ LOW[a,b]

Abbreviations: CI, confidence intervals; HT, hormone therapy; m, months; RR, risk ratio.
[a]High risk of bias due to lack of blinding; downgraded one level.
[b]Small sample size; downgraded one level.

References
Recurrence of pain and cysts: A12.

hirsuitism and/or acne, and five cases each of irregular vaginal bleeding, abnormal liver function, and menopausal symptoms.

Moxibustion plus hormone therapy versus hormone therapy

The study that compared moxibustion and HT also compared the combination of moxibustion plus HT with HT alone (A12). Low certainty evidence showed that the combination of moxibustion plus HT did not reduce the chance of recurrence of pain and cysts more than HT alone did (Table 7.5). The number of AEs was higher with HT alone than with moxibustion plus HT (36 versus 24, respectively). Adverse events with moxibustion plus HT were nine cases of hirsuitism and/or acne, five cases of menopausal symptoms, four cases of abnormal liver function, and three cases each of irregular vaginal bleeding and weight gain. Adverse events with gestrinone were 13 cases of weight gain, eight cases of hirsuitism and/or acne, and five cases each of irregular vaginal bleeding, abnormal liver function, and menopausal symptoms.

Table 7.5. GRADE: Moxibustion plus Hormone Therapy versus Hormone Therapy

Outcome	Absolute Effect		Relative Effect (95% CI) No. of Participants & Studies	Certainty of the Evidence (GRADE)
	With Moxibustion Plus HT	With HT		
Recurrence of pain and cysts Treatment duration: 6 m	2 per 100 Difference: 2 fewer per 100 patients (95% CI: 4 fewer to 16 more per 100 patients)	4 per 100	RR 0.52 (0.05 to 5.39) Based on data from 53 patients in 1 study	⊕⊕⊝⊝ LOW[a,b]

Abbreviations: CI, confidence intervals; HT, hormone therapy; m, months; RR, risk ratio.
[a]High risk of bias due to lack of blinding of participants and personnel; downgraded one level.
[b]Small sample size; downgraded one level.

References
Recurrence of pain and cysts: A12.

Safety of Moxibustion for Endometriosis

The safety of moxibustion was reported in one study (A12) and AEs have been reported in the section 'Assessment using Grading of Recommendations Assessment, Development and Evaluation'. The number of AEs was similar between moxibustion used alone and gestrinone, while fewer AEs were reported when moxibustion was used in combination with gestrinone.

Adenomyosis

Two studies focused on the role of acupuncture therapies for women with adenomyosis (A14, A15). Results for both studies were analysed and the findings are reported below.

Moxibustion

One RCT (A14) and one CCT (A15) conducted in mainland China reported employing moxibustion for the treatment of adenomyosis.

Randomised Controlled Trials of Moxibustion for Adenomyosis

The RCT provided three months of treatment with moxibustion or gestrinone for 50 Chinese women aged 30–49 with a CM diagnosis of *qi* stagnation and Blood stasis (A14). In the intervention group, ginger moxibustion was applied daily from the fifteenth day of the menstrual cycle for 10 days. The process for ginger moxibustion was to apply a paste made from ginger and other powdered herbs (including *ding xiang* 丁香 and *rou gui* 肉桂; 10 herbs in total) on top of mulberry paper along the Governor Vessel meridian while burning moxa cones on top. Ginger moxibustion was compared with gestrinone.

As a random number table was used to allocate women to groups and data were available for all participants, the study was assessed as having low risk of bias for sequence generation and incomplete outcome data. There was no information on blinding for participants, personnel, or outcome assessors (high risk), and the description of allocation concealment was inadequate (unclear risk). No trial registration or published protocol was located, so the study was evaluated as having unclear risk of bias for selective reporting. Overall, the methodological quality of this study was low.

The study documented one clinical outcome: dysmenorrhoea assessed using a VAS. At the end of treatment, the results showed that moxibustion provided a greater reduction in dysmenorrhoea than gestrinone did (50 women, MD −3.58 cm [−3.95, −3.21]).

Controlled Clinical Trials of Moxibustion for Adenomyosis

One CCT of moxibustion for adenomyosis met the eligibility criteria (A15). Sixty women with *qi* stagnation and Blood stasis and whose mean age ranged from 39.1 to 40.3 years were enrolled from a hospital outpatient department in China. The study assessed the effectiveness of moxibustion to CV4 *Guanyuan* 关元, CV3 *Zhongji* 中极, CV6 *Qihai* 气海, SP6 *Sanyinjiao* 三阴交, SP8 *Diji* 地机, SP10 *Xuehai* 血海, and LR3 *Taichong* 太冲. Treatment was provided for three months.

The CCT reported on dysmenorrhoea, assessed using the 1993 Guideline, and uterine volume. Compared with mifepristone, women who received moxibustion reported less severe dysmenorrhoea after three months of treatment than women who received mifepristone (MD −3.22 points [−3.87, −2.57]). Neither uterine volume (MD 1.29 cm^3 [−18.73, 21.31]) nor the maximum diameter of adenomyoma (MD 0.24 cm [−0.11, 0.59]) was statistically different between the two groups.

Safety of Moxibustion for Adenomyosis

The safety of moxibustion was reported in the CCT (A15). No AEs were reported in the moxibustion group, while 20 women in the control group reported weight gain, 13 women reported irregular vaginal bleeding, and nine women reported hot flushes.

Clinical Evidence for Commonly Used Acupuncture and Related Therapies

Acupuncture therapies are recommended in the contemporary clinical textbooks and guidelines described in Chapter 2. These interventions include acupuncture, ear acupuncture, abdominal acupuncture, and moxibustion. Studies included in this review investigated acupuncture, ear acupuncture (used in combination with other acupuncture techniques), and moxibustion. The role of abdominal acupuncture in alleviating symptoms of endometriosis and adenomyosis was not answered by this review, and it remains an area for further research.

Acupuncture was tested in 11 clinical studies and was clearly the most common technique evaluated in endometriosis research. All of the main points for manual acupuncture in the textbooks and guidelines included in Chapter 2 were used in multiple RCTs: CV4 *Guanyuan* 关元, CV3 *Zhongji* 中极, SP6 *Sanyinjiao* 三阴交, SP10 *Xuehai* 血海, ST36 *Zusanli* 足三里, and EX-CA1 *Zigong* 子宫. These points may be used whenever it is suitable for each woman's CM diagnosis.

Due to differences in comparisons and outcome measures, we were unable to conduct meta-analyses to estimate the effect of acupuncture, ear acupuncture, and moxibustion. Results from individual studies showed some benefits for acupuncture alone or in combination with other acupuncture therapies in reducing endometriosis-related pain and improving health-related quality of life.

Summary of Acupuncture and Related Therapies Clinical Evidence

While CHM remains an important treatment option for CM practitioners, there is a small but growing body of evidence suggesting that acupuncture therapies may offer pain relief for women with endometriosis and adenomyosis. Acupuncture was the most frequently evaluated intervention in studies included in this review and, in several cases, was combined with other acupuncture therapies, such as ear acupuncture and moxibustion. This scenario reflects clinical practice, where acupuncture and moxibustion are often used in combination.

Compared with CHM studies, it appeared that fewer acupuncture studies used CM diagnosis either as an inclusion criterion or to guide treatment. This finding is not surprising as the emphasis on syndrome differentiation is greater with CHM treatment. Studies that did describe CM syndromes were consistent with those described in Chapter 2, including concepts such as *qi* stagnation, cold congealing, and Blood stasis. This can reassure practitioners that the treatments in included studies are targeting the most common syndromes found in clinical practice.

The acupuncture points that were tested in clinical studies also reflect those used in clinical practice. Practitioners may wish to use acupuncture points CV4 *Guanyuan* 关元, CV3 *Zhongji* 中极, SP6 *Sanyinjiao* 三阴交, SP10 *Xuehai* 血海, ST36 *Zusanli* 足三里, and EX-CA1 *Zigong* 子宫 for women with endometriosis or adenomyosis and select supplementary points according to each woman's CM diagnosis.

While we planned to conduct meta-analyses in order to synthesise results from multiple studies, this was not possible due to differences in the interventions, comparators, and outcome measures used in included studies. Results favoured acupuncture over sham acupuncture in reducing dysmenorrhoea, pelvic pain, dyspareunia, and ovarian cyst diameter and improving health-related quality of life. Results did not favour acupuncture over HT for many of the selected outcomes. However, this should not be interpreted to mean that acupuncture is not effective, especially when HT treatments are already effective for endometriosis and adenomyosis.

Several studies examined the effects of acupuncture therapies after treatment had ceased. Acupuncture was more effective than sham acupuncture at reducing VAS scores for pelvic pain and dyspareunia after treatment had ceased and at improving the total score of the EHP-30 (but not individual domain scores). Furthermore, the combination of acupuncture, moxibustion, and ear electroacupuncture increased quality of life on the physical and social support domains of PedsQL at follow-up. However, neither acupuncture combined with moxibustion and electroacupuncture nor warm needle acupuncture showed significant benefits at follow-up. The varying effects observed highlight the lack of certainty about the long-term effects of acupuncture.

For chronic conditions like endometriosis and adenomyosis, clinical care typically involves an initial course of regular — perhaps weekly or more frequent — treatment to alleviate pain and other symptoms, followed by regular maintenance therapy. This pragmatic approach is difficult to test in clinical studies. In addition, the clinical course of endometriosis may include periods of relative stability punctuated by exacerbations of pain. Acupuncture therapies may also be effective in reducing acute exacerbations; however, there is currently insufficient evidence to support its use in ways that reflect clinical practice.

Like many complementary and alternative therapies, acupuncture is often considered a safe treatment option by patients. Studies included in this review reported minor and expected AEs, such as bruising and light-headedness, with similar numbers of AEs as controls. While this is reassuring, analysis of results identified two instances where women who received acupuncture therapies reported worse outcomes than controls. For example, women who received moxibustion had a higher chance of recurrence of pain or cysts than women who received HT, and some domains of the SF-36 were lower — indicating poorer health-related quality of life — with warm needle acupuncture than with goserelin. Practitioners should be mindful of the potential risks when providing treatment with acupuncture therapies.

References

1. 谢丽娟, 陈嘉欣. (2017) 针灸治疗子宫内膜异位症的系统评价. 中国妇幼保健 **32**(3): 635–638.
2. 肖小文, 周志刚, 王萍, et al. (2017) 针灸治疗子宫内膜异位症 Meta 分析. 江西中医药 **48**(410): 50–53.

3. Xu Y, Zhao W, Li T, *et al.* (2017) Effects of acupuncture for the treatment of endometriosis-related pain: A systematic review and meta-analysis. *PLoS One* **12**(10): e0186616.
4. Zhu X, Hamilton KD, McNicol ED. (2011) Acupuncture for pain in endometriosis. *Cochrane Database of Systematic Reviews* (9): 10.1002/14651858.CD007864.pub2.
5. 郑筱萸. (1993) *中药新药临床指导原则*. 北京: 中国医药科技出版社.
6. Jones G, Kennedy S, Barnard A, *et al.* (2001) Development of an endometriosis quality-of-life instrument: The Endometriosis Health Profile-30. *Obstet Gynecol* **98**(2): 258–264.
7. Ware JJ, Sherbourne C. (1992) The MOS 36-item short-form health survey (SF-36). I. Conceptual framework and item selection. *Med Care* **30**: 473–483.
8. Varni JW. (2020) The PedsQL™ measurement model for the Pediatric Quality of Life Inventory™. [cited 2020 19 May]. Available from: https://www.pedsql.org/index.html.

References for Included Acupuncture Therapies Clinical Studies

Study No.	Reference
A1	陈广贤. (2014) 穴位埋线疗法治疗子宫内膜异位症痛经疗效观察研究. 广州中医药大学.
A2	孙远征, 陈洪琳. (2006) 俞募配穴治疗子宫内膜异位症的对照研究. *中国针灸* **26**(12): 863–865.
A3	张靓裕. (2017) 针刺治疗血瘀型卵巢巧克力囊肿的临床观察. 黑龙江中医药大学.
A4	张晓云, 张春燕. (2014) 针药结合预防子宫内膜异位症腹腔镜手术后复发疗效观察. *中国针灸* **34**(2): 139–144.
A5	Chen L, Lin Y, Yuan LP, Huang HY. (2012) Abdominal acupuncture in treating 70 cases of endometriosis dysmenorrhea. *International Journal of Clinical Acupuncture* **21**(3): 100–102.
A6	de Sousa TR, de Souza BC, Zomkowisk K, da Rosa PC, Sperandio FF. (2016) The effect of acupuncture on pain, dyspareunia, and quality of life in Brazilian women with endometriosis: A randomized clinical trial. *Complement Ther Clin Pract* **25**: 114–121.

(Continued)

(Continued)

Study No.	Reference
A7	Rubi-Klein K, Kucera-Sliutz E, Nissel H, et al. (2010) Is acupuncture in addition to conventional medicine effective as pain treatment for endometriosis? A randomised controlled cross-over trial. *Eur J Obstet Gynecol Reprod Biol* **153**(1): 90–93.
A8	Wayne PM, Kerr CE, Schnyer RN, et al. (2008) Japanese-style acupuncture for endometriosis-related pelvic pain in adolescents and young women: Results of a randomized sham-controlled trial. *J Pediatr Adolesc Gynecol* **21**(5): 247–257.
A9	张鑫鑫, 李伟红. (2015) 电针治疗子宫内膜异位症疗效观察. 中国针灸 **35**(4): 323–326.
A10	沈群, 陆菁. (2017) 针灸治疗子宫内膜异位症临床观察. 上海针灸杂志 **36**(6): 711–714.
A11	Highfield ES, Laufer MR, Schnyer RN, et al. (2006) Adolescent endometriosis-related pelvic pain treated with acupuncture: Two case reports. *J Altern Complement Med* **12**(3): 317–322.
A12	袁红霞. (2009) 艾灸疗法用于中重度子宫内膜异位症术后治疗的临床研究. 广州中医药大学.
A13	张澎, 梁修朗, 范郁山. (2017) 隔药饼灸大椎穴与命门穴治疗子宫内膜异位症临床观察. 亚太传统医药 **13**(5): 121–123.
A14	宋宇惠, 师伟. (2012) 温督化瘀法治疗血瘀气滞型子宫腺肌病的临床观察. 中国保健营养(下旬刊) (2): 52.
A15	张瀚云. (2017) 艾灸治疗气滞血瘀型子宫腺肌症的临床研究. 广州中医药大学.

8

Clinical Evidence for Combination Therapies

OVERVIEW

Chinese medicine interventions are frequently used in combination in clinical practice. This chapter reviews the evidence from studies that tested combinations of Chinese medicine therapies. Combining Chinese herbal medicine with an acupuncture therapy was common among the 17 included clinical studies. Some promising benefits were seen in reducing dysmenorrhoea and dyspareunia, but more research is needed to confirm these findings.

Introduction

In Chinese medicine (CM) clinical practice, therapies are often used in combination. This chapter defines combination therapies as two or more CM interventions from different categories administered together. For example, Chinese herbal medicine (CHM) may be used in combination with acupuncture. The evidence from eligible clinical studies of combination therapies are reviewed in this chapter.

Identification of Clinical Studies

After a comprehensive search of English and Chinese language biomedical databases, 37,518 citations were identified. Duplicates were removed and the titles and abstracts were reviewed. The full text was retrieved to assess study eligibility against inclusion criteria. A total of 17 clinical studies were included: nine were randomised

Table 8.1. Summary of Interventions in Combination Therapies Studies

Combination Therapies	No. of Studies	Included Studies
CHM plus moxibustion	6	C1, C11, C13–C15, C17
CHM plus acupuncture	3	C9, C10, C12
CHM plus acupuncture and moxibustion	2	C2, C7
CHM plus acupuncture point stimulator	1	C4
CHM plus acupuncture, moxibustion, and plum-blossom needle therapy	1	C6
CHM plus acupuncture, tuina 推拿, and hormone therapy	1	C5
CHM plus ear acupressure	1	C8
CHM plus electroacupuncture	1	C3
CHM plus umbilical therapy	1	C16

controlled trials (RCTs), one was a non-randomised controlled clinical trial (CCT), and seven were non-controlled studies (Figure 8.1). All studies tested the combination of CHM with an acupuncture-related therapy, and the most common combination tested was CHM plus moxibustion (six studies; Table 8.1). Results of analyses are presented according to diagnosis of endometriosis, adenomyosis, or a combination of both.

Endometriosis

Eleven studies investigated the effects of various combinations of CM therapies in women with endometriosis. Six of these were RCTs (C1–C6), one was a CCT (C7), and four were non-controlled studies (C8–C11).

Randomised Controlled Trials of Combination Therapies for Endometriosis

The six RCTs included 608 adult women with endometriosis (C1–C6), two of which included three or more groups (C2, C3). The first

Clinical Evidence for Combination Therapies

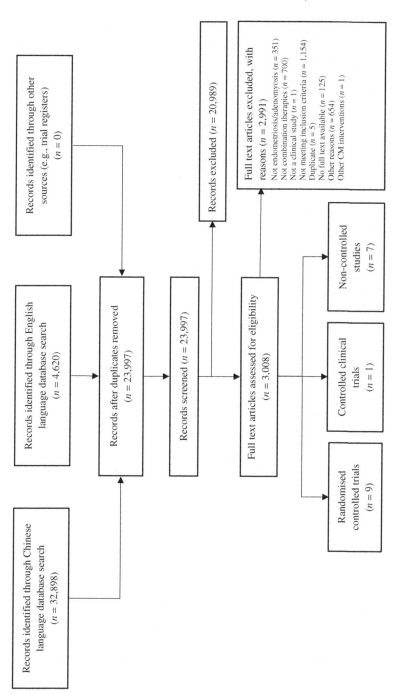

Figure 8.1. Flowchart of study selection process: Combination therapies.

study was a four-arm trial that compared CHM, acupuncture, and the combination of CHM plus acupuncture with gestrinone (C2). The results for the CHM and acupuncture arms have been included in Chapters 5 and 7, respectively. The second study compared women who received CHM and electroacupuncture with a control group who received mifepristone only and a second control group who received no treatment (C3). In this study, women in the treatment and active control groups underwent *in vitro* fertilisation (IVF) treatment after two months, while women in the no treatment group did not.

All studies were conducted in China, with women recruited from hospital inpatient or outpatient departments. In three RCTs, women underwent surgical treatment for endometriosis prior to commencing the trial (C2, C4, C5). Endometriosis was confirmed by laparoscopy in three studies (C2, C4, C5), and one study included women with disease stages II–III based on the revised American Society for Reproductive Medicine (rASRM) (C2). The median age of women was 33 years and the median duration of endometriosis was 3.7 years.

Two studies used CM syndrome as an inclusion criterion (C1, C5), and the syndrome *qi* stagnation and Blood stasis was common to both. The study by Sun and Liang (C5) also included women with Kidney deficiency and Blood stasis, phlegm-damp stasis, and *qi* deficiency and Blood stasis. Syndromes were also used to guide treatment. Two studies reported *qi* deficiency and Blood stasis and Kidney deficiency and Blood stasis (C2, C5), one reported phlegm and Blood stasis (C2), and one reported *qi* stagnation and Blood stasis and phlegm-damp stasis (C5).

Treatment was provided for two (C3) or three months (C1, C2, C4–C6), and all but one study (C6) conducted follow-up assessments after treatment ceased. Two studies tested a combination of CM therapies as an adjunct to conventional medical management (C3, C5). Three of the six RCTs used investigator-developed formulas (C3–C5), and there was no overlap in formulas used in the other three RCTs.

Analysis of herb ingredients showed that *dang gui* 当归, *gui zhi* 桂枝, and *wu ling zhi* 五灵脂 were the most used herbs (Table 8.2). Formulas were modified according to the stage of the menstrual

Clinical Evidence for Combination Therapies

Table 8.2. Frequently Reported Orally Used Herbs in Randomised Controlled Trials of Combination Therapies for Endometriosis

Most Common Herbs	Scientific Name	Frequency of Use
Dang gui 当归	*Angelica sinensis* (Oliv.) Diels	4
Gui zhi 桂枝	*Cinnamomum cassia* Presl	4
Wu ling zhi 五灵脂	*Trogopterus xanthipes* Milne-Edwards	4
Chi shao 赤芍	*Paeonia* spp.	3
Chuan xiong 川芎	*Ligusticum chuangxiong* Hort.	3
E zhu 莪术	*Curcuma* spp.	3
Pu huang 蒲黄	*Typha* spp.	3
San leng 三棱	*Sparganium stoloniferum* Buch. -Ham.	3
Tao ren 桃仁	*Prunus* spp.	3
Bai jiang cao 败酱草	*Patrinia scabiosaefolia* Fisch. Ex Link or *Patrinia villosa* Juss	2
Bai shao 白芍	*Paeonia lactiflora* Pall.	2
Dan shen 丹参	*Salvia miltiorrhiza* Bge.	2
Hong hua 红花	*Carthamus tinctorius* L.	2
Mo yao 没药	*Commiphora* spp.	2
Mu dan pi 牡丹皮	*Paeonia suffruticosa* Andr.	2
Shu di huang 熟地黄	*Rehmannia glutinosa* Libosch.	2
Shui zhi 水蛭	*Whitmania pigra* Whitman, *Hirudo nipponica* Whitman or *Whitmania acranulata* Whitman	2
Yan hu suo 延胡索	*Corydalis yanhusuo* W.T. Wang	2
Long xue jie 龙血竭	*Daemonorops draco* Bl.	2
Hong teng 红藤	*Sargentodoxa cuneata* (Oliv.) Rehd. & Wils.	2

Note: The use of some herbs may be restricted in some countries. Readers are advised to comply with relevant regulations.

cycle in three studies (C1, C3, C5). Analysis of acupuncture points found two points that were used in four RCTs: SP6 *Sanyinjiao* 三阴交 and CV4 *Guanyuan* 关元. EX-CA1 *Zigong* (Uterus) 子宫 was used in three RCTs, while CV3 *Zhongji* 中极, BL31 *Shangliao* 上髎, BL32 *Ciliao* 次髎, BL33 *Zhongliao* 中髎, and BL34 *Xialiao* 下髎 were used in two studies each.

Table 8.3. Risk of Bias of Randomised Controlled Trials: Combination Therapies for Endometriosis

Risk of Bias Domain	Low Risk n (%)	Unclear Risk n (%)	High Risk n (%)
Sequence generation	3 (50.0)	2 (33.3)	1 (16.7)
Allocation concealment	0 (0)	6 (100)	0 (0)
Blinding of participants	0 (0)	0 (0)	6 (100)
Blinding of personnel	0 (0)	0 (0)	6 (100)
Blinding of outcome assessors	0 (0)	6 (100)	0 (0)
Incomplete outcome data	5 (83.3)	1 (16.7)	0 (0)
Selective outcome reporting	0 (0)	6 (100)	0 (0)

Risk of Bias Assessment

All studies described using random allocation of participants to groups (Table 8.3). Three studies were judged as having low risk of bias for sequence generation as they used either a random number table (C1, C4) or block randomisation with stratification (C2). One study allocated participants according to the order of hospital registration and was judged as having high risk (C3). The remaining two studies were judged as having unclear risk as no details were provided about randomisation. None of the studies provided information about how group allocation was concealed (unclear risk). As neither participants nor personnel were blind to group allocation, all studies were judged as having high risk for these domains. Information about blinding of outcome assessors was not provided. Five studies reported no loss to follow-up and were judged as having low risk for incomplete outcome data (C1, C3–C6). One study was judged as having unclear risk for incomplete outcome data as the lack of missing data over the six-month trial period seemed unlikely (C2). None of the trials reported registering the trial protocol, and published trial protocols were not available.

Outcomes

Two outcomes were reported in multiple studies; three RCTs assessed the recurrence of cysts (C2, C4, C5) and two studies assessed dysmenorrhoea using a visual analogue scale (VAS) (C1, C5). One study each reported the number of women with dysmenorrhoea (C3) or dyspareunia (C3) at the end of treatment, and one study reported the pregnancy rate for women undergoing IVF (C3).

Clinical Evidence for Combination Chinese Medicine Therapies

Due to the variety of CM therapy combinations, it was not possible to conduct meta-analysis. Results for individual studies were analysed and are presented according to the intervention tested.

Chinese herbal medicine plus moxibustion

The combination of CHM and moxibustion was compared with ibuprofen in one study of 63 women (C1). This study found dysmenorrhoea measured on a VAS to be 1.10 cm lower at the end of treatment (95% confidence intervals [−1.79, −0.41]) and 1.60 cm lower at follow-up assessment in women who received combination CM therapies ([−2.55, −0.65]).

Chinese herbal medicine plus electroacupuncture

One three-arm study tested the combination of CHM and electroacupuncture in 180 women (C3). Among women with dysmenorrhoea at baseline, the number who continued to have dysmenorrhoea at the end of treatment was lower in the intervention group compared with the group who received mifepristone (RR 0.48 [0.30, 0.76]). Similarly, the number of women who continued to experience dyspareunia was lower in the intervention group at the end of treatment (RR 0.59 [0.42, 0.82]). Women in the intervention and control groups underwent IVF treatment, and the number of pregnancies was higher in the intervention group (RR 1.31 [1.02, 1.67]).

Compared with the no treatment control group, CHM plus electroacupuncture reduced the number of women with dysmenorrhoea (RR 0.33 [0.22, 0.49]) and dyspareunia (RR 0.52 [0.38, 0.71]) at the end of treatment. Women in the 'no treatment' control group did not undergo IVF treatment, so no comparison was made with the number of pregnancies.

Chinese herbal medicine plus acupuncture point stimulator

One study that used CHM and an acupuncture point stimulator measured cyst recurrence one year after surgery in 87 women (C4). There was no difference in the number of recurrence cases between women who received CHM plus acupuncture point stimulation and those who received danazol (risk ratio, RR, 0.98 [0.21, 4.58]).

Chinese herbal medicine plus acupuncture and moxibustion

The combination of CHM, acupuncture, and moxibustion was compared with gestrinone in one study of 60 women (C2). There was no statistical difference between groups in cyst recurrence three months after treatment (RR 1.00 [0.07, 15.26]) or six months after treatment (RR 0.11 [0.01, 1.98]).

Chinese herbal medicine plus acupuncture, tuina 推拿 and hormone therapy

Chinese herbal medicine was combined with acupuncture, tuina 推拿 (Chinese massage), and triptorelin acetate injection in one study with 80 women (C5). This combination resulted in a dysmenorrhoea VAS score that was 1.96 cm lower than in women who received triptorelin acetate injection ([−2.30, −1.62]). The combination was not statistically different from triptorelin acetate injection in reducing the number of women with cyst recurrence three months after treatment (RR 1.00 [0.21, 4.66]) or 12 months after treatment (RR 0.60 [0.30, 1.21]).

Chinese herbal medicine plus acupuncture, moxibustion, and plum-blossom needle therapy

In one study of 70 women, the combination of CHM, acupuncture, moxibustion, and plum-blossom needle therapy reduced the number of women with dysmenorrhoea among those with pain at baseline compared with danazol (RR 1.38 [1.01, 1.88]; C6). However, CM therapies did not reduce the number of women with dyspareunia (RR 0.50 [0.19, 1.33]).

Controlled Clinical Trials of Combination Therapies for Endometriosis

One CCT that included 132 women with endometriosis met the eligibility criteria (C7). Diagnosis was confirmed by laparoscopy, and adult women with rASRM stage I and II endometriosis were recruited after surgery from an inpatient hospital department in China. The average age of participants was 28.4 years and the average duration of endometriosis was 4.4 years. Treatment was provided for between three and six months, and the women were followed up for between three and 12 months.

The CM syndrome of Blood stagnation was used as an inclusion criterion. Two intervention groups were compared with a control group who received mifepristone. One intervention group tested the combination of CHM, acupuncture, and moxibustion, while the other tested this combination plus mifepristone. The formula *Dan e fu kang jian gao* 丹莪妇康煎膏 with herb ingredients including *chai hu* 柴胡, *dan shen* 丹参, *e zhu* 莪术, *san leng* 三棱, *dang gui* 当归, *yan hu suo* 延胡索, and *gan cao* 甘草 was used in the luteal phase of the menstrual cycle. Acupuncture and moxibustion were applied to acupuncture points CV3 *Zhongji* 中极, CV4 *Guanyuan* 关元, CV6 *Qihai* 气海, SP6 *Sanyinjiao* 三阴交, LR3 *Taichong* 太冲, EX-CA1 *Zigong* (Uterus) 子宫, KI13 *Qixue* 气穴, and KI3 *Taixi* 太溪, although each intervention was used at different times of the menstrual cycle.

Acupuncture was applied for 30 minutes daily for seven days, starting on the fifth day of the menstrual cycle. Moxibustion was commenced prior to the onset of pain and was used for less than three days.

The study evaluated dysmenorrhoea and recurrence. Dysmenorrhoea was assessed using the scale from the 1993 *Guideline for Clinical Research on New Chinese Herbal Medicine Drugs* (中药新药临床研究指导原则; 'the 1993 Guideline').[1] The combination of CM therapies resulted in a lower dysmenorrhoea score — indicating less pain — than mifepristone. This finding was seen when CHM, acupuncture, and moxibustion were used alone (MD −2.34 points [−3.70, −0.98]) or combined with mifepristone (MD −2.55 points [−3.92, −1.18]).

Recurrence was assessed in all participants, but the time at which recurrence was assessed was not specified. The combination of CHM, acupuncture, and moxibustion was no more likely to prevent recurrence when used alone (RR 1.09 [0.43, 2.74]) or as integrative medicine with mifepristone (RR 0.13 [0.02, 1.02]) than mifepristone.

Non-controlled Studies of Combination Therapies for Endometriosis

Four non-controlled studies assessed the combination of CM therapies in adult women with endometriosis (C8–C11). One study was a case series of 51 women from China (C8), one described a case report from a Chinese hospital outpatient department (C11), and two were case reports from community practices in the US (C9, C10). Two studies reported endometriosis durations of two (C9) or three years (C11). Endometriosis was confirmed by laparoscopy in one case report (C9), and none of the studies reported the rASRM stage of participants.

The treatment duration ranged from two months (C8) to one year (C11). One case report described the CM syndrome of *qi* stagnation and Blood stasis (C11), one described *qi* and Blood deficiency with heat (C10), and a third described multiple syndromes of Kidney *yang* deficiency, Liver *qi* and Blood stagnation, and Spleen *qi* deficiency (C9). All studies combined CHM with an acupuncture therapy, with the CHM modified according to the time of the menstrual cycle.

Two studies tested investigator-developed oral CHM formulas and CHM enema (C8, C11). CHM was combined with ear acupressure in the study by Xiang (C8), while Chen (C11) combined an investigator-developed formula with moxibustion. Moxibustion was applied to CV4 *Guanyuan* 关元 with a herb mixture as a medium. Traditional formulas were combined with acupuncture in the remaining two case reports. One study used *Yun nan bai yao* 云南白药 plus acupuncture (C10), while the other combined *Xiao yao san* 逍遥散 plus acupuncture. Both case reports tailored treatment according to the menstrual cycle.

Safety of Combination Therapies for Endometriosis

Safety was reported in four studies (C4, C6–C8). One case series reported that no adverse events occurred (C8). Eight adverse events were reported in the treatment groups, including three cases of acne, three cases of gastrointestinal discomfort, one case of local skin itch, and one case of weight gain. Eighty-seven adverse events were reported among women who received pharmacotherapy. These included 22 cases of weight gain, 15 cases of acne, 11 cases of abnormal liver function, 10 cases of tidal fever, eight cases of vaginal bleeding, seven cases of nausea and vomiting, five cases of amenorrhoea, five cases of breast distention, and four cases of nausea.

Adenomyosis

Five studies tested combinations of CM therapies in women with adenomyosis. Two were RCTs (C12, C13) and three were non-controlled studies (C14–C16).

Randomised Controlled Trials of Combination Therapies for Adenomyosis

The effects of combination CM therapies on adenomyosis was examined in two RCTs conducted in China involving 207 adult women (C12, C13). The median duration of disease was four years and the median age of participants was 35.7 years. Neither study reported using laparoscopy for diagnosis nor did they report surgical treatment prior to enrolment.

Chinese medicine syndrome was used as an inclusion criterion in one study that included women with the syndrome cold congealing and Blood stasis (C13). One study used CM therapies alone (C13) while the other combined CM therapies with conventional medical treatments. Treatment was provided for three months in both studies. All women completed the trials.

Treatment involved the combination of CHM with an acupuncture therapy. In one study, the formula *Nei yi xiao zheng tang* 内异消癥汤 with herb ingredients *dang gui* 当归, *huang qi* 黄芪, *mu li* 牡蛎, *bai zhu* 白术, *e zhu* 莪术, *fu ling* 茯苓, *chai hu* 柴胡, *jiang huang* 姜黄, *bai shao* 白芍, *shui zhi fen* 水蛭粉, and *gan cao* 甘草 was used from the twelfth day of the menstrual cycle (C12). This was combined with acupuncture to SP6 *Sanyinjiao* 三阴交, CV3 *Zhongji* 中极, ST36 *Zusanli* 足三里, ST25 *Tianshu* 天枢, and SP8 *Diji* 地机, administered daily from the eighth day of the menstrual cycle. Both groups received mifepristone and ibuprofen.

The second study used CHM with moxibustion (C13). The formula *Zi ni wen jing huo xue fang* 自拟温经活血方 included *dang gui* 当归, *chi shao* 赤芍, *chuan xiong* 川芎, *tao ren* 桃仁, *hong hua* 红花, *wu ling zhu* 五灵脂, *pu huang* 蒲黄, *yan hu suo* 延胡索, *gan jiang* 干姜, *ru xiang* 乳香, *mo yao* 没药, *xiao hui xiang* 小茴香, *gui zhi* 桂枝, *wu zhu yu* 吴茱萸, and *zhi gan cao* 炙甘草. The formula was modified seven days before menstruation to add *shui zhi* 水蛭, *wu gong* 蜈蚣, and *bie jia* 鳖甲 and was changed to *yan hu suo* 延胡索, *ru xiang* 乳香, *mo yao* 没药 with *tu si zi* 菟丝子, *nv zhen zi* 女贞子, and *du zhong* 杜仲 from the end of the period until the fourteenth day of the cycle. Moxibustion was applied to points on the Governor

Vessel meridian, from GV2 *Yaoshu* 腰俞 to GV14 *Dazhui* 大椎. Moxibustion involved the placement of a herbal paste made of herbs such as *fu zi* 附子, *rou gui* 肉桂, *gui zhi* 桂枝, *du zhong* 杜仲, *ding xiang* 丁香, *cu* 醋, and *yan hu suo* 延胡索 onto the skin, placing a slice of ginger on the paste, and a moxa cone on the ginger. Three cones were applied on the third day before menstruation and three days after the end of menstruation. Mifepristone was used as the comparator.

Risk of Bias Assessment

Both studies were assessed as having low risk of bias for sequence generation as both used a random number table for group allocation. Insufficient information was provided about group concealment, so this posed an unclear risk of bias. Neither study blinded participants or personnel, and were considered as having high risk of bias. All participants completed the studies with outcome data available. Neither study reported trial registration or published a trial protocol, and both were judged as having unclear risk of bias for selective outcome reporting.

Clinical Evidence for Combination Chinese Medicine Therapies

The results reported by included studies were subject to additional analysis. As interventions in the two studies were different, it was not possible to conduct meta-analysis. Results are presented separately.

Chinese herbal medicine plus acupuncture and hormone therapy

The study that tested CHM plus acupuncture as integrative medicine with hormone therapy reported on dysmenorrhoea as measured with a VAS and uterine volume (C12). The combination of CHM, acupuncture, mifepristone, and ibuprofen resulted in a score that was 0.97 cm lower on the VAS compared to mifepristone and ibuprofen alone

(82 women, [−0.97, −0.64]). Further, the uterine volume in women who received the combination of CM therapies with conventional treatment was lower than in women who received conventional treatment alone (82 women, MD −12.56 cm^3 [−16.93, −8.19]).

Chinese herbal medicine plus moxibustion

Dysmenorrhoea, assessed using the 1993 Guideline, and uterine volume were measured in one study (C13). Dysmenorrhoea was 2.58 points lower at the end of treatment among women who received CHM plus moxibustion compared with women who received mifepristone (125 women, [−3.30, −1.86]). Uterine volume was not statistically different between the two groups at the end of treatment (125 women, MD 2.57 mm^3 [−71.45, 76.59]).

Non-controlled Studies of Combination Therapies for Adenomyosis

Three non-controlled studies tested combination CM therapies in adult women with adenomyosis (C14–C16). Two case series involved 70 women with adenomyosis (C14, C16), and the third was a case report (C15). All studies were conducted in China, and two were in an outpatient department setting (C14, C15). The mean age of participants was 43.5 years in one case series (C14) and was not reported in other studies. The mean duration of adenomyosis was not specified in one study (C16), and was three years or greater in the other studies. None of the studies reported using laparoscopy for diagnosis or prior surgery for treatment.

All studies reported CM syndromes, which included *qi* and Blood stasis (C14), cold and dampness (C14), *qi* stagnation with cold congealing and Blood stasis (C15), and Kidney *yang* deficiency with Blood stasis (C16). Treatment ranged from three (C14, C16) to four months (C15). Chinese herbal medicine formulas were developed by study investigators in each study; these were administered according to the time of the menstrual cycle in two studies (C14, C15).

The case report (C15) tested moxibustion for three months plus oral CHM during menstruation (C15). In the first case series (C14), oral CHM and moxibustion were used during menstrual cycle days 12–16, and for one week before menstruation. The second case series (C16) used an investigator-developed oral CHM formula throughout the menstrual cycle, which was combined with umbilical therapy to the acupuncture point CV8 *Shenque* 神阙 using a variety of CHM herbs.

Safety of Combination Therapies for Adenomyosis

One of the five studies reported on safety (C12). Among women who received CHM plus acupuncture, adverse events included two cases of nausea and one case each of fatigue and dizziness. Adverse events in women who received mifepristone and ibuprofen included three cases of nausea, two cases of dizziness, and one case of fatigue.

Endometriosis and Adenomyosis

One RCT included women with either endometriosis, adenomyosis, or both conditions of 10 years duration (C17). The study, conducted in a hospital outpatient department in China, included 100 women with a mean age of 31 years. All participants received the same treatment, and the authors did not report CM syndromes.

Treatment with CHM and moxibustion was provided for three months. The formula *Gui zhi er chen tang* 桂枝二陈汤 was used for seven days starting one day before the menstrual period. Herb ingredients included *gui zhi* 桂枝, *chi shao* 赤芍, *bai fu ling* 白茯苓, *tao ren* 桃仁, *mu dan pi* 牡丹皮, *san leng* 三棱, *e zhu* 莪术, *shui zhi* 水蛭, *wei ling xian* 威灵仙, *mang xiao* 芒硝, *chen pi* 陈皮, *yu jin* 郁金, *ban xiao* 半夏, and *zhi gan cao* 炙甘草. Moxibustion was applied to EX-CA1 *Zigong* (Uterus) 子宫, CV3 *Zhongji* 中极, BL32 *Ciliao* 次髎, CV4 *Guanyuan* 关元, CV6 *Qihai* 气海, BL23 *Shenshu* 肾俞, ST36 *Zusanli* 足三里, ST40 *Fenglong* 丰隆, and SP6 *Sanyinjiao* 三阴交 for 15–20 minutes per day for seven days, starting one day before the menstrual cycle. The control group received 2.5 mg of gestrinone twice weekly for three months.

The study authors used a random number table to allocate participants to each group, and the study was judged as having low risk of bias for sequence generation. The method for concealing group allocation was unclear as insufficient information was provided. Neither participants nor personnel were blind to group allocation, posing high risk of bias. No information was provided as to whether outcome assessors were blinded to group allocation (unclear risk). All participants completed the study and there was no missing data, so the study was judged to pose low risk of bias for incomplete outcome data. As no trial protocol or trial registration was identified, the potential risk of selective outcome reporting was unclear.

Dysmenorrhoea severity was assessed using a 10 cm VAS. The mean VAS score at the end of three months was 2.7 cm lower among women who received the combination of CHM and moxibustion compared to gestrinone (100 women, [−3.28, −2.12]). The authors reported that no adverse events occurred during the trial.

Summary of Combination Therapies Evidence

This chapter summarised the use of two or more CM therapies in combination for endometriosis and/or adenomyosis. All studies used CHM and an acupuncture therapy as the intervention, with one study adding *tuina* 推拿 to the combination. Although the combined use of CHM and acupuncture therapies is common in clinical practice, there were few eligible clinical studies that have evaluated the combination in women with endometriosis and/or adenomyosis.

Many of the studies tested investigator-developed formulas that were modified according to the time of the menstrual cycle. While there was no overlap in formulas among the included studies, several herbs were used in multiple formulas: *dang gui* 当归, *gui zhi* 桂枝, and *wu ling zhi* 五灵脂. Acupuncture points SP6 *Sanyinjiao* 三阴交 and CV4 *Guanyuan* 关元 were also used in clinical studies; both points are recommended in clinical textbooks.[2]

Clinical Evidence for Combination Therapies

Results from individual studies suggest that the combination of CHM with acupuncture therapies may improve dysmenorrhoea and dyspareunia, but does not appear to reduce the risk of recurrence. As none of the studies were free from bias, the available evidence is insufficient to make recommendations for clinical practice. Further research that evaluates combination therapies for endometriosis and adenomyosis is needed.

Few adverse events were reported with combined CM therapies. Based on the available evidence, the combination of CHM and acupuncture therapies appear to be tolerated well by women with endometriosis or adenomyosis. Clinicians should consider the suitability of combined CM therapies for each individual patient.

References

1. 郑筱萸. (1993) 中药新药临床研究指导原则. 北京: 中国医药科技出版社.
2. 国家中医药管理局医政司. (2011) 24 个专业 105 个病种中医诊疗方案-癥瘕病 (卵巢巧克力样囊肿) 中医诊疗方案. 北京: 国家中医药管理局医政司.

References for Included Combination Therapies Clinical Studies

Study No.	Reference
C1	牛向馨, 牛乾, 王小蔓, *et al.* (2013) 平冲化瘀通络法联合灸法治疗子宫内膜异位症痛经32例的临床研究. 中国实验方剂学杂志 **19**(19): 329–332.
C2	张晓云, 张春雁. (2014) 针药结合预防子宫内膜异位症腹腔镜手术后复发疗效观察. 中国针灸 **34**(2): 139–144.
C3	于晓丽, 陈军, 孙伟. (2010) 针药对因子宫内膜异位症行体外受精患者妊娠结局的影响. 辽宁中医杂志 **37**(4): 731–733.
C4	姚琳琳. (2014) 中药加理疗防治卵巢子宫内膜异位囊肿术后复发的临床观察. 亚太传统医药 **10**(1): 95–96.
C5	孙红燕, 梁志超. (2018) 中医综合疗法治疗卵巢子宫内膜异位囊肿术后患者疗效观察. 现代中西医结合杂志 **27**(14): 1491–1493, 1496.

(Continued)

(Continued)

Study No.	Reference
C6	Xia T. (2006) Effect of acupuncture and traditional Chinese herbal medicine in treating endometriosis. *International Journal of Clinical Acupuncture* **15**(3): 145–150.
C7	雷换丽. (2014) 子宫内膜异位症腹腔镜术后中西医结合治疗的临床研究. 新乡医学院.
C8	向东方, 梁雪芳, 司徒仪. (2005) 中医多途径疗法治疗子宫内膜异位症痛经51例分析. *中医药学刊* **23**(9): 1616–1617.
C9	Handlin J. (2012) A case study on infertility due to endometriosis and advanced maternal age treated with traditional Chinese medicine. *American Acupuncturist* **61**: 26–40.
C10	Li Z. (2003) Regulating the Penetrating and Conception vessels to treat dysmenorrhoea: Two case histories. *Journal of Chinese Medicine* **73**: 13–15.
C11	陈光盛. (2006) 汪慧敏教授治疗子宫内膜异位症特色. *中医药学刊* **24**(5): 791–792.
C12	代学华, 叶永梅, 郭停. (2018) 扶正化瘀法联合西医疗法治疗子宫腺肌病的疗效观察. *世界临床药物* **39**(5): 334–337.
C13	王璐. (2016) 督灸联合温经活血方治疗寒凝血瘀型子宫腺肌症痛经的临床观察. *湖北中医杂志* **38**(6): 16–18.
C14	彭婧, 李娟, 朱赛英. (2015) 活血通络,化瘀止痛法配合穴位贴敷治疗子宫腺肌病32例临床观察. *实用中西医结合临床* (5): 47–48.
C15	詹明洁, 金颢璇. (2011) 汪慧敏教授治疗子宫腺肌病经验撷菁. *光明中医* **26**(8): 1545–1546.
C16	侣雪平, 刘欣彤, 姚艺, et al. (2014) 自拟补肾逐瘀汤配合脐疗治疗肾虚血瘀型子宫腺肌病痛经的临床观察. *中医药学报* **42**(6): 103–104.
C17	刘志霞, 刘志宏. (2016) 中药联合艾灸治疗子宫内膜异位症疗效观察. *陇东学院学报* **27**(03): 78–82.

9

Summary and Conclusions

OVERVIEW

Endometriosis and adenomyosis are chronic gynaecological conditions with a significant health burden. Surgery can alleviate symptoms, but recurrence is common. Women may look to Chinese medicine as a treatment option for long-term management of symptoms. This chapter provides a 'whole-evidence' analysis of CM treatments for signs and symptoms of endometriosis and adenomyosis. Treatments described in the contemporary and classical literature are compared with clinical studies, and the clinical efficacy and safety of CM treatments are described. The implications for clinical practice and research are highlighted.

Introduction

Endometriosis and adenomyosis are common gynaecological conditions in women of reproductive age.[1] Growth of endometrial-like tissue outside the uterus is associated with dysmenorrhoea, dyspareunia, chronic pelvic pain, low abdominal and back pain, fatigue, and impaired fertility.[2,3] The chronic nature of the condition requires a lifelong management plan that prioritises medical management over surgical treatment.[4] Women with endometriosis are more likely than those without endometriosis to seek treatment with complementary therapies, including Chinese medicine (CM) and acupuncture.[5]

This monograph provides a 'whole-evidence' analysis of CM treatments for the management of signs and symptoms of endometriosis and adenomyosis. Treatments recommended in clinical guidelines and textbooks include Chinese herbal medicine (CHM), acupuncture, ear acupuncture, abdominal acupuncture, and moxibustion (see Chapter 2). Management of signs and symptoms with CHM was a key focus in past eras (Chapter 3) and continues to be a focus in clinical research (Chapter 5). Acupuncture was less frequently described in classical literature and was evaluated in a small body of clinical studies (Chapter 7). Findings from meta-analyses of clinical studies showed promising effects of CHM for alleviating endometriosis-associated pain and reducing the chance of recurrence (Chapter 5).

Chinese Medicine Syndrome Differentiation

Syndrome differentiation is the cornerstone of CM treatment. Contemporary clinical textbooks and guidelines describe six syndromes that are common in women with endometriosis or adenomyosis: *qi* stagnation and Blood stasis 气滞血瘀, Kidney deficiency and Blood stasis 肾虚血瘀, cold congealing and Blood stasis 寒凝血瘀, *qi* deficiency and Blood stasis 气虚血瘀, phlegm and stasis binding 痰瘀互结, and dampness-heat and stasis obstructing the uterus 湿热瘀阻. While only three of the six syndromes — *qi* stagnation and Blood stasis 气滞血瘀, cold congealing and Blood stasis 寒凝血瘀, and dampness-heat and stasis obstructing the uterus 湿热瘀阻 — were specifically named in citations from the classical literature, the key concepts of these syndromes were mentioned. These included *qi* deficiency, Kidney deficiency, and Blood stasis.

Chinese medicine syndrome differentiation was a key feature of clinical studies. Among the biggest pool of CHM studies — oral CHM for endometriosis — 80 randomised controlled trials (RCTs) described using CM syndrome differentiation as an inclusion criterion or to guide treatment, with many RCTs describing multiple syndromes. The most frequently reported syndromes were Kidney deficiency with Blood stasis (24 studies) and *qi* stagnation and Blood stasis (23 studies). Other CM syndromes found three or more times among included studies were cold coagulation and Blood stasis (12 studies), *qi* deficiency and Blood stasis (eight studies), damp-heat stasis (four

Summary and Conclusions

studies), Liver *qi* stagnation (four studies), damp-heat (three studies), and phlegm-dampness (three studies).

Several syndromes described in Chapter 2 were also identified in clinical studies of acupuncture therapies. Both *qi* stagnation and Blood stasis (four studies) and Blood stasis (two studies) were described in multiple studies, while Kidney deficiency and Blood stasis as well as *qi* deficiency and Blood stasis were reported in one study each. Among studies that included combinations of CM treatments, four syndromes were reported in multiple studies: *qi* stagnation and Blood stasis (three studies), *qi* deficiency and Blood stasis (two studies), Kidney deficiency and Blood stasis (two studies), and phlegm-damp stasis (two studies). In addition, one study reported another syndrome described in Chapter 2: cold congealing and Blood stasis.

In addition to the syndromes described in Chapter 2, clinical studies described other syndromes, many of which included the same key concepts or different combinations of key concepts. *Yang* deficiency, phlegm, Spleen *qi* deficiency, and Liver *qi* stagnation were also seen in women with endometriosis and adenomyosis. Clinicians can be reassured that the syndromes reported in clinical studies are aligned with those reported in clinical guidelines, meaning that treatments being tested are likely to be relevant for clinical practice.

Chinese Herbal Medicine

This section summarises the findings from Chapters 2, 3, 5, and 8. Chinese herbal medicine is an important treatment option for the signs and symptoms of endometriosis and adenomyosis. Contemporary clinical textbooks and guidelines that informed the content in Chapter 2 describe both traditional formulas and manufactured products for each of the six key CM syndromes. In addition to the formulas for oral consumption, the contemporary literature also describes topical CHM products that can be applied to the abdomen or to acupuncture points, as well as CHM enemas.

Both oral and topical CHM have been used throughout the history of CM (Chapter 3). The earliest identified use of CHM for dysmenorrhoea was in the books *Hua Tuo Shen Fang* 华佗神方 and *Qian Jin Yi Fang* 千金翼方 (both c. 682 CE). Oral CHM was mentioned much more often than topical CHM, highlighting its relative importance. *Si wu tang* 四物汤 was the most frequently described oral CHM, a formula well known for treating gynaecological symptoms. *Si wu tang* 四物汤 consists of the herbs *dang gui* 当归, *bai shao* 白芍, *chuan xiong* 川芎, and *sheng di huang* 生地黄. *Dang gui* 当归, *bai shao* 白芍, and *chuan xiong* 川芎 were the three most common herbs, while *shu di huang* 熟地黄, sourced from the same plant as *sheng di huang* 生地黄, was the fourth. Topical preparations of CHM were also described throughout CM history, albeit less frequently, and were used as vaginal pessaries, applied as a paste to the umbilicus, or used as a genital wash.

Interest in CHM treatment of endometriosis and adenomyosis has continued throughout CM history and in contemporary clinical research. The majority of studies that met the inclusion criteria for this review were for oral CHM (Chapter 5); the popularity of oral CHM in clinical studies aligns with clinical practice. Of the 305 clinical studies that tested CHM for women with endometriosis, 268 tested oral CHM, 15 tested topical CHM, and 22 tested the combination of oral and topical CHM.

The number of studies that tested CHM in women with adenomyosis was smaller (96 clinical studies), but not insignificant; oral CHM was tested in 88 studies, topical CHM was evaluated in five studies, and the combination of oral plus topical CHM was used in three studies. Oral CHM was the main treatment method in studies that included either endometriosis or adenomyosis (or both), used in 28 of the 30 studies. Finally, oral CHM was the focus of an important group of studies that evaluated its potential role in reducing the side effects of gonadotropin-releasing hormone agonists (GnRHa).

Many clinical studies of CHM closely resembled practice: treatment was provided for between three and six months, follow-up assessments were conducted beyond the end of the initial treatment period, and investigators tailored treatment according to the time of

Summary and Conclusions

the menstrual cycle. These factors can reassure practitioners that the findings from included studies are relevant to clinical practice.

Results from RCTs and controlled clinical trials (CCTs) were analysed according to pre-specified outcomes and by comparison. Results of meta-analyses from RCTs, which are considered the highest level of evidence from clinical research, showed many positive effects of CHM.

In studies of women with endometriosis, oral CHM was superior to no treatment in reducing visual analogue scale (VAS) dysmenorrhoea scores, reducing the rate of recurrence beyond the end of treatment, increasing the pregnancy rate, and improving health-related quality of life on some domains of the general wellbeing scale Medical Outcome Study 36-Item Short-Form Health Survey (SF-36).[6] The formula *San jie zhen tong jiao nang* 散结镇痛胶囊 was better than no treatment in preventing recurrence two years after the end of treatment. In addition, oral CHM was better than placebo in reducing ovarian cyst diameter.

When compared with pharmacotherapy, meta-analyses showed that oral CHM used alone reduced dysmenorrhoea at the end of treatment and during follow-up; reduced recurrence of signs and symptoms, generally, and pain, specifically; increased the pregnancy rate in women trying to conceive; and improved health-related quality of life on some domains of the Endometriosis Health Profile 30-item scale (EHP-30)[7] and the abbreviated version of the World Health Organization Quality of Life Instruments (WHOQOL-BREF).[8] Evidence from one meta-analysis showed that the commercially manufactured product *San jie zhen tong jiao nang* 散结镇痛胶囊 reduced the chance of recurrence of signs and symptoms two years after the end of treatment.

When the combination of oral CHM and pharmacotherapy was compared with pharmacotherapy alone, the combination was more effective in reducing dysmenorrhoea at the end of treatment and at follow-up, reducing recurrence of signs and symptoms as well as cysts, reducing cyst diameter, increasing the pregnancy rate, and reducing the chance of miscarriage. Additionally, *Dan leng fu kang jian gao* 丹棱妇康煎膏 used in combination with pharmacotherapy was superior to pharmacotherapy alone in reducing dysmenorrhoea.

The most clinically important evidence of oral CHM for women with endometriosis was evaluated using the Grading of Recommendations Assessment, Development and Evaluation (GRADE) framework (see Chapter 4 for more detail). The strength and quality ('certainty') of the evidence was rated for each outcome. Analysis showed that oral CHM probably reduces dysmenorrhoea VAS scores compared to placebo (moderate certainty evidence). Oral CHM may slightly reduce dysmenorrhoea VAS scores and the total score for the EHP-30 (both low certainty evidence) compared to hormone therapy (HT). Oral CHM probably has little or no influence on live births compared to HT (moderate certainty evidence), and the true effect of oral CHM on VAS pelvic pain and dyspareunia scores is uncertain (low certainty evidence).

Assessments using the GRADE framework were also conducted for the combination of oral CHM and HT. There is uncertainty over whether the combination was more effective compared to HT alone in reducing VAS scores for dysmenorrhoea, pelvic pain, or dyspareunia scores (all very low certainty evidence). CHM plus HT may slightly reduce the recurrence of signs and symptoms at the end of treatment and at one year after surgery (both low certainty evidence). CHM plus HT probably makes little or no difference on live birth rates (moderate certainty evidence).

Analysis of formulas using the GRADE framework found that the combination of *Xue fu zhu yu tang* 血府逐瘀汤 and HT may slightly improve VAS pelvic pain scores and reduce recurrence of signs and symptoms at the end of treatment (both low certainty evidence), but the evidence for the effect of this combination on dysmenorrhoea or dyspareunia VAS scores and long-term chance of recurrence is uncertain (both very low certainty evidence). A second formula, *Gui zhi fu ling jiao nang* 桂枝茯苓胶囊, may slightly reduce the chance of recurrence of signs and symptoms two years after treatment when combined with HT (low certainty evidence); however, the effect of this combination on the recurrence of cysts one year after surgery was uncertain (low certainty evidence). When both of

Summary and Conclusions

these formulas were used alone, their effects in reducing the chance of recurrence compared with HT were also unclear (low certainty evidence).

In studies of adenomyosis, meta-analysis showed that oral CHM resulted in lower dysmenorrhoea VAS scores than did pharmacotherapy. Meta-analyses also showed that the combination of oral CHM was superior to HT alone in reducing dysmenorrhoea scores using a variety of measures and in reducing uterine and menstrual volume. Benefits were also seen for individual formulas in meta-analyses. When used with pharmacotherapy, *Gui zhi fu ling jiao nang/wan* 桂枝茯苓胶囊/丸, *Shao fu zhu yu tang/jiao nang* 少腹逐瘀汤/胶囊, and *San jie zhen tong jiao nang* 散结镇痛胶囊 all reduced dysmenorrhoea scores and uterine volume.

Meta-analyses of studies that included women with endometriosis, adenomyosis, or both endometriosis and adenomyosis did not indicate superiority of CHM. One meta-analysis of studies that examined the role of CHM in reducing the side effects of GnRHa showed that oral CHM plus pharmacotherapy reduced menopausal symptoms more than pharmacotherapy alone did.

While positive benefits were seen in the analyses described above, there were many other meta-analyses that showed no difference between intervention and control groups. In many cases, particularly those that compared CHM with pharmacotherapy, finding no difference between groups does not mean that CHM was ineffective — a result of no significant difference between CHM and pharmacotherapy suggests that CHM has not been shown to be less effective than the conventional medical treatments recommended in international clinical practice guidelines.

Chinese herbal medicines are often considered safe and natural. Like all drugs, the use of CHM may cause side effects. Reassuringly, the number of side effects reported in clinical studies was not higher in women who received CHM; in fact, when CHM was used in combination with pharmacotherapy, the number of adverse events was lower than with pharmacotherapy alone. This may suggest that CHM can have a preventative effect against the known side effects of conventional medical treatments.

Chinese Herbal Medicine Formulas in Key Clinical Guidelines and Textbooks, Classical Literature and Clinical Studies

The CHM formulas and products recommended in clinical guidelines and textbooks, described in the classical literature, and tested in clinical studies are diverse. A comparison of formulas was undertaken to identify consistencies across sources of evidence and over time. Table 9.1 summarises the traditional CHM formulas recommended in clinical guidelines and textbooks in Chapter 2, the formulas used in past eras in Chapter 3, and those tested in clinical studies in Chapters 5 and 8. Table 9.1 also includes formulas that were tested in 10 or more clinical studies, which may highlight emerging areas of research. Table 9.2 summarises the evidence for manufactured products.

Analysis of formula frequency was made according to the formula name and was not based on herb ingredients. Many clinical studies tested similar formulas, with the same or slightly different herb ingredients, but which were named differently. As such, it is possible that the number of uses of formulas in Tables 9.1 and 9.2 is actually higher than indicated here. Similarly, formulas come in a variety of preparation types — for example, *wan* 丸 (pills), *tang* 汤 (decoctions), and *san* 散 (powders) — only those of the preparation type included in Chapter 2 or used in 10 or more clinical studies are noted in these tables.

None of the traditional formulas included in Chapter 2 were found in the classical literature and only three of these were tested in multiple clinical trials: *Ge xia zhu yu tang* 膈下逐瘀汤 (three studies), *Shao fu zhu yu tang* 少腹逐瘀汤 (six studies), and *Xue fu zhu yu tang* 血府逐瘀汤 (seven studies) (Table 9.1). Both *Shao fu zhu yu tang* 少腹逐瘀汤 and *Xue fu zhu yu tang* 血府逐瘀汤 were used in capsule form in an additional one and three studies, respectively.

Although not recommended in the contemporary literature included in Chapter 2, *Dan leng fu kang jian gao* 丹棱妇康煎膏 was frequently used (11 studies). None of the traditional formulas from clinical guidelines and textbooks were tested in studies of combination CM therapies.

Summary and Conclusions

Table 9.1. Summary of Oral Chinese Herbal Medicine Traditional Formulas

Formula Name	Clinical Guidelines and Textbooks	Classical Literature (No. of Citations)	Clinical Studies (Chapter 5)			Combination Therapies (Chapter 8)
			RCTs (No. of Studies)	CCTs (No. of Studies)	Non-controlled Studies (No. of Studies)	
Cang fu dao tan wan 苍附导痰丸 plus Tao hong si wu tang 桃红四物汤	Yes	0	0	0	0	0
Ge xia zhu yu tang 膈下逐瘀汤	Yes	0	1	1	1	0
Gui shen wan 归肾丸 plus Tao hong si wu tang 桃红四物汤	Yes	0	0	0	0	0
Ju yuan jian 举元煎 plus Shi xiao san 失笑散 and san qi 三七	Yes	0	0	0	0	0
Ju yuan jian 举元煎 plus Tao hong si wu tang 桃红四物汤	Yes	0	0	0	0	0
Li chong tang 理冲汤	Yes	0	0	0	1	0
Qing re tiao xue tang 清热调血汤	Yes	0	1	0	0	0
Shao fu zhu yu tang 少腹逐瘀汤	Yes	0	4	0	2	0
Xue fu zhu yu tang 血府逐瘀汤	Yes	0	4	0	3	0
Dan leng fu kang jian gao 丹棱妇康煎膏	No	0	10	1	0	0

Abbreviations: CCTs: controlled clinical trials; RCTs: randomised controlled trials.

Commercially manufactured CHM products can also be useful to treat the signs and symptoms of endometriosis and adenomyosis; patients often find these preparation types more convenient than decoctions.[9] Four manufactured products were recommended in the guidelines and textbooks included in Chapter 2 (Table 9.2). Of these, *Ai fu nuan gong wan* 艾附暖宫丸 was the only formula recommended in clinical guidelines and textbooks that was also found in the classical literature. *Ai fu nuan gong wan* 艾附暖宫丸 was described in four citation, and the earliest citation was from the book *Ren Zhai Zhi Zhi Fang Lun* 仁斋直指方论 (c. 1264). Other citations were from the Ming and Qing dynasties. This formula was not evaluated in any of the included studies.

San jie zhen tong jiao nang 散结镇痛胶囊 was the most frequently tested formula among all clinical studies (26 studies). This finding was consistent with RCTs of oral CHM for endometriosis (Chapter 5, Part 1) and RCTs of women with either endometriosis, adenomyosis, or both (Chapter 5, Part 3). In RCTs of oral CHM for adenomyosis (Chapter 5, Part 2), *Gui zhi fu ling jiao nang* 桂枝茯苓胶囊 was tested

Table 9.2. Summary of Oral Chinese Herbal Medicine Manufactured Products

Formula Name	Clinical Guidelines and Textbooks	Classical Literature (No. of Citations)	Clinical Studies (Chapter 5)			Combination Therapies (Chapter 8)
			RCTs (No. of Studies)	CCTs (No. of Studies)	Non-controlled Studies (No. of Studies)	
Ai fu nuan gong wan 艾附暖宫丸	Yes	4	0	0	0	0
Dan e kang fu jian gao 丹莪妇康煎膏	Yes	0	0	0	0	1
Gui zhi fu ling jiao nang 桂枝茯苓胶囊	Yes	0	5	3	1	0
San jie zhen tong jiao nang 散结镇痛胶囊	Yes	0	21	4	1	0

Abbreviations: CCTs: controlled clinical trials; RCTs: randomised controlled trials.

in five RCTs, with an additional five RCTs using different preparation types (e.g., *Gui zhi fu ling wan* or *wan fang* 桂枝茯苓丸/丸方). *Dan e kang fu jian gao* 丹莪妇康煎膏 was only tested in one study where it was combined with both acupuncture and moxibustion.

The clinical textbooks and guidelines in Chapter 2 describe formulas that focus on treating endometriosis and adenomyosis, thereby alleviating signs and symptoms. An important group of formulas are not included in Chapter 2 — those with actions to reduce the side effects of conventional medical treatments; in particular, GnRHa. Side effects of GnRHa are due to a low level of oestrogen, and resulting signs and symptoms include those typically associated with menopause: hot flushes, night sweats, and mood changes.

Chinese medicine textbooks and guidelines recommend the traditional formula *Zuo gui wan* 左归丸[10,11] and the manufactured product *Kun tai jiao nang* 坤泰胶囊,[10-12] among others, for menopausal symptoms, and both of these formulas have been tested in multiple clinical studies for menopause.[13] Both *Zuo gui wan* 左归丸 and *Kun tai jiao nang* 坤泰胶囊 were evaluated in three RCTs included in Chapter 5. *Zuo gui wan* 左归丸 improved scores on some domains of the EHP 5-item version[14] and reduced menopausal symptoms as measured with the Kupperman Index,[15] a global measure of menopause symptom severity. Results for *Kun tai jiao nang* 坤泰胶囊 were included in meta-analysis with other CHM formulas and were not reported separately as part of this review. Practitioners may consider these formulas for women who report menopausal symptoms following GnRHa treatment.

Acupuncture and Related Therapies

This section summarises the evidence from Chapters 2, 3, 7, and 8. While acupuncture therapies have not been evaluated as thoroughly as CHM, they remain an important treatment option, especially considering that acupuncture is known to be effective in reducing various types of pain. Four acupuncture therapies were recommended in the clinical guidelines and textbooks on which the content of Chapter 2 was based: acupuncture, ear acupuncture, abdominal acupuncture, and moxibustion. Both acupuncture and moxibustion were described as treatments for endometriosis-like symptoms in the classical literature (Chapter 3).

The number of clinical studies that evaluated the clinical effects of acupuncture therapies (Chapter 7) was much smaller than for CHM. Acupuncture was the key intervention tested and was used in 11 of the 15 included studies. Several studies used different combinations of acupuncture therapies (e.g., acupuncture plus moxibustion or acupuncture, moxibustion, and ear electroacupuncture), which is a common approach in clinical practice.

Due to differences in interventions, comparators, and outcome measures, results from studies could not be pooled for meta-analysis. Results of individual studies were analysed and, where possible, assessments of the certainty of the evidence were made according to the GRADE framework. Analysis showed that acupuncture probably improves pelvic pain (moderate certainty evidence) and dyspareunia (moderate certainty evidence) compared to sham acupuncture, but there is less certainty about its effect in reducing VAS scores for dysmenorrhoea (low certainty evidence). Acupuncture was equally as effective as HT in reducing the chances of having dysmenorrhoea or dyspareunia at the end of treatment (evidence not graded).

Included studies reported minor and expected adverse events with acupuncture therapies, such as bruising, discomfort, and minor burns with moxibustion. Of note, women who received moxibustion reported a higher likelihood of recurrence of pain or cysts, while women who received warm needle acupuncture (moxibustion on top of acupuncture needles) scored worse on some domains of quality of life scales than women who received HT. As moxibustion was common to both findings, practitioners may consider the appropriateness of this intervention for women with endometriosis and adenomyosis.

Acupuncture Therapies in Key Clinical Guidelines and Textbooks, Classical Literature and Clinical Studies

Consistency in the use of acupuncture therapies was examined across different sources of evidence. Many of the clinical studies

Summary and Conclusions

included in Chapters 7 and 8 combined different acupuncture therapies — for example, acupuncture plus moxibustion — and each intervention is counted separately in Table 9.3. This meant that the sum of the number of studies for each intervention is greater than the number of included studies. Further, studies that used electroacupuncture were counted in the group 'acupuncture', as acupuncture needles must be inserted through the skin in order to apply electrical stimulation. One exception to this was for a study that used ear electroacupuncture and was included in the group 'ear acupuncture'.

Acupuncture techniques recommended in clinical guidelines and textbooks included in Chapter 2 and those found in classical literature and evaluated in clinical studies are summarised in Table 9.3. Both acupuncture and moxibustion are recommended in contemporary literature (Chapter 2), were found in classical literature citations (Chapter 3), and have been evaluated in clinical studies, alone or in combination with other CM therapies.

Developed in the 1950s, ear acupuncture is a relatively new acupuncture technique.[16] As such, we would not have expected to find references to ear acupuncture in classical literature. Only one RCT used ear acupuncture or, more specifically, ear electroacupuncture, despite ear acupuncture being recommended in textbooks and

Table 9.3. Summary of Acupuncture and Related Therapies

Intervention	Clinical Guidelines and Textbooks (Chapter 2)	Classical Literature (Chapter 3) (No. of Citations)	Clinical Studies (Chapter 7)*			Combination Therapies (Chapter 8)
			RCTs (No. of Studies)	CCTs (No. of Studies)	Non-controlled Studies (No. of Studies)	
Acupuncture	Yes	3	8	2	1	7
Ear acupuncture	Yes	0	1	0	0	0
Abdominal acupuncture	Yes	0	0	0	0	1
Moxibustion	Yes	5	5	1	1	8

*Some studies used more than one intervention (e.g., acupuncture plus moxibustion). These are counted separately in this table.
Abbreviations: CCTs: controlled clinical trials; RCTs: randomised controlled trials.

guidelines. This may be due to the small number of studies that met the inclusion criteria for review.

Like ear acupuncture, abdominal acupuncture is a recently developed acupuncture microsystem that uses both meridian and extra points to treat disease. Abdominal acupuncture is recommended in textbooks and guidelines for the treatment of endometriosis and adenomyosis. Abdominal acupuncture as a system was not tested in included studies; however, one non-controlled study combined umbilical therapy (a system of treatment using points on and around the umbilicus) with CHM, while other studies used points on the abdomen (some of which are also used in abdominal acupuncture) as part of treatment using local and distal points.

In addition to comparing the interventions used across evidence sources, analysis was also conducted to identify the acupuncture points that have been used consistently throughout CM history and those that are frequently tested in clinical studies. Results are summarised in Table 9.4. As highlighted above, the abdominal acupuncture microsystem was not specifically tested in any of the

Table 9.4. Summary of Acupuncture Points

Intervention	Clinical Guidelines and Textbooks (Chapter 2)	Classical Literature (Chapter 3) No. of Citations)	Clinical Studies (Chapter 7)*			Combination Therapies (Chapter 8)*
			RCTs (No. of Studies)	CCTs (No. of Studies)	Non-controlled Studies (No. of Studies)	
Acupuncture						
CV4 Guanyuan 关元	Yes	1	5	1	1	5
CV3 Zhongji 中极	Yes	1	6	1	0	3
SP6 Sanyinjiao 三阴交	Yes	2	7	2	1	7
SP10 Xuehai 血海	Yes	0	4	1	1	2
EX-CA1 Zigong 子宫	Yes	0	2	0	0	2

Summary and Conclusions

Table 9.4. (*Continued*)

Intervention	Clinical Guidelines and Textbooks (Chapter 2)	Classical Literature (Chapter 3) No. of Citations	Clinical Studies (Chapter 7)*			Combination Therapies (Chapter 8)*
			RCTs (No. of Studies)	CCTs (No. of Studies)	Non-controlled Studies (No. of Studies)	
ST36 *Zusanli* 足三里	Yes	0	3	0	1	2
Ear acupuncture						
TF2 *Zigong* 子宫	Yes	0	0	0	0	0
TF2 *Luanchao* 卵巢	Yes	0	0	0	0	0
CO18 *Neifenmi* 内分泌	Yes	0	0	0	0	0
TF4 *Shenmen* 神门	Yes	0	0	0	0	0
AT4 *Pizhixia* 皮质下	Yes	0	0	0	0	0
CO12 *Gan* 肝	Yes	0	0	0	0	0
CO10 *Shen* 肾	Yes	0	0	0	0	0
Abdominal acupuncture						
CV3 *Zhongji* 中极	Yes	0	0	0	0	0
ST26 *Wailing* 外陵	Yes	0	0	0	0	0
Xiafengshidian 下风湿点	Yes	0	0	0	0	0
Moxibustion						
CV8 *Shenque* 神阙	Yes	1	1	0	0	1
CV4 *Guanyuan* 关元	Yes	0	2	1	0	3
SP6 *Sanyinjiao* 三阴交	Yes	0	2	0	1	5

*Some studies used more than one intervention (e.g., acupuncture plus moxibustion). These are counted separately in this table.
Abbreviations: CCTs: controlled clinical trials; RCTs: randomised controlled trials.

included studies, while one study that applied electroacupuncture to ear points did not specify which points were used. As such, there is no data from the included studies about which acupuncture points of the abdominal acupuncture microsystem, and which points stimulated with electroacupuncture, could relieve signs and symptoms of endometriosis and adenomyosis.

Four acupuncture points that are recommended in the contemporary literature were found in classical texts: CV4 *Guanyuan* 关元, CV3 *Zhongji* 中极, SP6 *Sanyinjiao* 三阴交 (all used with acupuncture), and CV8 *Shenque* 神阙 (used with moxibustion). Among those recommended in the contemporary literature, the most frequently tested acupuncture point in clinical trials was SP6 *Sanyinjiao* 三阴交, followed by CV4 *Guanyuan* 关元. Practitioners may consider these points as the main acupuncture points for women with endometriosis or adenomyosis, and may select supplementary points according to each individual's CM syndrome differentiation.

Limitations of Evidence

The information included in this monograph has been identified using a rigorous and comprehensive approach. While every effort has been made to ensure the accuracy of the contents of this monograph, the information described herein is not exhaustive. Many CM textbooks on gynaecology and specialist textbooks on endometriosis exist, so it is possible that other textbooks and guidelines may describe different CM syndromes, CHM formulas, acupuncture techniques, and other CM therapies for endometriosis and adenomyosis. The information included in Chapter 2 should not be considered exhaustive, and clinicians should continue to expand their clinical knowledge by reading widely to provide the best quality care for women with endometriosis and adenomyosis.

Classical Literature

The database used to identify possible citations of endometriosis in classical CM literature, the *Zhong Hua Yi Dian* 中华医典,[17] contains

Summary and Conclusions

a collection of more than 1,100 books that are considered to be representative of CM historical development.[18,19] Several challenges arose while searching for possible cases of endometriosis or adenomyosis. Neither of these conditions have unique identifying features to confidently determine their likelihood of being endometriosis or adenomyosis. The characteristic symptoms — dysmenorrhoea, pelvic pain, and to a lesser extent, infertility — are common to many other gynaecological and non-gynaecological conditions.

Search terms were selected based on key symptoms. Criteria were developed to select citations that displayed either some or most of the common symptoms, but this was based on the assumption that the characteristic symptoms of endometriosis in the contemporary literature were the same as those in the classical literature. As over half of all included citations were identified with the combination of search terms for dysmenorrhoea and *fu tong* 腹痛 (abdominal pain; 415 citations), this may suggest a different view of endometriosis and adenomyosis in past eras. Further, as some women may not experience symptoms from these diseases,[20] any cases of women with asymptomatic endometriosis in the classical literature would not have been identified.

The selection of search terms and inclusion criteria were developed in consultation with experienced clinicians and researchers; however, the use of other search terms and inclusion criteria may produce different results. Assessment of the likelihood of each citation being cases of endometriosis or adenomyosis involved reading each citation and carefully interpreting what they mean. Classical books were written in a different style to contemporary texts and language has changed over time. These factors may have resulted in judgements that are open to debate.

Just as language has changed over time, the names of CHM formulas have also changed. Formulas with similar names were grouped to identify the most frequently used formulas in past eras. It is possible that formulas with similar (or the same) herb ingredients but with different names were included in the dataset. Due to the complexities of determining the similarity of herb ingredients in differently named formulas, we did not seek to group formulas by herb ingredients.

As such, the frequency of formulas described in Chapter 3 may be an over- or under-estimate of the actual frequency among included citations.

Oral CHM was the main treatment used for endometriosis-like symptoms in past eras, but other treatments were also used. A small number of citations described treatment with topical CHM, acupuncture, or moxibustion. It is possible that symptoms of endometriosis were managed using these treatments more frequently than the results of our analyses suggest, or that symptoms were managed with other treatments. Accordingly, the absence of information about treatments in included citations should not be interpreted as lack of use.

Clinical Studies

A large number of clinical studies published in both English and Chinese language journals have evaluated the role of CM therapies for women with endometriosis or adenomyosis. While some studies used clinical trial methods that limit potential sources of bias, the majority of studies either used methods likely to introduce bias or reported limited trial details such that it was difficult to determine the potential for bias. Further, reporting of the safety of CM interventions was typically limited to the nature and number of events, with very few studies reporting the severity of adverse events or determining the likelihood of the event being due to the intervention.

Laparoscopy is required for definitive diagnosis of endometriosis;[21] however, not all women will undergo laparoscopic surgery. The key symptoms of chronic pelvic pain, dysmenorrhoea, dyspareunia, dyschezia, and subfertility can be suggestive of endometriosis in the absence of laparoscopy,[22] with advanced imaging techniques now often considered definitive for diagnosis. Approximately half of all clinical studies used laparoscopy to confirm the diagnosis. Planned subgroup analyses to evaluate evidence from studies with laparoscopically confirmed endometriosis could not be conducted for all outcomes, which limits certainty about the effectiveness of CM therapies for endometriosis.

Summary and Conclusions

The vast majority of studies included adult women with endometriosis or adenomyosis, with few studies including adolescents with these conditions. As such, it is difficult to determine whether the results of analyses are applicable to adolescents. Another less common, but equally important, subgroup is endometriosis outside the pelvic cavity. Only three of the 466 included studies tested the role of CM therapies for endometriosis outside the pelvic cavity, and all were non-controlled studies for which the results were not subject to analysis. No statements can be made about the role of CM therapies for these less prevalent types of endometriosis.

Substantial statistical heterogeneity was common in meta-analyses for patient-reported outcomes, such as dysmenorrhoea and pelvic pain, but not for other outcomes, such as pregnancy outcomes and some analyses of recurrence. There is greater potential for variation in subjective outcome measures, which may have contributed to the statistical heterogeneity seen in meta-analyses.

While pain and recurrence were measured frequently, very few studies reported on fatigue or health-related quality of life. Given the chronic nature of endometriosis and adenomyosis and their significant health burden throughout a woman's reproductive years, it is important to evaluate the role of CM treatments on these outcomes. The current evidence is insufficient to make any statements about the role of CM therapies in reducing fatigue and improving health-related quality of life.

Many clinical studies adapted CHM and acupuncture therapy treatments according to the menstrual cycle, which reflects clinical practice. However, when analysing the results of such studies, it is not possible to determine the relative contributions of each formula to the overall treatment effect. The same can be said for meta-analyses of CHM overall. Where possible, additional meta-analyses were conducted to identify the effectiveness of specific formulas, which may provide some guidance for practitioners.

Finally, no clinical studies of other CM therapies, such as cupping or exercise therapies comprising *taichi* 太极 or *qigong* 气功, met the eligibility criteria for this review. This was not surprising as CHM and acupuncture therapies are used more frequently in clinical practice.

However, given the chronic nature of endometriosis and the reduction in health-related quality of life, some exercise or meditation therapies may be of value to women.

Experimental Studies

The experimental studies summarised in Chapter 6 provide an overview of the potential actions of some of the key herbs used for endometriosis and adenomyosis. Studies were identified by searching several English language databases. There is a wealth of research on CM therapies conducted in China and published in Chinese language journals. It is possible that some herbs included in Chapter 6 have other relevant actions for endometriosis apart from those highlighted. Thus, the information contained in Chapter 6 provides the reader with an overview of the potential actions of herbs, and practitioners who wish to learn more about these herbs are advised to search for studies more broadly.

Implications for Practice

The contemporary and classical literature as well as clinical studies have described many of the same concepts for the signs and symptoms of endometriosis: *qi* stagnation, Blood stasis, cold congealing, and *qi* deficiency. This should reassure clinicians that there has been some degree of consistency in syndrome diagnosis throughout CM history.

The formulas *San jie zhen tong jiao nang* 散结镇痛胶囊 and *Gui zhi fu ling jiao nang* 桂枝茯苓胶囊 are both recommended in clinical textbooks and guidelines and have been tested in clinical studies. Both formulas reduced the chance of recurrence when used alone for women with endometriosis, and both reduced dysmenorrhoea scores and uterine volume when used in combination with pharmacotherapy for women with adenomyosis. While these results are promising, statistical heterogeneity was detected in several meta-analyses, which lowers confidence in the results.

Summary and Conclusions

Treatments examined in clinical studies were generally tested for the same amount of time as would be used in clinical practice. Given the chronic nature of the condition, however, many women may seek regular, ongoing maintenance treatments rather than a shorter, finite period of treatment to resolve symptoms. That said, the evidence base for conventional medical treatments is notoriously lacking in the evaluation of long-term treatment effects, with 12 months regarded as 'long term'.[23,24] Understanding patient expectations and values while communicating risks and benefits effectively is critical to forming a successful therapeutic relationship between patient and clinician.

Meta-analyses could not be conducted for acupuncture therapies due to diversity in the included studies. Meta-analyses showed benefits with CHM for several outcomes, although considerable statistical heterogeneity lowered confidence in some of the results. When other factors relating to the strength and/or quality of the evidence were considered, there were few results that allowed for confident statements about the evidence; most results were considered to come from low to very low certainty evidence. It seems unlikely that the addition of new studies in the future will substantially change confidence in the results, but practitioners should keep abreast of the latest research to maintain an evidence-based approach to the treatment of women with endometriosis and adenomyosis.

Results of meta-analyses showed positive effects of oral CHM used alone or in combination with HT for endometriosis in reducing pain, preventing recurrence, reducing uterine volume and ovarian cyst size, and increasing pregnancy outcomes. Analysis of treatments tested in the studies included in these meta-analyses found that the most frequently used herbs were *dang gui* 当归, *e zhu* 莪术, *yan hu suo* 延胡索, *tao ren* 桃仁, *gan cao* 甘草, *dan shen* 丹参, and *dang shen* 党参. Similarly, studies of oral CHM for women with adenomyosis showed positive effects in meta-analyses for dysmenorrhoea and sonographic measures, and the most frequently used herbs in studies included in these meta-analyses were *dang gui* 当归, *yan hu suo* 延胡索, *wu ling zhi* 五灵脂, *bai shao* 白芍, and *chi shao* 赤芍.

Several of these herbs have been found to have anti-inflammatory and analgesic actions, as well as regulatory effects on the hormonal and immune systems (see Chapter 6). Understanding the actions of these herbs may help practitioners to select formulas that use these herbs, or to modify formulas to include these herbs, for patients with endometriosis or adenomyosis.

As no study of other CM therapies met the inclusion criteria for this review, practitioners should use caution and their clinical judgement about the appropriateness of these treatments given the lack of clinical evidence on their effectiveness. Further, results from individual studies showed that women who received moxibustion alone or with acupuncture reported worse outcomes for recurrence of pain or cysts, as well as on some domains of the SF-36, than women who received HT. Practitioners should consider the appropriateness of these interventions and continue to keep up-to-date when more evidence becomes available.

Implications for Research

Many systematic reviews have examined the role of CM treatments for endometriosis and adenomyosis (see Chapters 5 and 7). These reviews highlight the methodological shortcomings of existing research and frequently conclude that more research is required. While that may be true, it is perhaps more pertinent that research is focused on the interventions and outcomes that are important to women.

As part of a concerted effort to improve endometriosis research, Duffy et al. (2020)[25] developed a core outcome set by group consensus and nominal group process. Three key outcomes were selected for intervention trials for pain and symptoms of endometriosis: overall pain, improvement in the most bothersome symptom, and quality of life. An additional eight pregnancy-related outcomes were selected for trials of interventions for infertility due to endometriosis. Regardless of the focus, adverse events and patient satisfaction should be assessed. Future research using these core outcomes will increase the ability to synthesise results from multiple studies;

however, the benefits of having a core outcome set will not be seen for several years. In the interim, CM clinical trials should prioritise validated outcome scales and include assessments of patient satisfaction with treatment.

It is important for clinical trials to test treatments using outcomes that reflect clinical practice, which ultimately results in improved patient care.[26] Management of gynaecological conditions with CM frequently involves tailoring the treatments for each individual according to the phase of the menstrual cycle. Testing this approach in clinical trials, such as pragmatic RCTs, is limited to providing broad statements about the effectiveness of CM therapies, rather than the effectiveness of specific formulas or acupuncture points, and does not allow for meaningful translation of treatments into practice. Conversely, testing one treatment for all women regardless of the menstrual phase — as is the approach in the 'gold standard' double-blind RCT — disregards CM theory and, one may argue, negates the valuable knowledge, skills, and experience that CM physicians have developed over many years of study and practice. This paradox presents a quandary for researchers, for which there is no easy solution. Schnyer et al.[27] posit that 'manualisation' (the provision of a treatment manual for the implementation of treatment algorithms in clinical trials) may provide a potential solution, for trials of acupuncture at least, and have implemented such a manual in an RCT of Japanese acupuncture for endometriosis-related chronic pelvic pain in young women.[28]

Furthermore, the assumption that tailored treatment — such as targeted intervention at specific times of the menstrual cycle — improves clinical outcomes also needs to be tested. A review by Armour et al.[29] found high variability in the 'dose' of acupuncture provided in RCTs for primary dysmenorrhoea, and two studies that provided acupuncture before menses showed greater short-term pain relief than others that provided treatment at the start of menses. Armour et al.'s subsequent RCT[30] found no additional improvement in primary dysmenorrhoea with an intensive course of acupuncture prior to menstruation compared to regular treatments throughout the menstrual cycle. There is a clear need to examine factors related to tailoring treatment in clinical studies to allow practitioners to make evidence-informed choices about the care they provide.

These challenges aside, there are several areas of CM research that require further consideration. There is limited research evaluating the potential benefits of topical CHMs for endometriosis and adenomyosis. Topical treatments may be easier for women to administer at home, and greater adherence to treatment may improve outcomes. Diagnosis confirmed by laparoscopy will allow for a more accurate assessment of recurrence. There is limited evidence for CM therapies other than CHM and acupuncture techniques, particularly for CM exercise-based therapies, which may provide benefits for outcomes such as fatigue and health-related quality of life.

Trial reporting was identified as an area for improvement in this review. Many studies either used inappropriate methods for sequence generation and allocation concealment or reported insufficient detail to allow the potential for bias to be determined. Blinding remains a challenge in studies evaluating CM, particularly those conducted in China where CM therapies are an accepted mainstream treatment, meaning that the most appropriate comparison is with conventional medicine.

Registering clinical trials in searchable regional and international registers increases transparency in trial conduct. Researchers should follow the Consolidated Standards of Reporting Trials (CONSORT)[31] and extensions for acupuncture,[32] CHM formulas,[33] and moxibustion[34] when reporting trial results. Trials of CHM should document the results of authentication of formulas and herb ingredients as part of the quality insurance process. Further, quantification of the various compounds within herbs and formulas will improve understanding of their relevant biological actions.

Finally, adequate reporting of adverse events is critical to ensuring that treatments are safe and allows for more accurate assessments of the benefits and risks of CM treatments. Many CM studies of endometriosis and adenomyosis have documented the number and nature of adverse events. Additional assessment of severity and assignment of causality will enhance evaluation of the potential risks with treatment. In addition, some CM treatments have shown worse outcomes than pharmacotherapy. While this finding is based on results from individual studies, there is a need to ensure that such treatments are safe and do not negatively affect clinical outcomes.

References

1. Johnson NP, Hummelshoj L. (2013) Consensus on current management of endometriosis. *Hum Reprod* **28**(6): 1552–1568.
2. Sinaii N, Plumb K, Cotton L, *et al.* (2008) Differences in characteristics among 1,000 women with endometriosis based on extent of disease. *Fertil Steril* **89**(3): 538–545.
3. Schenken R. Endometriosis: Pathogenesis, clinical features and diagnosis 2019 [cited 2019 28th July]. Available from: https://www.uptodate.com/contents/endometriosis-pathogenesis-clinical-features-and-diagnosis.
4. Practice Committee of the American Society for Reproductive Medicine. (2014) Treatment of pelvic pain associated with endometriosis: A committee opinion. *Fertil Steril* **101**(4): 927–935.
5. Fisher C, Adams J, Hickman L, *et al.* (2016) The use of complementary and alternative medicine by 7427 Australian women with cyclic perimenstrual pain and discomfort: A cross-sectional study. *BMC Complement Altern Med* **16**: 129.
6. Ware JJ, Sherbourne C. (1992) The MOS 36-item short-form health survey (SF-36). I. Conceptual framework and item selection. *Med Care* **30**: 473–483.
7. Jones G, Kennedy S, Barnard A, *et al.* (2001) Development of an endometriosis quality-of-life instrument: The Endometriosis Health Profile-30. *Obstet Gynecol* **98**(2): 258–264.
8. World Health Organization. Division of Mental Health. WHOQOL-BREF: Introduction, administration, scoring and generic version of the assessment: Field trial version. Available from: https://apps.who.int/iris/handle/10665/63529: World Health Organization; 1996.
9. Coyle ME, Yu JJ, Zhang AL, *et al.* (2020) Patient experiences of using Chinese herbal medicine for psoriasis vulgaris and chronic urticaria: A qualitative study. *J Dermatolog Treat* **31**(4): 352–358.
10. 中华中医药学会. (2012) 中医妇科常见病诊疗指南. 北京: 中国中医药出版社.

11. 罗颂平, 刘雁峰. (2017) 中医妇科学 ('十二五'普通高等教育本科国家级规划教材). 第3版. 北京: 人民卫生出版社.
12. 中华医学会妇产科学分会绝经学组. (2013) 绝经期管理与激素补充治疗临床应用指南. *中华妇产科杂志* **48**(10): 795–799.
13. Coyle ME, Liu J, Zhang AL, *et al.* (2020) Menopause. In: Xue CC, Lu C, eds. *Evidence-based Clinical Chinese Medicine*: World Scientific Publishing Co. Pte. Ltd.
14. Jones G, Jenkinson C, Kennedy S. (2004) Development of the short form endometriosis health profile questionnaire: The EHP-5. *Qual Life Res* **13**(3): 695–704.
15. Kupperman HS, Wetchler BB, Blatt MH. (1959) Contemporary therapy of the menopausal syndrome. *J Am Med Assoc* **171**: 1627–1637.
16. Gori L, Firenzuoli F. (2007) Ear acupuncture in European traditional medicine. *Evid Based Complement Alternat Med* **4**(Suppl 1): 13–16.
17. Hu R. (2000) *Encyclopedia of Traditional Chinese Medicine*. Hunan Electronic and Audio-Visual Publishing House, Changsha.
18. May B, Lu C, Xue C. (2012) Collections of traditional Chinese medical litearture as resources for systematic searches. *J Altern Complement Med* **18**(12): 1101–1107.
19. May B, Lu Y, Lu C, *et al.* (2013) Systematic assessment of the representativeness of published collections of the traditional literature on Chinese medicine. *J Altern Complement Med* **19**(5): 403–409.
20. Rawson JM. (1991) Prevalence of endometriosis in asymptomatic women. *J Reprod Med* **36**(7): 513–515.
21. Vercellini P, Vigano P, Somigliana E, *et al.* (2014) Endometriosis: Pathogenesis and treatment. *Nat Rev Endocrinol* **10**(5): 261–275.
22. Kuznetsov L, Dworzynski K, Davies M, *et al.* (2017) Diagnosis and management of endometriosis: Summary of NICE guidance. *BMJ* **358**: j3935.
23. Surrey E, Taylor HS, Giudice L, *et al.* (2018) Long-term outcomes of elagolix in women with endometriosis: Results from two extension studies. *Obstet Gynecol* **132**(1): 147–160.
24. Taylor HS, Giudice LC, Lessey BA, *et al.* (2017) Treatment of endometriosis-associated pain with elagolix, an oral GnRH antagonist. *N Engl J Med* **377**(1): 28–40.
25. Duffy J, Hirsch M, Vercoe M, *et al.* (2020) A core outcome set for future endometriosis research: An international consensus development study. *BJOG* **127**(8): 967–974.

26. Duffy JMN, Ziebland S, von Dadelszen P, et al. (2019) Tackling poorly selected, collected, and reported outcomes in obstetrics and gynecology research. *Am J Obstet Gynecol* **220**(1): 71.e1–71.e4.
27. Schnyer RN, Allen JJ. (2002) Bridging the gap in complementary and alternative medicine research: Manualization as a means of promoting standardization and flexibility of treatment in clinical trials of acupuncture. *J Altern Complement Med* **8**(5): 623–634.
28. Schnyer RN, Iuliano D, Kay J, et al. (2008) Development of protocols for randomized sham-controlled trials of complex treatment interventions: Japanese acupuncture for endometriosis-related pelvic pain. *J Altern Complement Med* **14**(5): 515–522.
29. Armour M, Smith CA. (2016) Treating primary dysmenorrhoea with acupuncture: A narrative review of the relationship between acupuncture 'dose' and menstrual pain outcomes. *Acupunct Med* **34**(6): 416–424.
30. Armour M, Dahlen HG, Zhu X, et al. (2017) The role of treatment timing and mode of stimulation in the treatment of primary dysmenorrhea with acupuncture: An exploratory randomised controlled trial. *PloS One* **12**(7): e0180177–e0180177.
31. Schulz K, Altman D, Moher D. (2010) CONSORT 2010 statement: Updated guidelines for reporting parallel group randomised trials. *PLoS Med* **7**(3): e1000251.
32. MacPherson H, Altman D, Hammerschlag R, et al. (2010) Revised STandards for Reporting Interventions in Clinical Trials of Acupuncture (STRICTA): Extending the CONSORT statement. *J Evid Based Med* **3**(3): 140–155.
33. Cheng CW, Wu TX, Shang HC, et al. (2017) CONSORT extension for Chinese Herbal Medicine formulas 2017: Recommendations, explanation, and elaboration. *Ann Intern Med* **27**(2): 112–121.
34. Cheng C, Fu S, Zhou Q, et al. (2013) Extending the CONSORT statement to moxibustion. *J Integr Med* **11**(1): 54–63.

Glossary

Terms	Acronym	Definition	Reference
95% confidence interval	95% CI	A measure of the uncertainty around the main finding of a statistical analysis. Estimates of unknown quantities, such as the odds ratio comparing an experimental intervention with a control, are usually presented as a point estimate and a 95% confidence interval. This means that if someone were to keep repeating a study in other samples from the same population, 95% of the confidence intervals from those studies would contain the true value of the unknown quantity. Alternatives to 95%, such as 90% and 99% confidence intervals, are sometimes used. Wider intervals indicate lower precision; narrow intervals, greater precision.	https://training.cochrane.org/handbook
Acupuncture	—	The insertion of needles into humans or animals for remedial purposes.	WHO International Standard Terminologies of Traditional Medicine in the Western Pacific Region. World Health Organization; 2007.

(*Continued*)

(*Continued*)

Terms	Acronym	Definition	Reference
Allied and Complementary Medicine Database	AMED	Alternative medicine bibliographic database.	https://www.ebsco.com/products/research-databases/allied-and-complementary-medicine-database-amed
Australian New Zealand Clinical Trial Registry	ANZCTR	Clinical trial registry based in Australia.	www.anzctr.org.au/
China National Knowledge Infrastructure	CNKI	Chinese language bibliographic database.	www.cnki.net
Chinese Biomedical Literature Database	CBM	Chinese language bibliographic database.	www.imicams.ac.cn
Chinese Clinical Trial Registry	ChiCTR	Chinese clinical trial registry.	http://www.chictr.org.cn/
Chinese herbal medicine	CHM	Chinese herbal medicine.	—
Chinese medicine	CM	Chinese medicine.	—
Chongqing VIP Information Company	CQVIP	Chinese language bibliographic database.	www.cqvip.com
ClinicalTrials.gov	—	Clinical trial registry based in the United States of America.	https://clinicaltrials.gov/
Cochrane Central Register of Controlled Trials	CENTRAL	Bibliographic database that provides a highly concentrated source of reports of controlled trials.	https://community.cochrane.org/editorial-and-publishing-policy-resource/overview-cochrane-library-and-related-content/databases-included-cochrane-library/cochrane-central-register-controlled-trials-central

Glossary

(*Continued*)

Terms	Acronym	Definition	Reference
Combination therapies	—	Two or more Chinese medicines from different therapy groups (e.g. Chinese herbal medicine, acupuncture therapies or other Chinese medicine therapies) administered together.	—
Controlled clinical trials	CCT	A study in which people are allocated to different interventions using methods that are not random.	https://training.cochrane.org/handbook
Convention on International Trade in Endangered Species of Wild Fauna and Flora	CITES	International convention aimed at preventing or regulating trade in threatened and endangered species of plants and animals.	https://www.cites.org/eng/disc/text.php
Cumulative Index of Nursing and Allied Health Literature	CINAHL	Bibliographic database.	https://www.ebscohost.com/nursing/products/cinahl-databases
Effect size	—	A generic term for the estimate of the effect of a treatment in a study.	http://handbook.cochrane.org/
Electroacupuncture	—	Electric stimulation of the acupuncture needle following insertion.	WHO International Standard Terminologies of Traditional Medicine in the Western Pacific Region. World Health Organization; 2007.
Endometriosis Health Profile	EHP	Quality of life scale for endometriosis. The full version includes 30 items (EHP-30), while the shortened version includes five items (EHP-5).	Jones G, Kennedy S, Barnard A, *et al.* (2001) Development of an endometriosis quality-of-life instrument: The Endometriosis Health Profile-30. *Obstet Gynecol* **98**(2): 258–264.

(*Continued*)

(Continued)

Terms	Acronym	Definition	Reference
			Jones G, Jenkinson C, Kennedy S. (2004) Development of the Short Form Endometriosis Health Profile Questionnaire: The EHP-5. *Qual Life Res* **13**(3): 695–704.
European Union Clinical Trials Register	EU-CTR	European clinical trial registry.	https://www.clinicaltrialsregister.eu
Excerpta Medica database	Embase	Bibliographic database.	http://www.elsevier.com/solutions/embase
Grading of Recommendations Assessment, Development and Evaluation	GRADE	Approach used to grade quality of evidence and strength of recommendations.	http://www.gradeworkinggroup.org/
Health related quality of life	HR-QoL	A conceptual or operational measurement that is commonly used in a health care setting as a means to assess the impact of disease on the person.	
Heterogeneity	—	Used in a general sense to describe the variation in, or diversity of, participants, interventions, and measurement of outcomes across a set of studies, or the variation in internal validity of those studies. Used specifically, as statistical heterogeneity, to describe the degree of variation in the effect estimates from a set of studies. Also used to indicate the presence of variability among studies beyond the amount expected due solely to the play of chance.	https://training.cochrane.org/handbook

Glossary

(*Continued*)

Terms	Acronym	Definition	Reference
Homogeneity	—	Used in a general sense to mean that the participants, interventions, and measurement of outcomes are similar across a set of studies. Used specifically to describe the effect estimates from a set of studies where they do not vary more than would be expected by chance.	https://training.cochrane.org/handbook
I^2	—	A measure of study heterogeneity; indicates the percentage of variance in a meta-analysis.	https://training.cochrane.org/handbook
Integrative medicine	—	Chinese herbal medicine combined with pharmacotherapy or other conventional therapy.	
Mean difference	MD	In meta-analysis: A method used to combine measures on continuous scales, where the mean, standard deviation, and sample size in each group are known. The weight given to the difference in means from each study (e.g., how much influence each study has on the overall results of the meta-analysis) is determined by the precision of its estimate of effect; mathematically this is equal to the inverse of the variance. This method assumes that all of the trials have measured the outcome on the same scale.	https://training.cochrane.org/handbook

(*Continued*)

(*Continued*)

Terms	Acronym	Definition	Reference
Medical Outcome Study 36-Item Short-Form Health Survey	SF-36	A scale used to measure general wellbeing.	Ware JJ, Sherbourne C. (1992) The MOS 36-item short-form health survey (SF-36). I. Conceptual framework and item selection. *Med Care* 30: 473–83.
Meta-analysis	—	The use of statistical techniques in a systematic review to integrate the results of included studies. Sometimes misused as a synonym for systematic reviews, where the review includes a meta-analysis.	—
Moxibustion	—	A therapeutic procedure involving ignited material (usually moxa) to apply heat to certain points or areas of the body surface for managing disease.	WHO International Standard Terminologies of Traditional Medicine in the Western Pacific Region. World Health Organization; 2007.
Non-controlled studies	—	Observations made on individuals, usually receiving the same intervention, before and after the intervention but with no control group.	https://training.cochrane.org/handbook
Other Chinese medicine therapies	—	Other Chinese medicine therapies include all traditional therapies except Chinese herbal medicine and acupuncture therapies, such as *taichi, qigong, tuina*, and cupping.	
PubMed	PubMed	Bibliographic database.	http://www.ncbi.nlm.nih.gov/pubmed

Glossary

(*Continued*)

Terms	Acronym	Definition	Reference
Randomised controlled trial	RCT	Clinical trial that uses a random method to allocate participants to treatment and control groups.	—
Risk of bias	—	Assessment of clinical trials to indicate if the results may overestimate or underestimate the true effect because of bias in study design or reporting.	https://training.cochrane.org/handbook
Risk ratio (relative risk)	RR	The ratio of risks in two groups. In intervention studies, it is the ratio of the risk in the intervention group to the risk in the control group. A risk ratio of one indicates no difference between comparison groups. For undesirable outcomes, a risk ratio that is less than one indicates that the intervention was effective in reducing the risk of that outcome.	https://training.cochrane.org/handbook
Standardised mean difference	SMD	In meta-analysis: A method used to combine results for continuous scales which measure the same outcome, but in different ways (e.g., with different scales). The results of studies are standardised to a uniform scale to allow data to be combined.	https://training.cochrane.org/handbook
Summary of findings	SoF	Presentation of results and rating the quality of evidence based on the GRADE approach.	http://www.gradeworkinggroup.org/

(*Continued*)

(Continued)

Terms	Acronym	Definition	Reference
Tuina 推拿	—	Chinese massage: Rubbing, kneading, or percussion of the soft tissues and joints of the body with the hands, usually performed by one person on another, especially to relieve tension or pain.	WHO International Standard Terminologies of Traditional Medicine in the Western Pacific Region. World Health Organization; 2007.
Visual analogue scale	VAS	Scale frequently used to measure pain. Scored 0–10 cm or 0–100 mm, lower scores indicate less severe pain.	—
Wanfang database	Wanfang	Chinese language bibliographic database.	www.wanfangdata.com
World Health Organization	WHO	The World Health Organization is the directing and coordinating authority for health within the United Nations system. It is responsible for providing leadership on global health matters, shaping the health research agenda, setting norms and standards, articulating evidence-based policy options, providing technical support to countries, and monitoring and assessing health trends.	http://www.who.int/about/en/
World Health Organization Quality of Life Instruments	WHOQOL-BREF	A generic health-related quality of life scale.	World Health Organization. Division of Mental Health. WHOQOL-BREF: Introduction, administration, scoring and generic version of the assessment: Field trial version. https://apps.who.int/iris/handle/10665/63529: World Health Organization; 1996.

Glossary

(Continued)

Terms	Acronym	Definition	Reference
Zhong Hua Yi Dian 中华医典	ZHYD	The *Zhong Hua Yi Dian* ('Encyclopaedia of Traditional Chinese Medicine') is a comprehensive series of electronic books on compact disk. The collection was put together by the Hunan electronic and audio-visual publishing house. It is the largest collection of Chinese electronic books and includes the major Chinese ancient works, many of which are from rare manuscripts and are the only existing copies. These books cover the period from ancient times up to the period of the Republic of China (1911–1948).	Hu R, ed. (2000) *Zhong Hua Yi Dian [Encyclopaedia of Traditional Chinese Medicine]*. 4th ed. Hunan Electronic and Audio-Visual Publishing House, Chengsha.
Zhong Yi Fang Ji Da Ci Dian 中医方剂大辞典	ZYFJDCD	Compendium of Chinese herbal formulae with over 96,592 entries derived from classical Chinese books. The Nanjing Chinese Medicine Institute compiled the *Zhong Yi Fang Ji Da Ci Dian* and first published it in 1993.	Peng HR, ed. (1994) *Zhong Yi Fang Ji Da Ci Dian [Great Compendium of Chinese Medical Formulae]*, 1st ed. People's Medical Publishing House, Beijing.

Index

abdominal acupuncture, 34, 36, 37, 389
acupuncture, 35, 65, 329–331, 333–347, 352, 354–358, 389
adverse events, 72, 75, 76, 82
Ai fu nuan gong wan 艾附暖宫丸, 30, 240, 241

bai shao 白芍, 50, 54–56, 59–61, 64, 68, 155
Ba wu tang 八物汤, 56
Ba zhen tang 八珍汤, 56
BL23 *Shenshu* 肾俞, 35, 334, 347
BL32 *Ciliao* 次髎, 35, 348, 363, 373

Cang fu dao tan wan 苍附导痰丸, 31, 240, 241
chi shao 赤芍, 100, 155, 168, 187, 211, 292, 293, 314
chuan xiong 川芎, 64, 292, 295, 314
cold congealing and Blood stasis, 24, 25, 27, 29, 35, 38, 379
CV3 *Zhongji* 中极, 35, 334, 363, 367, 370, 373, 392
CV4 *Guanyuan* 关元, 35, 363, 367, 369, 373, 374, 392
CV6 *Qihai* 气海, 334, 346–348, 353

CV8 *Shenque* 神阙, 37, 65, 391, 392

dampness-heat and stasis obstructing uterus, 24, 25, 27, 32, 378
Dan e kang fu jian gao 丹莪妇康煎膏, 28, 240, 241
dang gui 当归, 58, 100, 300, 362, 363, 367, 370, 374
dang shen 党参, 397
Dan leng fu kang jian gao 丹棱妇康煎膏, 147, 381, 384, 385
dan shen 丹参, 292, 298
diagnosis, 1–4, 9–11
dysmenorrhoea, 2, 9

ear acupuncture, 34, 36, 389
EHP-5, 75, 80
EHP-30, 75, 79
Endometriosis Health Profile, 75, 79
EX-CA1 *Zigong* 子宫, 35, 334, 346, 348, 354, 355
e zhu 莪术, 100, 292, 302

gan cao 甘草, 292, 304
Ge xia zhu yu tang 膈下逐瘀汤, 28, 240, 241, 384

gonadotropin-releasing hormone agonists, 13
Grading of Recommendations Assessment, Development and Evaluation (GRADE), 84–86
Gui jing liang an tang 归经两安汤, 60, 64
Gui shen wan 归肾丸, 26, 29, 385
gui zhi 桂枝, 362, 363, 371, 373, 374
Gui zhi fu ling jiao nang 桂枝茯苓胶囊, 30, 93, 94, 146, 147, 148, 156, 201, 202, 208, 240, 249–251, 253, 256, 257, 386
Gui zhi fu ling jiao nang/wan 桂枝茯苓胶囊/丸, 383
Gui zhi fu ling wan 桂枝茯苓丸, 315

hu po san 琥珀散, 55–57

infertility, 1–3, 11, 13

Ju yuan jian 举元煎, 30, 240, 241

KI, 81
KI3 Taixi 太溪, 35, 367
Kidney deficiency and Blood stasis, 24–26, 28, 35, 378
Kun tai jiao nang 坤泰胶囊, 387
Kupperman Index, 75, 81

LI4 Hegu 合谷, 334, 346
Li chong tang 理冲汤, 30, 240, 244
LR3 Taichong 太冲, 35, 334, 346, 353

miscarriage rate, 75, 77, 79
moxibustion, 37, 65, 329, 331, 333, 338, 339, 341–344, 347–356, 388

pelvic pain, 2, 8, 9
phlegm and stasis binding, 27, 25, 31, 35
pregnancy rate, 75, 77, 79
prevalence, 1, 3, 5

qi deficiency and Blood stasis, 25, 30, 378
Qing re tiao xue tang 清热调血汤, 32, 244, 385
qi stagnation and Blood stasis, 30, 24–27, 35, 38, 378

recurrence, 75, 76, 78

San jie zhen tong jiao nang 散结镇痛胶囊, 28, 93, 95, 147, 149, 155, 156, 161, 188, 193–196, 198, 199, 201–204, 208, 210, 218, 220, 240, 245–249, 253, 256, 257, 386
San leng 三棱, 292, 307
SF-36, 75, 80
Shao fu zhu yu tang 少腹逐瘀汤, 30, 134, 135, 142, 201, 240, 243, 244, 384
Shao fu zhu yu tang/jiao nang 少腹逐瘀汤/胶囊, 383
Shi xiao san 失笑散, 30, 240, 241
shu di huang 熟地黄, 54, 55, 56, 59–61, 64, 68
Shun jing tang 顺经汤, 51, 60, 64
Si wu tang 四物汤, 54, 56, 63–65, 67, 68, 380

SP6 *Sanyinjiao* 三阴交, 35, 363, 367, 370, 373, 374, 392
SP8 *Diji* 地机, 35, 370
SP10 *Xuehai* 血海, 35, 334, 346–348, 353–355
ST36 *Zusanli* 足三里, 35, 334, 347, 354, 355
surgical management, 11, 12

Tao hong si wu tang 桃红四物汤, 26, 27, 30, 31
tao ren 桃仁, 292, 308

visual analogue scale (VAS), 75, 77

Wen jing tang 温经汤, 56, 57
wu ling zhi 五灵脂, 362, 363, 374, 397

xiang fu 香附, 292, 310
Xue fu zhu yu tang 血府逐瘀汤, 28, 134, 135, 142–144, 146, 239, 240, 242, 243, 256, 384

yan hu suo 延胡索, 312, 397

Zuo gui wan 左归丸, 387

Evidence-based Clinical Chinese Medicine

(*Continued from page ii*)

Vol. 12 *Post-Stroke Shoulder Complications*
Lead Authors: Claire Shuiqing Zhang and Shaonan Liu

Vol. 13 *Post-Stroke Spasticity*
Lead Authors: Claire Shuiqing Zhang and Shaonan Liu

Vol. 14 *Unipolar Depression*
Lead Authors: Yuan Ming Di and Lingling Yang

Vol. 15 *Chronic Heart Failure*
Lead Authors: Claire Shuiqing Zhang and Liuling Ma

Vol. 16 *Atopic Dermatitis*
Lead Authors: Meaghan Coyle and Junfeng Liu

Vol. 17 *Colorectal Cancer*
Lead Authors: Brian H May and Yihong Liu

Vol. 18 *Cancer Pain*
Lead Authors: Brian H May and Yihong Liu

Vol. 20 *Chronic Cough*
Lead Authors: Johannah Shergis and Yuanbin Chen

Vol. 22 *Urinary Tract Infection*
Lead Authors: Meaghan Coyle and Xindong Qin

Vol. 23 *Episodic Migraine*
Lead Authors: Claire Shuiqing Zhang and Shaohua Lyu

Vol. 24 *Menopause*
Lead Authors: Meaghan Coyle and Jian Liu

Vol. 28 *Endometriosis*
Lead Authors: Meaghan Coyle and Yongxia Wang

Vol. 29 *Cervical Radiculopathy*
Lead Authors: Claire Shuiqing Zhang and Dihui Zhang

Forthcoming

Vol. 21 *Type 2 Diabetes Mellitus*
Lead Authors: Yuan Ming Di and Lu Sun

Vol. 25 *Rhinosinusitis*
Lead Authors: Brian H May and Wenmin Lin

Made in United States
Orlando, FL
05 September 2025